Extending Medicare Coverage for Preventive and Other Services

Marilyn J. Field, Robert L. Lawrence, and
Lee Zwanziger, *Editors*

Committee on Medicare Coverage Extensions

Division of Health Care Services

INSTITUTE OF MEDICINE

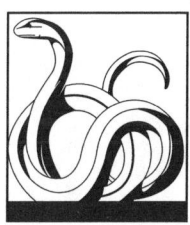

NATIONAL ACADEMY PRESS
Washington, D.C.

NATIONAL ACADEMY PRESS • 2101 Constitution Avenue, N.W. • Washington, DC 20418

NOTICE: The project that is the subject of this report was approved by the Governing Board of the National Research Council, whose members are drawn from the councils of the National Academy of Sciences, the National Academy of Engineering, and the Institute of Medicine. The members of the committee responsible for the report were chosen for their special competences and with regard for appropriate balance.

Support for this project was provided by the Department of Health and Human Services (Contract Number 500-98-0275). The views presented are those of the Institute of Medicine Committee and are not necessarily those of the funding organization.

International Standard Book Number 0-309-06889-4

Extending Medicare Coverage for Preventive and Other Services is available for sale from the National Academy Press, 2101 Constitution Avenue, N.W., Box 285, Washington, DC 20055. Call (800) 624-6242 or (202) 334-3313 (in the Washington metropolitan area), or visit the NAP on-line bookstore at **www.nap. edu.** The full text of this report is available on line at **www.nap.edu.**

For more information about the Institute of Medicine, visit the IOM home page at **www.iom.edu.**

Printed in the United States of America

The serpent has been a symbol of long life, healing, and knowledge among almost all cultures and religions since the beginning of recorded history. The serpent adopted as a logotype by the Institute of Medicine is a relief carving from ancient Greece, now held by the Staatliche Museen in Berlin.

THE NATIONAL ACADEMIES

National Academy of Sciences
National Academy of Engineering
Institute of Medicine
National Research Council

The **National Academy of Sciences** is a private, nonprofit, self-perpetuating society of distinguished scholars engaged in scientific and engineering research, dedicated to the furtherance of science and technology and to their use for the general welfare. Upon the authority of the charter granted to it by the Congress in 1863, the Academy has a mandate that requires it to advise the federal government on scientific and technical matters. Dr. Bruce M. Alberts is president of the National Academy of Sciences.

The **National Academy of Engineering** was established in 1964, under the charter of the National Academy of Sciences, as a parallel organization of outstanding engineers. It is autonomous in its administration and in the selection of its members, sharing with the National Academy of Sciences the responsibility for advising the federal government. The National Academy of Engineering also sponsors engineering programs aimed at meeting national needs, encourages education and research, and recognizes the superior achievements of engineers. Dr. William A. Wulf is president of the National Academy of Engineering.

The **Institute of Medicine** was established in 1970 by the National Academy of Sciences to secure the services of eminent members of appropriate professions in the examination of policy matters pertaining to the health of the public. The Institute acts under the responsibility given to the National Academy of Sciences by its congressional charter to be an adviser to the federal government and, upon its own initiative, to identify issues of medical care, research, and education. Dr. Kenneth I. Shine is president of the Institute of Medicine.

The **National Research Council** was organized by the National Academy of Sciences in 1916 to associate the broad community of science and technology with the Academy's purposes of furthering knowledge and advising the federal government. Functioning in accordance with general policies determined by the Academy, the Council has become the principal operating agency of both the National Academy of Sciences and the National Academy of Engineering in providing services to the government, the public, and the scientific and engineering communities. The Council is administered jointly by both Academies and the Institute of Medicine. Dr. Bruce M. Alberts and Dr. William A. Wulf are chairman and vice chairman, respectively, of the National Research Council.

COMMITTEE ON MEDICARE COVERAGE EXTENSIONS

ROBERT S. LAWRENCE, M.D. (*Chair*), Associate Dean for Professional Education and Programs and Professor of Health Policy, Johns Hopkins University School of Hygiene and Public Health, Baltimore

JACK C. EBELER, Senior Vice President and Director, Robert Wood Johnson Foundation, Princeton, N.J.

MARTHE R. GOLD, M.D., Arthur C. Logan Professor and Chair, Department of Community Medicine, City University of New York Medical School

BERTRAM L. KASISKE, M.D., Director, Division of Nephrology, Hennepin County Medical Center and Professor of Medicine, University of Minnesota

LAUREN L. PATTON, D.D.S., Associate Professor of Dental Ecology, University of North Carolina School of Dentistry, Chapel Hill (from May 1999)[*]

STEPHEN G. PAUKER, M.D., Vice Chairman for Clinical Affairs, Department of Medicine, New England Medical Center, and Sara Murray Jordan Professor of Medicine, Tufts University School of Medicine

ROBERT S. STERN, M.D., Professor of Dermatology, Harvard University Medical School at Beth Israel Deaconess Medical Center, Boston

Staff

MARILYN J. FIELD, Ph.D., Study Director and Deputy Director, Health Care Services

LEE L. ZWANZIGER, Ph.D., Senior Program Officer

DEE SUTTON, Administrative Assistant

---

[*]Dr. Patton replaced Robert J. Genco, D.D.S., Ph.D., distinguished professor and chairman, Department of Oral Biology, and distinguished professor of microbiology, Schools of Dentistry and Medicine, State University of New York (SUNY) at Buffalo, who was unable to continue his service on the committee.

Acknowledgments

In developing this report, the committee benefited from the expertise and experience of many individuals. In particular, it learned much from the presenters and participants in three workshops held in May and June 1999. Appendix A lists the workshop participants, presenters, and agendas.

The authors of the commissioned background papers presented in Appendixes B (Mark Helfand, Karen Eden, and Susan Mahon), C (Alex White, James Lipton, William Kohn, and Lauren Patton), D (Robert Gaston), and E (Jesse Kerns, Al Dobson, and Joan Da Vanzo) made essential contributions to this report through their evidence reviews and their extensive discussions with committee members and staff. Their ability to develop the evidence reviews on a tight schedule for discussion at the workshops was especially appreciated.

At the Health Care Financing Administration, project officer Katharine Pirotte and medical adviser Joseph Chin were always helpful. Paul Eggers provided information and guidance for developing estimates of the cost of extending Medicare coverage of immunosuppressive drugs. Others at the agency who provided information and explanations about policies and practices included John Whyte, Peter Hickman, Joan Stieber, Odette Cohen, Willam Larson, Dorothy Honemann, and Lauren Geyer.

The committee and staff likewise appreciate the assistance of David Atkins at the Agency for Health Care Policy and Research in developing a cooperative strategy for a background paper on skin cancer screening that could be used both by the committee and by the U.S. Preventive Services Task Force (consistent with provisions of the legislation providing for this study). The Task Force will be publishing clinical practice recommendations on skin cancer screening and other topics early in 2000.

The committee and staff also benefited from information provided by a number of other individuals and organizations including Greg Raab of the Health Industry Manufacturers Association, Andrew Swire of the Pharmaceutical Research and Manufacturers of America, Dolph Chianchiano and Troy Zimmerman of the National Kidney Foundation, Julia Christensen of the Congressional Budget Office, Charles (Bud) Conklin of Carilion Dental Care, Alan Geller of Boston University, Ira Parker of the University of California at San Diego, Geoffrey Cook of Novartis, Bill Leinhos of Fero Pharmaceuticals, Robert Spieldenner of the United Network for Organ Sharing, John Rutkauskas of the American Academy of Pediatric Dentistry (formerly of the Federation of Special Care Organizations in Dentistry), and Cheryl Jacobs, Marilyn Leister, and Melissa Kamps, all of Fairview University Transplant Services.

At the Institute of Medicine, study staff appreciate the assistance of Claudia Carl, Mike Edington, Sue Barron, Sally Stanfield, Ellen Johnson, Barbara Rice, Janice Mehler, Kay Harris, and Linda Kilroy among others. Florence Poillon helped in copy editing the report.

REVIEWERS

This report has been reviewed in draft form by individuals chosen for their diverse perspectives and technical expertise, in accordance with procedures approved by the National Research Council's Report Review Committee. The purpose of this independent review is to provide candid and critical comments that will assist the Institute of Medicine in making the published report as sound as possible and to ensure that the report meets institutional standards for objectivity, evidence, and responsiveness to the study charge. The review comments and draft manuscript remain confidential to protect the integrity of the deliberative process. The committee wishes to thank the following individuals for their participation in the review of this report:

James D. Bader, D.M.D., School of Dentistry, University of North Carolina at Chapel Hill

David R. Challoner, M.D., Institute for Science and Health Policy, University of Florida

Chester W. Douglass, D.D.S., Department of Oral Health Policy and Epidemiology, Harvard University School of Dental Medicine

Robert J. Genco, Ph.D., D.D.S., Department of Oral Biology, School of Dental Medicine, University at Buffalo, State University of New York

Bernard J. Gersh, M.B., Ch.B., D. Phil., Mayo Clinic, Cardiovascular Diseases Division, Rochester, Minnesota

Barbara A. Gilchrest, M.D., Department of Dermatology, Boston University

Thomas A. Gonwa, M.D., Dallas Nephrology Associates, Dallas, Texas

Roland E. (Guy) King, Ernst & Young, Annapolis, Maryland

Peter B. Lockhart, D.D.S., Department of Oral Medicine, Carolinas Medical Center, Charlotte, North Carolina

Lorelei Mucci, M.P.H., Department of Oral Health Policy and Epidemiology, Harvard School of Dental Medicine

Joseph P. Newhouse, Ph.D., Department of Health Policy and Management, Harvard University, Cambridge

Len Nichols, Ph.D., Health Policy Center, The Urban Institute, Washington, D.C.

Arthur J. Sober, M.D., Department of Dermatology, Massachusetts General Hospital, Boston

George E. Thibault, M.D., Partners HealthCare System, Inc., Boston

Although the individuals listed above have provided constructive comments and suggestions, it must be emphasized that responsibility for the final content of this report rests entirely with the authors and the Institute of Medicine.

Preface

When Congress created the Medicare program over three decades ago, no one could anticipate the dramatic improvements in diagnostic and therapeutic measures that would emerge in subsequent years. Nor was there any expectation that health care costs would so steadily outpace the annual increase in the cost of living and cause the Medicare budget to grow so rapidly. Pressures to expand the original coverage limitations have become a regular feature of debates about the Medicare budget. The original concept of providing health insurance for those age 65 or over to protect them from the substantial costs of medical care, especially that requiring hospitalization for unexpected illnesses, was first changed to include coverage of some younger individuals with disabilities or permanent kidney failure. In 1980, the first preventive service was added when pneumococcal vaccine was covered.

Our committee was asked to analyze the possible extension of Medicare coverage for three very different conditions: skin cancer screening, medically necessary dental services, and elimination of time limits on coverage of immunosuppressive drugs for certain transplant recipients. The committee commissioned background papers for review of the evidence published in peer-reviewed scientific papers, heard from interested specialty organizations and patient advocacy groups, and contracted with consultants for estimates of the cost to Medicare of various coverage scenarios. In the course of our work we were struck by the advances in the methods for reporting clinical research, reviewing scientific evidence, and assessing the effectiveness of health care services. At the same time, we saw that continued work was needed to improve these methods and to employ them consistently to guide decisions and recommendations about clinical care and coverage policy. We include in this report our observations of these systemic problems with coverage decision making and offer some examples of different approaches for the Congress to consider.

Robert S. Lawrence, M.D.
Chair

Contents

BOXES, FIGURES, AND TABLES

Boxes

Figures

Tables

Extending Medicare Coverage for Preventive and Other Services

Summary

Congress created the Medicare program in 1965 to provide health insurance for Americans age 65 or over. It later extended coverage to some individuals with disabilities or permanent kidney failure. From the outset, the program has focused on coverage for hospital, physician, and certain other services that are "reasonable and necessary for the diagnosis or treatment of illness or injury or to improve the functioning of a malformed body member." With certain exceptions, Congress explicitly excluded Medicare coverage for preventive services, outpatient prescription drugs, and dental care.

Most sessions of Congress see proposals to expand Medicare coverage to some currently excluded services. With Medicare spending growth having far exceeded 1960s' projections, however, the added cost of such expansions has often discouraged change. Moreover, Congress has set budget rules for itself requiring that decisions to increase most types of federal spending must be accompanied by explicit decisions to reduce spending elsewhere or to raise taxes. These rules underscore the reality that expanding Medicare coverage involves making trade-offs in the face of resource constraints.

In the Balanced Budget Act of 1997 (Public Law 105-33), Congress called for the Department of Health and Human Services to arrange for the National Academy of Sciences (NAS) to analyze "the short- and long-term benefits, and costs to Medicare" of extending coverage for certain preventive and other services. The services were screening for skin cancer; medically necessary dental services; elimination of time restrictions on coverage for immunosuppressive drugs after transplants; routine patient care costs in clinical trials; and nutrition therapy.

This report, which was developed by an expert committee of the Institute of Medicine, reviews the first three services listed above.[1,2] It is intended to assist policymakers by providing syntheses of the best evidence available about the effectiveness of these services and by estimating the cost to Medicare of covering them. For each service or condition examined, the committee commissioned a review of the scientific literature that was presented and discussed at a public workshop.

As requested by Congress, this report includes explicit estimates only of costs to Medicare, not costs to beneficiaries, their families, or others. It also does not include cost-effectiveness analyses. That is, the extent of the benefits relative to the costs to Medicare—or to society generally—is not evaluated for the services examined.

The method for estimating Medicare costs follows the generic estimation practices of the Congressional Budget Office (CBO). The objective was to provide Congress with estimates that were based on familiar procedures and could be compared readily with earlier and later CBO estimates. For each condition or service, the estimates are intended to suggest the order of magnitude of the costs to Medicare of extending coverage, but the estimates could be considerably higher or lower than what Medicare might actually spend were coverage policies changed. The estimates cover the five-year period 2000–2004.

In addition to the conclusions about specific coverage issues, the report examines some broader concerns about the processes for making coverage decisions and about the research and organizational infrastructure for these decisions. It also briefly examines the limits of coverage as a means of improving health services and outcomes and the limits of evidence as a means of resolving policy and ethical questions.

EVIDENCE AND COST ESTIMATES FOR SELECTED SERVICES

Skin Cancer Screening

The three major kinds of skin cancers are melanoma, basal cell carcinoma, and squamous cell carcinoma. The latter two are often grouped together as non-melanoma skin cancers. Melanoma accounts for less than 5 percent of reported cases of skin cancer but about 80 percent of deaths. Squamous cell carcinoma accounts for most of the rest.

---

[1]For the other services, see *Extending Medicare Reimbursement in Clinical Trials* and *The Role of Nutrition Therapy in Maintaining the Health of the Nation's Elderly: Evaluating Coverage of Nutrition Services for Medicare Beneficiaries,* both available from the National Academy Press (www.nap.edu).

[2]As this report was being completed, Congress extended coverage of immunosuppressive drugs for up to eight months (subject to expenditure limits) for transplant recipients eligible for Medicare by reason of age or disability (P.L. 106-113).

Melanoma is primarily a disease of fair-skinned people. White men have a 0.38 percent lifetime risk of dying from the disease. For white women the comparable risk of dying is 0.28 percent. In comparison, the lifetime risks for white men of dying from lung or prostate cancer are 6.94 percent and 3.09 percent, respectively. For white women, the lifetime risks of dying from lung cancer or invasive breast cancer are 4.77 percent and 3.47 percent, respectively.

Clinical screening is defined as the examination of the skin of an asymptomatic person by a physician or other trained individual. The main goal of a new program of skin cancer screening would be to improve survival for people with melanoma. It is the most lethal skin cancer, and treatment is not very successful for late-stage disease. Cure rates are already very high for people with basal cell carcinoma and squamous cell carcinoma, which grow slowly and rarely spread to other organs.

Current Coverage

Unless explicitly authorized by Congress, Medicare does not cover screening, immunizations, and similar preventive services. In recent years, Congress has approved coverage under certain circumstances for several preventive services including screening for breast cancer and colorectal cancer.

Clinical screening of asymptomatic people for skin cancer is not explicitly authorized. Medicare does, however, cover a physician visit initiated by a patient concerned about, for example, a change in the color of a mole or a new skin growth. Similarly, if a physician notices a suspicious skin condition during a visit for another purpose and extends the visit to investigate further, Medicare may pay more for that visit if it meets certain criteria. In either situation, if the physician refers the patient to a dermatologist, the referral visit is also covered, as are any skin biopsies.

Evidence Review, Conclusions, and Cost Estimates

The committee concluded that *the evidence for the effectiveness of skin cancer screening is insufficient to support positive or negative conclusions about a new program of clinical screening of asymptomatic Medicare beneficiaries.* Direct evidence of the effectiveness of clinical screening for skin cancer is lacking rather than negative or ambiguous. No controlled clinical trials have tested the assumption that cancers detected through clinical screening of asymptomatic people have better outcomes than those found by patients or by physicians who discover them during visits for other purposes. A 10-year trial of screening is now underway in Australia, where skin cancers are much more common than in the United States.

The indirect evidence for skin cancer screening is suggestive but not conclusive. Physicians, especially dermatologists, tend to detect thinner melanomas than patients and are more accurate in distinguishing malignant from benign skin conditions. Studies of survival following surgery indicate that thinner melanomas are associated with better survival. These indirect data point to the value of early detection and treatment of skin cancer, but they are not the equivalent of direct evidence from controlled studies showing that detecting thinner melanomas through screening—compared to detection through usual care by alert health care professionals—improves survival. Clinical screening of asymptomatic people might simply (1) extend the time between diagnosis and death (lead-time bias) without improving outcomes or (2) discover many nonaggressive tumors that exist for long periods of time without causing harm, while missing fast-growing, more lethal tumors that arise between screenings (length bias). These biases are important because screening invites healthy people to put themselves at risk for untoward effects (e.g., false positive results that lead to unnecessary further testing and treatment).

For a new program of skin cancer screening, the estimated net five-year cost to Medicare could range from about $150 million to nearly $900 million, depending on the screening approach adopted. The more successful a strategy was in focusing on a smaller group of higher-risk people, the less costly—and the more cost-effective—it would be.

Because indirect evidence does support the benefits of early detection and early treatment as part of usual medical care, clinicians and patients should continue to be alert to the common signs of skin cancer and to investigate suspicious signs further. Medicare already covers skin examination and testing prompted by patient concern about a skin abnormality or by incidental physician discovery of an abnormality.

In addition, *dermatology and other organizations should continue educational programs including programs that encourage people to limit sun exposure (especially children and adolescents) and inform themselves about skin cancer risk factors.* Perhaps the major challenge related to the Medicare population is identifying and implementing better ways of reaching the group at highest risk of death from skin cancer—older white males. Although evidence about the effectiveness of skin self-examination in improving health outcomes is limited, some evidence indicates that women are more likely to self-identify melanomas than men and that men are more likely than women to have a melanoma identified by a family member. It may be useful to investigate further the value of education programs that emphasize the role of family members and close friends in noticing and encouraging professional evaluation of abnormal-appearing areas of skin.

Medically Necessary Dental Services

In discussions about insurance coverage, the term "medically necessary dental services" has been used narrowly to mean care that occurs as the direct result of an underlying medical condition or its treatment or that has a direct effect on such a condition. Under this definition, care for serious periodontal disease would not be "medically necessary" unless, for example, it threatened the health of someone with leukemia or was caused by the disease or its treatment (and could otherwise be health threatening if untreated). Such a restrictive definition may suggest that periodontal or other tooth-related infections are somehow different from infections elsewhere and imply that the mouth can be isolated from the rest of the body, notions neither scientifically based nor constructive for individual or public health. Therefore, this report refers to "medically necessary dental services," using quotation marks as a reminder of the term's specialized and restricted meaning in this discussion of Medicare coverage policy.

Given the resources available, the number of conditions that the committee could review was limited. Based on earlier analyses by others, the committee identified five conditions for examination: (1) head and neck cancer, (2) leukemia, (3) lymphoma, (4) organ transplants, and (5) heart valve repair or replacement. In general, a common link is the risk of oral infection affecting or caused by the medical condition or its treatment.

Current Coverage

From its beginning, the Medicare program has excluded coverage for dental care to treat, fill, remove, or replace teeth or to treat the gums and other structures directly supporting the teeth. A narrow exception allows payments in connection with the provision of dental services incidental to a covered medical procedure, for example, the repair of a fractured jaw. Otherwise, the Health Care Financing Administration (HCFA) has approved Medicare coverage in two situations. One is the extraction of teeth prior to radiation therapy to the jaw, which may be appropriate for patients with extensive periodontal disease and dental abscesses but not for others whose problems can be treated with less drastic interventions. HCFA has also approved coverage for an oral examination as part of patient preparation for kidney transplantation.

Evidence Review, Conclusions, and Cost Estimates

The direct evidence to support coverage for "medically necessary dental services" varies depending on the medical condition to which dental services are related. No randomized clinical trials have investigated outcomes of dental care for head and neck cancer patients receiving radiation therapy to the jaws. Small retrospective studies provide limited direct evidence that replacing aggressive tooth-extraction protocols with tooth-preserving protocols prior to radiation can reduce radiation-related caries and tooth extractions that place patients at high risk for osteoradionecrosis. (Osteoradionecrosis involves bone cell death that can lead to infection, serious disfigurement, and functional impairment). Other retrospective analyses show higher rates of osteoradionecrosis for patients with inadequate dental care and preradiation extractions. Extractions are, however, appropriate for some patients. *Given this limited evidence, the severe consequences of radiation-induced osteoradionecrosis, and Medicare's investment in treating patients with head and neck cancer, it is reasonable for Medicare to cover both tooth-preserving care and extractions.* Patients should be referred for dental examinations as appropriate by their oncologist.

Weak direct evidence suggests that the provision of dental care to prevent or eliminate acute oral infection for leukemia patients prior to chemotherapy can prevent or reduce subsequent episodes of septicemia and prevent or reduce severe oral complications of treatment. *Given this limited evidence, the severe consequences of septicemia and other complications of chemotherapy, and Medicare's investment in treating leukemia patients, it is reasonable for Medicare to cover a dental examination, cleaning of teeth, and treatment of acute infections of the teeth or gums for a leukemia patient prior to chemotherapy.* Again, patients should be referred to a dentist as appropriate by their physician.

The committee concluded that *the evidence is insufficient to support positive or negative conclusions about dental services for patients with lymphoma, organ transplants, and heart valve repair or replacement.* Indirect evidence and biologic plausibility are suggestive but not conclusive that health outcomes may be improved by eliminating oral sources of infection that may cause septicemia in immunosuppressed lymphoma or organ transplant patients or endocarditis in patients with a diseased, abnormal, or surgically repaired or replaced heart valve. The committee notes, however, that widely accepted clinical protocols for identifying and eliminating all infections and potential sources of infection before organ transplantation and certain other procedures are based largely on biological principles, animal studies, and clinical experience, not direct evidence from controlled trials.

For head and neck cancer patients receiving radiation therapy, the estimated net five-year cost to Medicare for covering a limited set of dental services would be $12.9 million. For leukemia patients undergoing chemotherapy, the net cost would be $20.9 million. The estimated five-year net costs to Medicare would be $32.3 million for beneficiaries being treated for lymphoma, $24.2 for those receiving a solid organ transplant, and $117.5 million for those undergoing heart valve replacement or repair. These estimates generally assume, on average, two visits per patient with teeth.

Although the evidence base for "medically necessary dental services" is limited, the committee is concerned about interpretations of the current law that might preclude further coverage exceptions for dental services that are effective in reducing infections in high-risk patients. Given therapeutic advances since the creation of Medicare and these concerns about coverage interpretation, the committee concludes that it is reasonable for Congress to update statutory language to clearly allow coverage of these kinds of dental services. Specifically, the committee suggests that *Congress should direct the Health Care Financing Administration (with assistance as appropriate from the Agency for Health Care Policy and Research and the National Institutes of Health) to develop recommendations—on a condition-by-condition basis—for coverage of effective dental services needed in conjunction with surgery, chemotherapy, radiation, or pharmacological treatment for a life-threatening medical condition.* The phrase "in conjunction with" would limit the window of coverage to a specified period before or after surgery or other treatment but would not require that the services be provided as an immediate part of a medical procedure. This minimal revision in the 1965 statute would not alter Medicare's basic focus on treatment of acute illness or injury.

Eliminating the Time Limit on Coverage of Immunosuppressive Drugs for Transplant Recipients

Successful transplantation of human organs is one of the most dramatic achievements of modern medicine. From the 1950s through the 1970s, organ transplantation was restricted by the limited effectiveness of treatment to control the body's rejection of grafted organs. When effective immunosuppressive drugs became available in the 1980s, transplantation became an accepted treatment for an increasing number of deadly diseases. Over 20,000 transplants were performed in 1998, and estimates of the number of people living with a functioning graft range up to 125,000.

Today, a major limit on transplantation is the shortage of donated organs. Nearly 65,000 people were registered on waiting lists for organ transplantation in 1998, and more than 4,500 were removed from waiting lists due to death. The high cost of immunosuppressive drugs, which may total from $5,000 to $16,000 each year, means most transplant recipients need financial assistance to pay for them.

Current Coverage

Immunosuppressive drugs prescribed for transplant recipients represent one of the few exceptions to Medicare's exclusion of coverage for self-administered outpatient drugs. Coverage of the drugs is limited to three years following a transplant, an increase from the one year of coverage originally authorized in 1986. Except for kidney transplant recipients (who are covered under special legislation for people with end-stage renal disease [ESRD]), transplant recipients must qualify for Medicare by reason of age or disability.

Evidence Review, Conclusions, and Cost Estimates

Good evidence supports patients' continued need for immunosuppressive therapy and their increased risk of graft loss if they cannot follow their prescribed drug regimen. Although people who lose coverage often find other options for securing sufficient drugs to maintain immunosuppression, experience and limited evidence suggest that some transplant recipients eventually lose their grafts for lack of coverage. Some return to dialysis or receive a second transplant, but others die. *Given this evidence and the existing Medicare policy of supporting organ transplants, the rationale for eliminating the current time limits for coverage of immunosuppressive drugs for all solid organ transplant recipients is strong.*

The estimated five-year net cost to Medicare of completely eliminating the three-year limit on coverage would be approximately $778 million if coverage were limited to those qualifying for Medicare by reason of age or disability.[3] If coverage were also extended to kidney transplant recipients who have qualified for Medicare based on ESRD diagnosis alone (and who lose all Medicare coverage after three years), the estimated net cost would rise to approximately $1.06 billion.

In addition to the economic and possible clinical consequences of time-limited drug coverage for transplant recipients, current policy has societal implications. Organs are a scarce resource for which demand far outstrips supply. Every graft failure that results in retransplantation is a special burden on this limited supply. Beyond those immediately affected, others have a strong interest in the successful maintenance of grafts to protect their potential access or that of their loved ones.

Nonetheless, the case of immunosuppressive drugs highlights the ethical dilemmas and other complexities that policymakers can encounter in trying to develop rational, consistent, and fair coverage policies for all Medicare beneficiaries. This report does not examine such issues in depth, but it does look at a few broad questions about coverage decisionmaking for preventive and other services.

DECIDING COVERAGE FOR PREVENTIVE AND OTHER SERVICES

Medicare coverage decisions range from very broad-based decisions about whole categories of services to very narrow decisions about whether a specific service will be covered for a specific individual. In between are decisions about the general circumstances under which a specific service will be covered (e.g., that bone marrow transplant will be covered for certain cancers and not others). In general, these kinds of decisions are made at three different levels, with

- Congress making broad decisions about categories of coverage and coverage exceptions,
- HCFA focusing on the general circumstances under which a new or established service will be covered, and
- private contractors that administer Medicare claims for the government deciding whether specific services billed for a specific beneficiary are covered and also establishing policies for services and circumstances for which HCFA has no policy.

One criticism of Congress's service-by-service approach to coverage decisions about preventive services and other generally excluded categories of care

---

[3]As this report was being completed, Congress approved an extension of coverage for eight months for this group of beneficiaries.

is that this approach may favor services for high-profile conditions and technologies that have strong lobbying groups but not necessarily a strong evidence base. Another criticism is that the focus on winning coverage for specific services, especially services of questionable effectiveness, can distract policymakers, advocates, and clinicians from nonfinancial barriers to the widespread use of preventive services and other interventions known to be effective.

Linking Evidence to Medicare Coverage:
The Case of Preventive Services

During the first three decades following the establishment of Medicare, Congress appeared to be sensitive to issues of clinical effectiveness and cost-effectiveness. For example, at the behest of Congress, the now-defunct Office of Technology Assessment undertook analyses of the cost-effectiveness of several preventive services. Congress also authorized the Department of Health and Human Services (DHHS) to undertake preventive services demonstration projects that included assessments of cost-effectiveness. A study of congressional coverage decisions from 1965 to 1990 identified evidence of favorable cost-effectiveness ratios as one factor differentiating preventive services approved for coverage from those not approved.

A comparison of the preventive services now covered by Medicare with those recommended by the United States Preventive Services Task Force (USPSTF) for asymptomatic people over age 64 shows that Medicare excludes some services that were recommended by the Task Force and includes some that were not recommended. The Task Force is charged with making evidence-based recommendations about the use of clinical preventive services as part of a periodic health examination; it does not make coverage recommendations.

Of the eight screening services recommended by USPSTF for those over age 64, Medicare does not explicitly cover blood pressure testing, height and weight checks, and screening for vision and hearing impairment and problem drinking. Of the 15 recommended counseling and education services, Medicare explicitly covers only diabetes education. Some recommended services, in particular, blood pressure tests, are routine parts of patient visits for many older people who see a physician or nurse practitioner for a variety of reasons including screenings covered by Medicare. About 90 percent of Medicare beneficiaries have at least one physician visit a year.

In 1997, Congress approved coverage for two screening services that were not among those recommended by the USPSTF. Specifically, the Task Force judged the evidence insufficient to recommend for or against osteoporosis screening by bone densitometry. Further, it judged the evidence sufficient to recommend that men not be screened for prostate cancer. To the extent that Medicare covers such services, it gives them a "stamp of approval." It could thereby help divert patients, clinicians, and others from focusing on more beneficial care and from adequately weighing the potential of some services to harm healthy people who have false positive screening results and then undergo unnecessary further testing and treatment.

Given the improved methods for systematically assessing scientific evidence about what works and does not work in medical care, it may be useful for decisionmakers to consider more explicit processes for linking coverage of services to evidence of their effectiveness and cost-effectiveness. For example, as suggested above, Congress could direct the HCFA to develop evidence-based recommendations for covering dental care in conjunction with certain serious medical conditions and treatments. Similarly, for the preventive services recommended by the USPSTF based on reviews of relevant evidence, Congress could direct the Health Care Financing Administration to assess these services in the context of the Medicare program and then make coverage recommendations. Such recommendations would provide Congress systematic analyses of the potential benefits, harms, costs, and cost-effectiveness of covering additional dental or preventive services. These tasks would require new resources. Adding to HCFA's workload without adding new resources could do more harm than good, for example, if the agency simply rerouted resources from quality monitoring or other important administrative responsibilities.

The Infrastructure for Making Coverage Decisions

The committee's work reinforced its view that evidence-based review of new and existing health services can be a powerful tool for guiding clinical and policy decisions. Such an approach helps make clear the extent to which there is good evidence about the benefits and harms of a particular intervention and points those who conduct and fund research toward important health problems for which good evidence does not exist. It puts pressure on clinicians to abandon practices that are clearly not beneficial and to apply and recommend practices that have been identified as worthwhile. It likewise supports governments and others who pay for care in revising coverage, reimbursement, quality assessment, and related policies to discourage nonbeneficial services and encourage effective care.

The analyses reported here also make clear the value of public and private efforts to build a stronger knowledge infrastructure for clinical, public health, and other health care decisions. This "infrastructure" includes

1. Clinical, epidemiological, health services, and other research that helps clinicians, consumers, and policymakers compare the potential benefits and harms of different health care strategies;

2. Methods and tools that are needed to conduct and present valid and useful research; and

3. Organizational structures and procedures that must exist to initiate and manage knowledge-building efforts, effectively apply knowledge to clinical and policy decisions, and then monitor results to guide future activities.

Although this report did not comprehensively examine the infrastructure for coverage decisionmaking, certain weaknesses became evident in the course of this study. One weakness relates to the still-limited use in much clinical research of outcomes measures that are meaningful to patients. Physiological measures are important and convenient but not sufficient for assessing whether interventions improve health as people actually experience it.

Much is assumed but relatively little is known about how individuals perceive the possible benefits and harms of different health services. Without assessments of individual and societal preferences for the outcomes of different health interventions, the usefulness of cost-effectiveness analyses and comparisons may be diminished. For example, the calculation of quality-adjusted life years or similar summary measures of health status depends not only on evidence about the benefits and harms of interventions but also on information about how people value these outcomes.

Another weakness is that, despite steps taken by public and private organizations to improve information and processes for clinical and coverage decisionmaking, no common standards of evidence govern the multiple decisionmakers now involved. This is particularly true for the early stages when innovative technologies first come to the attention of health plans.

Further, despite calls for health plans and other organizations to be more rigorous and open about their criteria and evidence for making recommendations or decisions, organizational practices and statements are highly variable. The committee's review of statements by other organizations revealed both substantive disagreement and differences in the extent to which recommendations were accompanied by descriptions of their development process and supporting evidence. All use some degree of expert judgment and consensus, but the role of evidence in informing judgment is not clear in many cases. This makes it difficult to judge the basis for inconsistent recommendations and identify gaps in biomedical, clinical, and health services research.

The uneven consideration of cost-effectiveness and costs is a further concern. Currently, congressional decisions about extending coverage for now-excluded care are governed by budget neutrality rules that favor services projected to save the Medicare program money. Even if excluded services are more cost-effective—that is, have greater benefits relative to costs—than some already covered services, they face a high hurdle to acceptance. On the administrative side, HCFA has tried but largely failed in its efforts to include cost-effectiveness among the explicit criteria for coverage decisions.

To tackle these and other weaknesses in the infrastructure for coverage decisionmaking and improve the value of Medicare spending will require resources. As noted above, adding new tasks for HCFA without adding new resources could do more harm than good. Although additional resources for infrastructure improvements would be minuscule compared to the total budget for Medicare or the National Institutes of Health, they nonetheless could be difficult to commit under current budget rules.

BEYOND COVERAGE

The Medicare program has undoubtedly helped millions of Americans obtain needed health services. Still, even those individuals fortunate enough to have coverage from Medicare or other sources do not necessarily receive recommended care. In some cases, beneficiaries fail to seek these services or their physicians fail to provide or recommend them. That coverage fails to guarantee the use of effective services is not, of course, an argument for not covering them. It is, however, an argument for paying attention to other obstacles to care.

Many organizations, including Congress and DHHS, have recognized such obstacles to implementing recommended clinical preventive measures and supported public and private actions to overcome them. For some services and populations, community-based prevention programs may be more successful (and less expensive) in getting services to high-risk groups than coverage, which involves a physician visit. Such programs—particularly those involving quick, noninvasive services such as immunizations—may seek people out in workplaces, shopping centers, and similar places.

As is true for health care services themselves, the effectiveness of organizational efforts to improve the delivery of services cannot be assumed. Although evaluation is expensive and often difficult, especially when controlled studies are attempted, organizational initiatives also need to be evaluated.

BEYOND EVIDENCE

The conclusions summarized above reflect the limited evidence available to support clinical or coverage decisions about many health care services. In addition, each service presents policy and ethical questions that were beyond the scope of this report.

For example, decisions about coverage of immunosuppressive drugs take place in the context of a complicated set of distinctions about what (and who) Medicare does and does not cover. Thus, the availability and scope of coverage varies for people with and without an ESRD diagnosis; for ESRD patients on dialysis versus those who receive kidney transplants; for kidney versus other transplant candidates or recipients; and for Medicare-covered transplant recipients versus other beneficiaries needing expensive prescription drugs. Are these distinctions fair? Should government attempt to eliminate or reduce such major disparities in coverage?

Evidence cannot usually resolve such fundamental political and ethical questions. It can, however, often clarify the rationales and potential consequences of different answers. It can also help policymakers assess the actual consequences—for good and ill—of their decisions.

1

Introduction

Congress created the Medicare program in 1965 to provide health insurance for Americans age 65 or over. It later extended coverage to some individuals with disabilities or permanent kidney failure. From the outset, the program has focused on coverage for hospital, physician, and certain other services that are "reasonable and necessary for the diagnosis or treatment of illness or injury or to improve the functioning of a malformed body member" (section 1862 of the Social Security Act). With certain exceptions, Congress explicitly excluded coverage for preventive services, outpatient prescription drugs, dental care, and long-term nursing home care and other supportive services for people with chronic disabling conditions.

Most sessions of Congress see proposals to expand Medicare coverage for one or more of the services that are currently excluded. For example, while this report was being drafted, Congress was debating the addition of outpatient drug benefits, which even under the most limited proposals would add substantially to the program's costs. With growth in Medicare spending and health care costs having far exceeded 1960s' estimates, the increased cost of additional services has generally discouraged coverage expansions. Moreover, Congress has set budget rules for itself requiring that decisions to increase most types of federal spending must be accompanied by explicit decisions to reduce spending elsewhere or to raise taxes. These rules underscore the reality that expanding Medicare coverage involves making trade-offs in the face of resource constraints.

In the Balanced Budget Act of 1997 (Public Law 105-33), Congress called for the Department of Health and Human Services to arrange for the National

Academy of Sciences (NAS) to analyze "the short- and long-term benefits, and costs to Medicare" of extending Medicare coverage for certain preventive and other services. These services were screening for skin cancer; medically necessary dental services; elimination of time restrictions on coverage for immunosuppressive drugs for transplant recipients; nutrition therapy; and routine patient care for beneficiaries enrolled in approved clinical trials.

This request from Congress reflects two significant developments since Medicare's beginnings: an accelerating pace of technological innovation and— partly as a consequence—a greater than anticipated escalation of program expenditures and overall health care costs. Scientific and technological advances have clearly led to a multitude of new medical procedures, drugs, devices, and other services that prolong life, protect physical and mental functioning, prevent disease, and otherwise improve people's health and well-being. Of course, not all innovations perform as promised. Moreover, most new—and established—technologies have risks that have to be weighed against expected benefits. Cost constraints also require that trade-offs be made.

The 1980s and 1990s saw increasing recognition that the knowledge base for clinical practice and health policy was more limited than had previously been acknowledged (e.g., see IOM, 1992; OTA, 1994; PPRC, 1989). For example, those developing clinical practice guidelines often found little or no sound research to inform many of the specific decisions faced in the course of caring for people with a particular health problem. A number of public and private sector initiatives have tackled this knowledge deficit. Some have focused on primary clinical research, and others on systematically assessing the results of past research. Each of the services examined in this report highlights different challenges in using available research and analytic methods to guide decisions.

This report, prepared by a committee appointed by the Institute of Medicine (IOM; part of the NAS), analyzes the evidence base for three of the five areas listed in the Balanced Budget Act: (1) skin cancer screening, (2) medically necessary dental services, and (3) elimination of time limits on coverage of immunosuppressive drugs for certain transplant recipients.[1] In addition to examining the expected clinical effectiveness and the expected cost to Medicare of covering these services, the IOM also examined more generally the processes and organizational infrastructure for making decisions about Medicare coverage of preventive and other services.

The analyses and conclusions presented here are intended to assist policymakers by providing a synthesis of the best evidence available about the effec-

---

[1]The other two areas are covered by separate reports developed by other IOM committees, *Extending Medicare Reimbursement in Clinical Trials* and *The Role of Nutrition Therapy in Maintaining the Health of the Nation's Elderly: Evaluating Coverage of Nutrition Services for Medicare Beneficiaries,* which are available from the National Academy Press (www.nap.edu).

tiveness of the services and the cost to Medicare of covering these interventions. The conclusions do not include detailed coverage recommendations for Medicare, nor are they specific enough to constitute practice guidelines that physicians, dentists, nurse practitioners, or other clinicians could use to inform day-to-day clinical decisions. The analyses are, however, meant to be credible to clinicians as well as policymakers.

The next sections of this chapter briefly summarize the evolution of the Medicare program and review current processes for determining what services Medicare will cover. This discussion provides context for the remainder of the report.

THE MEDICARE PROGRAM

Historical Background

When Congress—following years of debate—created Medicare as Title XVIII of the Social Security Act (SSA), it was responding to the growing availability of effective medical services and the difficulty faced by older people in either paying for these services directly or obtaining private health insurance.[2] At the same time, Congress also created the federal–state Medicaid program (Title XIX of the SSA), which provided health insurance for certain categories of low-income individuals (primarily low-income mothers and children and low-income aged, blind, or disabled people). Reflecting the needs of these lower-income beneficiaries, Medicaid covers a generally broader array of services than Medicare (e.g., well-baby visits, extended nursing home care). It also provides states some flexibility in deciding what to cover (e.g., certain dental services, outpatient prescription drugs). Certain low-income people, called "dual eligibles," qualify for full or partial Medicaid benefits as well as regular Medicare coverage. Their Medicaid benefits cover many of the Medicare program's cost-sharing requirements and "fill in" some of the gaps in Medicare benefits. In 1972, Congress expanded Medicare to cover certain disabled persons and created a unique entitlement to coverage for people who suffer from end-stage kidney disease (ESRD).[3]

Continuing a division that had emerged earlier in private health insurance, the Medicare program as initially created had two parts: hospitalization insurance, also known as HI or Part A, and supplementary medical insurance for physician and certain other services, also known as SMI or Part B.[4] Part A, which is

---

[2]This discussion draws on Ball, 1995; Feingold, 1966; Harris, 1969; Marmor, 1973; Somers and Somers, 1961, 1967, 1977a,b; Starr, 1982; and Stevens, 1989.

[3]Appendix D briefly reviews the history of the ESRD benefit. See also IOM, 1991.

[4]In 1997, as part of the Balanced Budget Act, Congress created Part C (known as Medicare+Choice), which restructured and expanded options for Medicare beneficiaries to enroll in approved health maintenance organizations and other private health insurance plans. These plans, which are paid a fixed monthly amount per enrolled beneficiary, must provide Medicare-covered services but may also offer additional benefits.

financed by payroll taxes (1.45 percent paid by employers and employees), covers inpatient hospital care subject to an annual deductible set at $768 in 1999 and a per-day copayment after 60 days. It also covers (subject to various time limitations, cost-sharing requirements, and other restrictions) services provided by other institutional providers including skilled nursing facilities and hospices. One rationale for covering these kinds of services and providers has been that such coverage may encourage the use of alternatives to more expensive hospital care. Part B covers physician and certain other professional services provided in the hospital, office, and selected other settings. It also covers a number of additional services such as outpatient dialysis services, clinical laboratory tests, durable medical equipment, ambulance services and, since 1997, most home health care services. For Part B coverage, beneficiaries pay a monthly premium (set to cover 25 percent of Part B expenditures or $45.50 per beneficiary in 1999) and coinsurance of 20 percent for most services. Part A coverage is virtually automatic for those eligible, but enrollment in Part B is voluntary, although nearly all those eligible do enroll.

As noted above, the legislation creating Medicare excluded coverage for services not deemed "reasonable and necessary" for the diagnosis or treatment of an illness or injury or to improve the functioning of a malformed body member. Preventive services, dental care (except in very limited situations related to serious medical problems), and outpatient prescription drugs were among the services categorically excluded in 1965.

One rationale for excluding preventive services from Medicare was that they did not fit the traditional insurance model of providing coverage for expenses that are unpredictable (and thus cannot be budgeted) and substantial (and thus are a serious financial burden to individuals and families). When Medicare was created, hospitalization and other major expenses related to care for acute illnesses fit the model; expenses for most preventive services, outpatient prescription drugs, and dental care did not. In addition, insurance principles also discouraged coverage for "broad and ill-defined" services such as routine physicals and health education or counseling (Breslow and Somers, 1977; OTA, 1990b).

Since 1965, Congress has authorized a few exceptions to the coverage exclusions just described. After rejecting 350 bills to make one or more exceptions to Medicare's exclusion of preventive services, Congress approved its first exception—for pneumococcal pneumonia vaccine—in 1980 (Schauffler, 1993). More exceptions have followed. As discussed in Chapter 6, Congress has waived the application of the Part B deductible and coinsurance provisions for some covered preventive services.

Although the significance and cost of drug therapies have increased substantially since 1965, Congress has approved very few exceptions to its exclusion of coverage for prescription drugs. In 1986, Congress authorized time-limited coverage of self-administered immunosuppressive drugs for Medicare-covered transplant patients, and it has since added a handful of further exceptions for other prescription drugs that patients self-administer on an outpatient basis.

Congress has made no additional exceptions to the original coverage exclusion related to dental care. As discussed in Chapter 4, the Health Care Financing Administration (HCFA) has ruled that very few services meet the limited exception provided in the 1965 legislation.

Because of gaps in Medicare coverage, about 80 percent of beneficiaries purchase or otherwise obtain some form of supplemental coverage to help pay for certain excluded services, deductibles, and copayments or coinsurance (HCFA, 1998a). This coverage may be provided through an employer-sponsored program, an individually purchased "Medigap" policy, or a state Medicaid program. Medicare beneficiaries covered by health maintenance organizations (HMOs) may be eligible for additional preventive and other services, sometimes by paying an additional premium, but HMOs vary greatly in the extent to which they offer benefits not required by Medicare (Kaiser Family Foundation, 1998).

Enrollment and Expenditure Trends

Since the program was implemented, the number of Medicare beneficiaries has roughly doubled, from 19.1 million when the program took effect in 1966 to approximately 38.4 million in 1997 (about 4.8 million of whom qualify for Medicare due to disability and about 0.3 million due to a diagnosis of end-stage renal disease [HCFA, 1999a]). The growth in Medicare enrollment will accelerate as the baby boom generation begins to reach age 65 (and becomes eligible for coverage) in 2011. By 2015, the population age 65 years and over is projected to reach 56.3 million. Unless age or other eligibility requirements change, virtually all will be covered by Medicare. Those qualifying because of disability or end-stage renal disease are expected to constitute a somewhat larger fraction of the total beneficiary population by 2015 (about 16 percent compared to 13 percent in 1997).

Initial forecasts of program spending proved to be gross underestimates of actual spending. While the number of beneficiaries was doubling, Medicare net outlays grew from $2.7 billion in 1967 (the program's first full year) to $174.2 billion in 1996 (U.S. House of Representatives, 1997, 1998). (In constant 1995 dollars, 1967 expenditures would amount to about $10 billion.)

Current debates about Medicare's future revolve primarily around predictions that Part A of the program will become insolvent (spending will exceed revenues) early in the 21st century. Projections of long-term Medicare program costs—and health care costs more generally—have many uncertainties (White, 1999). Nonetheless, concerns about the federal spending and program solvency have prompted discussions of major and controversial program changes such as raising the age of eligibility, instituting some kind of means testing, directing more beneficiaries into capitated managed care plans, and establishing a formula for the government's contribution to program costs that would shift more of the risk for continued health care cost escalation to beneficiaries. A major component of the Balanced Budget Act of 1997 was a set of measures to slow the growth in program spending and at least delay the date at which Medicare spending is projected to exceed revenues (Kahn and Kuttner, 1999).[5] Solvency concerns are also shaping reactions to less comprehensive changes of the kind considered in this report.

As mentioned earlier, congressional budget rules require that certain decisions to increase federal government spending in one area be offset with actions to reduce spending in other areas or to increase taxes or other revenues. For example, higher estimated net spending for covering new preventive or dental services or outpatient drugs would usually have to be matched by increased taxes or reduced spending either elsewhere in the Medicare program (e.g., through lower payment rates for health care providers) or in other areas (e.g., Medicaid).

MEDICARE COVERAGE DECISIONS

Medicare coverage decisions range from very broad-based decisions about whole categories of services to very narrow decisions about whether a specific service will be covered for a specific individual. In between are decisions about the general circumstances under which a specific service will be covered (e.g., that bone marrow transplant will be covered for certain cancers and not others). For the most part, these kinds of decisions are made at three different levels, with

- Congress making broad decisions about categories of coverage and coverage exceptions,
- HCFA focusing on the circumstances under which a new or established service will be covered, and
- private contractors that administer Medicare claims for the government deciding whether specific services billed for a specific beneficiary are covered and also establishing policies for services and circumstances for which HCFA has no policy.

Congress

Congress establishes the broad categories of covered and excluded services. It may also make coverage exceptions for individual services in otherwise ex-

---

[5]As this report was being completed, Congress extended coverage of immunosuppressive drugs for up to eight months (subject to expenditure limits) for transplant recipients eligible for Medicare by reason of age or disability (P.L. 106-113).

cluded categories. In considering legislative proposals to extend coverage, Congress may hold hearings to solicit expert advice (including assessments of scientific evidence) and the views of patients, families, clinicians, health industry manufacturers, administrators, and other interested groups. Until it was terminated in 1995, the congressional Office of Technology Assessment (OTA) responded to congressional requests for assessments of clinical preventive measures, immunosuppressive drugs, and other services. The OTA analyses considered scientific and clinical issues but were also explicitly intended to provide guidance to policymakers by examining the cost-effectiveness of clinical interventions, possible costs to Medicare of extending coverage, and other policy issues.

For categories of covered services, Congress has authorized HCFA to establish procedures for making more specific coverage decisions about individual services within the broad categories established legislatively. It could also authorize HCFA (which is part of the Department of Health and Human Services) or a quasi-public body either to make coverage exceptions or recommend exceptions for services that now fall in the categories of generally excluded services. For example, the early 1990s discussion of health care reform saw various proposals for delegating decisions about preventive services (OTA, 1993).

Health Care Financing Administration

Within the broad coverage categories established by Congress, more specific determinations about what services are or are not covered are the responsibility of the Health Care Financing Administration (Bagley and McVearry, 1998). HCFA also provides detailed guidance to Medicare contractors regarding the application of its coverage rules and the development of local contractor medical policies for situations not dealt with by such rules.

Altogether, HCFA has issued about 700 national coverage policy decisions (personal communication, John Whyte, July 1999). These decisions typically involve either new services and technologies or new indications (clinical circumstances) for the use of technologies that had previously been covered for a limited set of indications. Some determinations restrict coverage of an already covered service—usually because new evidence suggests the service is unsafe or ineffective.

The coverage determination process may involve reviews of the scientific evidence, consultations with clinical experts, and comparisons with similar technologies. For those outpatient drugs (e.g., immunosuppressants for transplant patients) that fall under congressionally established coverage categories or exceptions, HCFA usually requires, among other conditions, that drugs have final marketing approval by the Food and Drug Administration, meaning they are considered safe and effective for the indications specified on the label.[6]

Some technology assessments are conducted by HCFA staff, whereas others are referred to different governmental or private organizations including the federal Agency for Health Care Policy and Research (AHCPR) and its Evidence-Based Practice Centers (EPCs). Created by Congress in 1989, AHCPR supports an array of activities intended to increase and evaluate the evidence base for health care services. The EPCs—many of which are consortia or partnerships of universities and other institutions—produce evidence reports and technology assessments on topics as requested. If nongovernmental parties request a coverage determination from HCFA, they are expected to provide supporting documentation including reviews and analyses of the scientific evidence, unless they lack the resources to do so.

In making coverage determinations, HCFA must follow federal rule-making procedures and requirements. After criticism that agency procedures violated federal open government rules, HCFA created a new Medicare Coverage Advisory Committee, for which administrative procedures are being developed and reviewed.[7] Because the services considered in this report are explicitly excluded by statute from current coverage categories, they would not normally be candidates for consideration by this new committee.

HCFA has interpreted the congressional requirement that services be covered only if "reasonable and necessary" for the diagnosis or treatment of an illness or injury to mean that they must be (1) safe and effective, (2) provided in an appropriate setting, and (3) not experimental or investigational (HCFA, 1989). The criteria and processes for determining what services are medically necessary have been the subject of much debate and dissatisfaction (e.g., see Anderson et al., 1998; Bergthold, 1995; Cunningham, 1999; IOM, 1992; NHPF, 1998, 1999).

In January 1989, and as recently as 1996, HCFA proposed to consider the cost-effectiveness of technologies as part of the coverage review process (HSR, 1997). The proposal provoked considerable controversy and was never adopted. HCFA should shortly be issuing a new *Federal Register* notice proposing national coverage criteria.

---

[6]In establishing specific coverage policies, HCFA does not necessarily restrict coverage to the so-called labeled indications. For decisions about off-label uses, HCFA provides that its administrative contractors may consider authoritative medical literature and "accepted standards of medical practice" (*Carriers Manual,* section 2049.4 [HCFA, 1999b]).

[7]This committee will operate under the Federal Advisory Committee Act (*Federal Register [FR]* Vol. 63, No. 239, December 14, 1998, p. 68780). HCFA has also published a notice explaining the new process of making national coverage decisions (*FR* Vol. 64, No. 80, April 27, 1999, pp. 22619–22625). A notice on proposed coverage criteria is expected by the end of 1999.

Because individual coverage determinations by HCFA are not directly governed by the "budget neutrality" rules of Congress, new services that fit within established coverage categories face different hurdles to coverage approval than do services that require congressional action. The last chapter of this report returns to this and other issues related to the role of effectiveness, cost, and cost-effectiveness analyses in coverage decisions.

Administrative Contractors

In practice, many coverage determinations—perhaps 90 percent (HIMA, 1999)—are made not by HCFA but by the 60-plus private contractors that the agency uses to administer payment of Medicare claims on a state, substate, or multistate basis. On the Part A side, these organizations are called "intermediaries." For Part B, which generates nearly all coverage questions, they are known as "carriers." HMOs and other private health plans approved by Medicare to serve beneficiaries must follow intermediary and carrier policies, but they also must make their own coverage determinations in the absence of such policies.

Frequently, it is the private carriers that first encounter questions about new medical services or services for which coverage is sought beyond the uses originally recognized. Their determinations are codified in the form of local medical review policies. Local medical policies may also specify more precisely the appropriate indications for established technologies for which excessive use is suspected. This is consistent with HCFA's description of medical review policy as a "program integrity" tool intended to protect the program from fraud and abuse (*Program Integrity Manual,* section 7501.2 [HCFA, 1999b]).

Carriers make decisions about payment after services have been provided. HCFA uses another group of contractors, Peer Review Organizations (PROs), to conduct prior reviews of certain surgical procedures and engage in other activities intended to improve the quality of care provided Medicare beneficiaries. Contractors administering provider claims for payment must coordinate with the appropriate PROs to assure that payments are made consistent with the PROs' decisions (*Carriers Manual,* section 4170 [HCFA, 1999b]).

HCFA's new procedures for national coverage decisionmaking make clear that local medical policy decisions cannot conflict with a national decision by HCFA. Other HCFA policies direct carriers to base policies on the best evidence available, cite the basis and references for local medical policies, submit the policies to their Carrier Advisory Committees, publish them in their provider bulletins, and consider comments submitted in response (*Carriers Manual,* section 7501 [HCFA, 1999b]). Carriers may conduct their own assessments of new or established services and technologies, or they may rely on others, for example, ECRI (originally the Emergency Care Research Institute) or the Technical

Evaluation Center of the Blue Cross and Blue Shield Association (both of which are designated EPCs).

Carrier coverage policies are generally prompted by the need to make determinations about coverage of a service provided to a specific individual rather than by, for example, a request for a policy or by the anticipation of claims related to an emerging technology. When the judgments are negative, such case-by-case negative decisions may readily evoke images of big, impersonal bureaucracies refusing to pay for innovative treatments that provide the last hope for desperately ill individuals. Controversies about such negative coverage decisions—and conflicting decisions from different carriers—may then prompt HCFA on its own initiative or at the request of others to develop a uniform national policy. In addition to revising procedures for national coverage decision-making and clarifying the role of local organizations in the coverage process, HCFA has a contractor examining variation in local medical policies.

COVERAGE, ACCESS TO CARE, AND OUTCOMES

Rationales for Extending Medicare Coverage

The conditions and services examined in this report illustrate the range of arguments—which may or may not be supported by evidence—for altering statutory coverage exclusions. For screening services, which are directed at people without symptoms, the argument in favor of Medicare coverage typically assumes that coverage will encourage the use of services (especially among low-income beneficiaries) by reducing the cost barrier to care. It is argued further that increased use of screening services will mean that problems will be caught earlier and that this will permit more successful treatment. A related claim in support of screening is that it will save Medicare money by reducing the use of expensive late-stage care.

For "medically necessary dental services," the argument is that dental care is one part of appropriate care for many people with serious medical problems, particularly those vulnerable to life-threatening systemic infections. Excluding coverage for these services unreasonably adds to the physical, emotional, or financial burden of illness and may increase Medicare costs for treating avoidable complications of the medical conditions.

Finally, for immunosuppressive drugs, the argument is that eliminating the three-year coverage limit will reduce the financial and emotional burdens on transplant patients (especially those without other financial resources) and will improve patient access and adherence to drug regimens that are effective in reducing graft rejection and mortality. Reduced rejection of grafts will then reduce Medicare spending for retransplantation or dialysis. Extended coverage might also reduce incentives for some beneficiaries to stay qualified for disability benefits rather than try to return to work. More generally, because organs are a scarce resource for which demand far outstrips supply, the larger society of citizens has a strong interest in the successful maintenance of grafts.

In each example above, one assumption is that Medicare coverage will increase the use of beneficial health care by reducing the cost to the beneficiary. Certainly, as an insurance program, Medicare has sought both to increase access to appropriate health care and to reduce the financial burden of ill health.

Insurance and the Use of Health Care Services

Health services research suggests that insurance coverage encourages the use of preventive and other health services (e.g., see Cohen et al., 1997; Faulkner and Schauffler, 1997; German et al., 1995; Lave et al., 1996; Marquis and Long, 1996; Powell-Griner et al., 1999). Research also suggests that lack of financial access is not the only barrier to the provision or use of preventive and other services (e.g., see CDC, 1997; Chan et al., 1999; Lave et al., 1996; Lieu et al., 1994; Schauffler and Rodriguez, 1993; Weese and Krauss, 1995). Other barriers may include lower levels of education or information, rural or inner city residence, language difficulties, physical or cognitive disabilities, transportation difficulties, and health care organizational or system problems. The latter problems include long waiting times for appointments, poor coordination of services, requirements for advance approval of services by health plans, and lack of reminder and follow-up systems for both patients and clinicians.

Thus, although health insurance supports access to care, it cannot guarantee it. Moreover, some studies suggest that insurance may be more effective in encouraging use of preventive services among higher-income, lower-risk people than among those more at risk (e.g., see Amonkar et al., 1999; Roos et al., 1999; Solberg et al., 1997; Taira et al., 1997). As discussed further in Chapter 6, policymakers, public health officials, and others have worked to develop additional strategies to deliver needed care to the latter groups.

Another problem has been highlighted by research that links insurance to greater use of both appropriate and inappropriate care, and conversely, the application of some cost management strategies to reductions in the use of both categories of care (e.g., see Foxman et al., 1987; Kahn et al., 1990; Keeler et al., 1985; Lohr et al., 1986; Shaughnessy et al., 1994; Siu et al., 1986). Inappropriate care may be informally defined as care that evidence or expert judgment indicates will be ineffective given a patient's condition. Such care wastes scarce resources and may endanger patients. It is, consequently, a prime target of many educational, financial, administrative, and other strategies that attempt to both control the costs and improve the quality of health care.

Even appropriate care may be subject to coverage limits based on traditional insurance principles that target coverage for events or services that are (1) unpredictable for the insured individual but predictable for large groups, (2) outside the control of the insured individual, (3) precisely definable and measurable, (4) too expensive for most people to budget, but (5) not so expensive that the cost of coverage is unacceptable to the insurance purchaser (Donabedian, 1976; Faulkner, 1940; IOM, 1993; MacIntyre, 1962). One or more of these restrictions can be cited to justify exclusions for many preventive and dental services, and prescription drugs.

Nonetheless, as the broader social implications of insurance principles and programs have been recognized, insurers as well as governments have weighed these principles against other values and found occasions to make health insurance programs less restrictive. For example, as evidence has grown of the effectiveness of services such as screening mammography, Pap smears, and immunizations, public and private insurers have extended coverage to a variety of preventive services—including some for which the evidence is inconclusive or inadequate (see Chapter 6).

OVERVIEW OF THE REPORT

To develop this report, the Institute of Medicine, part of the National Academy of Sciences, created a seven-member committee of clinical and health policy experts that met five times between February 1999 and August 1999. This committee engaged consultants to develop background papers on each of the services it was examining, and other consultants assisted the committee in developing cost estimates. Appendix A includes more information about study activities.

Most of this report focuses on two questions. One is whether evidence indicates that the services examined here will be effective in improving the health and well-being of Medicare beneficiaries. The other is what extending coverage to these services would cost Medicare. Whether coverage itself can be linked to better health outcomes is considered primarily in relation to immunosuppressive drugs. For skin cancer screening, a key issue is whether coverage of screening—even if evidence indicates that screening can improve outcomes—would effectively attract those at highest risk: older white males.

Given the constraints of the committee's charge and resources, formal cost-effectiveness analyses are not included, and equity issues are not considered in any depth. Nonetheless, each of the categories of services reviewed raises different concerns about how resources are allocated through the Medicare program. Screening presents questions about the political saliency of different health problems and the importance of scientific evidence in decisions about which preventive services Medicare should cover. Proposals to extend the coverage of immunosuppressive drugs raise questions of why one disease or organ gets differential priority (i.e., immediate Medicare coverage of dialysis or kidney transplants for persons with renal failure) and why coverage has been extended to a few expensive lifesaving outpatient drugs but not others. The near-total exclusion of coverage for dental services raises the question of why some parts of the body are considered less germane to the health of Medicare beneficiaries than others.

Chapter 2 reviews the methods and principles that guided the committee in its assessment of the "benefits and costs to Medicare" of extending coverage. More specific information about methods is provided in the chapters and appendixes examining specific coverage topics.

Chapters 3, 4, and 5 focus, respectively, on screening for skin cancer, medically necessary dental services, and immunosuppressive drugs for transplant patients. Each is written with the expectation that it might be read with little or no reference to this introduction or to other chapters of the report, so some background material that might otherwise have been included in this chapter (e.g., definitions) is deferred and some material is repeated in all three chapters. These three chapters review current Medicare coverage; provide background information on the clinical problems being considered and the burden of illness they cause; describe the specific clinical interventions that were analyzed; and summarize the literature on the benefits and harms of the interventions. They also present estimates of the five-year cost to Medicare of covering the interventions.

Chapter 6 compares current Medicare coverage of preventive services with the recommendations on clinical preventive services published by the U.S. Preventive Services Task Force. It more generally considers the processes for making coverage decisions about preventive and other services and the adequacy of the scientific, procedural, and organizational infrastructure for coverage decisionmaking.

Finally, Appendixes B, C, and D include background papers commissioned by the committee to provide detailed reviews of the scientific literature related to the topics considered in Chapters 3, 4, and 5. Appendix E provides a more detailed discussion of the Medicare cost estimates used by the committee.

2

Objectives, Principles, and Methods

Advances in biomedical research and clinical innovations have greatly expanded the array of medical interventions available to prevent or manage disease or injury. Keeping track of these advances and the scientific evidence about their potential benefits and harms has become increasingly difficult for busy clinicians and for payers and policymakers who want to cover beneficial care while limiting payments for ineffective or harmful services. One result has been increased demand for more systematic evaluations of the benefits and harms of health services. Another result has been a demand for improvements in the methods for conducting and reporting clinical research. Under the labels of technology assessment and evidence-based medicine, researchers, caregivers, payers, policymakers, and others have been seeking agreement on criteria, procedures, and techniques for evaluating evidence and reaching valid and credible conclusions about what works and what does not work in medical care.

This chapter reviews the committee's principles for reaching conclusions and its analytic strategy for assessing evidence and estimating coverage costs. The chapters and appendixes on the different services assessed by the committee provide more specific details.

OBJECTIVES AND PRINCIPLES

Given its charge, the committee's primary objective was to provide analyses that could help Congress make decisions about Medicare coverage for skin cancer screening, medically necessary dental services, and the elimination of the three-year time limit on the coverage of immunosuppressive drugs for transplant recipients. The committee also intended that its findings and conclusions should be credible to practicing clinicians, patients, and the public. Several principles guided the committee's work within the limits of existing evidence, time, and resources:

- Findings and conclusions should be consistent with available knowledge; apparent departures from the evidence should be explained.
- Health outcomes meaningful to patients or consumers—not only changes in physiological measures—should be emphasized in assessments. Meaningfulness relates to the kinds of benefits and harms identified, the magnitude of the effect of an intervention on an outcome, and the preferences of individuals about different outcomes.
- The quality, strength, and limits of the evidence for findings and conclusions should be assessed and described. Evidence about effectiveness (results in usual clinical practice) as well as efficacy (results under controlled research conditions) should be considered.
- The role of expert judgment and experience in assessing evidence and making judgments about the effectiveness of services should be identified.
- Key analytic choices—such as the specification of the health care intervention, the identification of target populations, and the selection of data and methods for cost analyses—should be explained.
- The limitations of analytic methods should be described. In this report, for example, a notable limitation is a cost estimation strategy that (consistent with the committee's charge) focused on costs to the Medicare program rather than costs or cost-effectiveness from a societal perspective.

The committee's task was not to craft statements that were precise and detailed enough to serve as legislative or regulatory language or clinical practice guidelines. (See Eddy et al. [1992] and IOM [1990a] for discussions of principles and criteria for development of practice guidelines.) While acknowledging their importance, the committee also did not examine the full range of ethical, economic, cultural, political, and other issues relevant to decisions about Medicare coverage policies or other options for achieving health goals.

Criteria and Trade-Offs

For each intervention examined, the committee found it helpful to consider a version of the "evidence pyramid" that Figure 2-1 depicts for a generic health care intervention. In this pyramid, each lower tier represents a condition to be met before the next-higher tier is considered. This generic pyramid has been modified to fit the special characteristics of the interventions examined in the next three chapters.

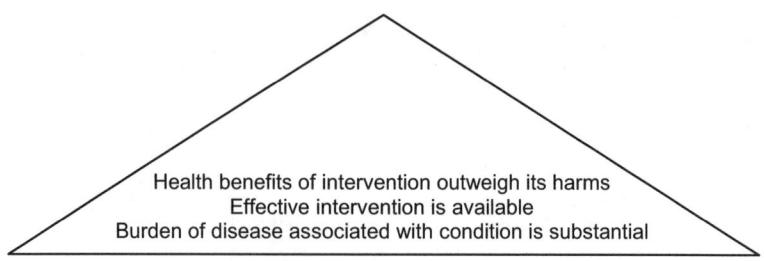

FIGURE 2-1 Evidence pyramid for assessing a health care intervention. SOURCE: Adapted from IOM/NRC, 1999, p. 89.

In brief, someone applying the criteria depicted above must first establish that a health problem exists. Because this report considers a public program, Medicare, the problem should affect Medicare beneficiaries. The next question is whether anything can be done about the problem, that is, whether effective treatment is available. Further, because treatment can be effective but still have significant side effects or harms, the balance of benefits relative to harms must be favorable.

Figure 2-2 modifies the evidence pyramid to illustrate how similar criteria could be applied to coverage decisions. Consistent with the discussion in Chapter 1, Chapters 3, 4, and 5 each discuss why the effectiveness of coverage in achieving desired health goals cannot be assumed.

In practice, the application of the criteria represented in the evidence pyramids involves other trade-offs besides the weighing of benefits against harms. For example, if a health problem affects many people, the benefits of an intervention are great, and the risks of the intervention are minimal, then weaker evidence may be tolerated in assessing options for patients (USPSTF, 1996). In contrast, if the condition is uncommon, the health risks of the intervention are significant, and the benefits are modest, then stronger evidence is usually required before an intervention is recommended. Some argue that preventive services should face stricter scrutiny than treatment services because rather than responding to sick people who need medical care, they invite healthy people to receive care.

Furthermore, even for an intervention that meets all the criteria in Figures 2-1 and 2-2, the extent of the benefits relative to the cost to Medicare, a health plan, or society generally would still have to be considered. In addition, the decision to implement an intervention would need to take into account various practical and cultural issues such as whether groups most at risk are likely to seek or be otherwise identified for care.

As noted throughout this report, the committee developed explicit estimates only of costs to Medicare, not costs to patients, families, or others. It did not

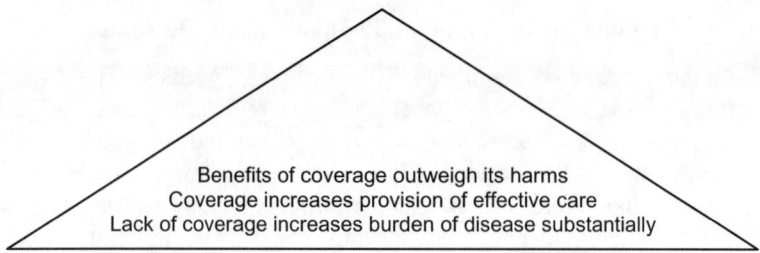

FIGURE 2-2 Evidence pyramid for assessing a coverage policy. SOURCE: Adapted from IOM/NRC, 1999, p. 89.

generate formal cost-effectiveness analyses for each of the interventions considered. For example, the analysis of eliminating the three-year limit on Medicare coverage of immunosuppressive drugs for transplant patients does not compare the estimated cost per life year gained from eliminating the limit with a similar estimate for extending coverage to outpatient antihypertensive drugs.

ANALYTIC STRATEGY

With the assistance of its consultants, the committee employed an analytic strategy that included several steps: (1) defining the intervention, population, and outcomes; (2) identifying and assessing the research literature; (3) linking the evidence to conclusions; (4) estimating costs to Medicare of extending coverage; and (5) considering benefits and costs together. These steps, in general, follow a set of broadly accepted methods for identifying and making use of the best available evidence.[1]

---

[1]For general overviews and selected applications, see CDC, 1996; Eckman et al., 1998; Eddy, 1991; Eddy et al., 1992; Gold et al., 1996; Guyatt et al., 1998; IOM, 1985, 1992; Kassirer et al., 1987; Mulrow and Cook, 1998; Mulrow and Oxman, 1997; OTA, 1994; Pauker and Kassirer, 1997; Pauker and Kopelman, 1994; Sackett et al., 1997; and USPSTF, 1996. The *Journal of the American Medical Association* has been publishing a series of articles—users' guides to the medical literature—developed for practicing physicians by the Evidence-Based Medicine Working Group. In providing guidance on a topic such as how to use a clinical decision analysis or how to assess the soundness of practice guidelines, each article reviews basic principles and methods for evaluating evidence. See, for example, Barratt et al., 1999 (using screening guidelines); Dans et al., 1998 (using clinical trial results); Drummond et al., 1997, and O'Brien et al., 1997 (using an economic analysis); Guyatt et al., 1995 (grading health care recommendations); and Guyatt et al., 1999 (using treatment recommendations). An ongoing series of articles under the heading "Clinical Problem Solving" in the *New England Journal of Medicine* provides many examples of systematic uses of scientific literature and analytic tools in clinical practice.

Defining the Intervention, Population, and Outcomes

Both the topics to be examined by the Institute of Medicine (IOM) and the population of interest (Medicare beneficiaries) were determined by the request from Congress. For each topic, one important step in the committee's analysis was to define more fully and explicitly the intervention to be assessed. For example, as explained more fully in Chapter 3 and Appendix B, screening is defined as involving only people without symptoms. This definition thus excludes a skin examination conducted by a physician during a visit sought by a patient concerned about recent growth of a mole or other physical change. It likewise excludes a physician's incidental discovery and further investigation of a suspicious mole during a visit for some other purpose.

In addition to identifying the tests, procedures, treatments, or other elements that characterize the intervention to be assessed, analysts must also specify the target population and the possible outcomes of the intervention. The target population for this report was generally those age 65 or over, who constitute the substantial majority of Medicare beneficiaries. The evidence reviewed was not, however, restricted to this age group. Clinical studies have sometimes excluded older patients, included too few for meaningful analysis, or not reported results by age. In the case of transplant-related interventions, the relevant population also includes a significant proportion of younger people who have qualified for Medicare by virtue of disability or diagnosis of permanent kidney failure. Clinical studies of transplant patients generally do not describe their Medicare status.

As discussed above, the committee was especially interested in health outcomes that would be directly meaningful to patients or consumers, including mortality, morbidity, and health-related quality of life. In identifying such outcomes for assessment, analysts need to consider possible harms as well as benefits. Although some interventions have little potential for harm, others have the potential to do considerable harm. Chapters 3, 4, and 5 consider benefits and harms relevant to the services and conditions being examined.

To reach conclusions specific enough to guide clinicians and policymakers, analysts also have to assess information about additional elements of an intervention—in particular, how frequently a screening test should be used. Evidence on which to base recommendations about frequency is scarce.

The committee and its consultants often found various tabular and graphic tools useful in analyzing the quite different kinds of clinical problems and interventions examined here.[2] These tools helped the committee and consultants to

---

[2]See, for example, Detsky et al., 1997; Eddy et al., 1992; Owens et al., 1997; and Scheinkopf, 1999. Although this report omits a detailed discussion of the varied graphic and tabular tools used at intermediate stages of the committee's work, some that proved helpful included probability trees, decision trees, evaporating clouds, influence diagrams, current and future reality trees, and Venn diagrams.

(1) identify missing or ambiguous aspects of the definition of the intervention, target population, outcomes, or costs to Medicare of covering the intervention; (2) clarify underlying assumptions or expectations about the causal pathway linking the intervention and outcomes; (3) identify uncertainties related to different links in the causal pathway that might temper the interpretation of evidence and the formulation of conclusions; (4) guide the literature search for direct and indirect evidence; and (5) understand the assumptions that underlie conflicts in analytic strategies and conclusions. Where tables and graphics are useful in presenting information, explanations, and conclusions, they are included in the report text or the background papers. Had the data available to the committee been more extensive and solid, some of these tools would have been employed further to guide mathematical modeling of the relationships between interventions and outcomes.

Identifying and Assessing the Scientific Literature

Given the definition of the intervention (and sometimes its redefinition in light of additional information and discussion), the next step was to identify available evidence about its effectiveness. The literature search strategies (including search terms, criteria for inclusion or exclusion in the analysis, databases consulted) are described in more detail in Appendix B for skin cancer screening and Appendix C for dental services. (Appendix D on immunosuppressive therapy for transplant patients was intended more as an overview than as a full and systematic evaluation of the literature.)

For the literature that met the criteria for further assessment, the next questions concerned the quality, relevance, and consistency of the evidence. Some studies employ stronger research designs that allow more confidence in their findings than studies using weaker designs. Ideally, analysts would locate evidence directly relating the intervention to the outcomes of interest, for example, multiyear, properly randomized, controlled trials that followed people over age 65 who had been screened or not screened for skin cancer and then reported consistent findings. Often, however, analysts must rely on chains of indirect evidence, for example, one set of studies of the stage of cancer identified during screening versus "usual" care and another set relating the stage of cancer to health outcomes. Analysts also may find that results of different studies are contradictory and cannot be explained by obvious differences in study methods or populations.

In general, the assessment of evidence here follows that of the U.S. Preventive Services Task Force (USPSTF [1996], adapted from the Canadian Task Force on the Periodic Health Examination [CTFPHE, 1979]). Unlike the USPSTF, the committee did not rate the quality of the evidence numerically but, rather, described the types of evidence available (e.g., multicenter randomized clinical trial, small case-control studies) for each topic examined.[3]

If multiple studies are available, they will often differ sufficiently in their focus, methods, and results, so that overall conclusions are not obvious. The technique of meta-analysis is sometimes employed to synthesize the results of such studies, although experts still debate techniques for conducting and interpreting these analyses (Bailar, 1997; Blettner et al., 1999; Lau et al., 1997; Moher and Pham, 1999; Mulrow and Oxman, 1997; Sutton et al., 1998). The evidence identified in the course of this study did not warrant formal meta-analyses. Instead, the background papers included in Appendixes B, C, and D generally present tables describing relevant studies and their results.

Linking Evidence to Conclusions

For some interventions, the evidence will be sufficient in quality, relevance, clarity, and consistency to justify positive or negative conclusions about an intervention, at least under certain circumstances. For many interventions, however, analysts may find little or no direct evidence of efficacy or effectiveness, and useful indirect evidence may also be very limited. Even if analysts identify potentially relevant studies, they may be inconclusive, conflicting, or poorly designed. At this point, an analysis may essentially stop with the conclusion that there is insufficient evidence to justify a positive or negative conclusion about either clinical practice or coverage.[4]

Alternatively, the assessment process may tap professional expertise and experience to see whether a consensus can be reached about what clinical practice or insurance coverage should be in the absence of adequate evidence. Proc-

---

[3]Major types of research designs include randomized clinical trials (which compare outcomes for study subjects randomly allocated between an intervention group and a control group); case-control studies (which compare a group that has a specific condition or characteristic of interest with a group that does not); cohort studies (which follow a group over time to compare outcomes among subgroups with different treatment or other characteristics); and multiple time-series studies (which compare outcomes at multiple points before and after adoption of an intervention).

[4]For example, the Clinical Efficacy Assessment Program of the American College of Physicians, a leader in developing the principles and practices of evidence-based medicine, limited its conclusions to those supported by acceptable evidence. In two of its reports, *Common Diagnostic Tests: Use and Interpretation* (Sox, 1987) and *Common Screening Tests* (Eddy, 1991), the text includes reviews of the evidence on the efficacy of tests such as blood cultures for infectious diseases and mammography for breast cancer screening. Appendixes, which were developed in collaboration with the Blue Cross and Blue Shield Association using a formal process of evidence assessment and expert judgment, provided recommendations on the use of these tests in clinical practice.

esses for reaching these kinds of consensus-based conclusions range from informal and implicit to formal and explicit (e.g., see IOM, 1985, 1990b,c, 1995b).

As methods for systematically reviewing and reporting research have developed, so have ways of describing the strength of conclusions or recommendations about an intervention. One approach used by the USPSTF (also adapted from the Canadian Task Force) takes into account the quality of the evidence, the direction and importance of reported effects (both benefits and harms), and the burden of disease associated with the condition in question. Again, the committee did not assign explicit ratings to its conclusions but rather described the strength or sufficiency of the evidence to support conclusions about the services it investigated.

Another way of summarizing the strength of a recommendation has been proposed for use by those developing clinical practice policies or guidelines (Eddy et al., 1992). It relies partly on the strength of the evidence base and partly on the degree of understanding and agreement about the outcomes associated with an intervention. This approach reserves the term *standard* for statements for which the health and economic consequences are reasonably well understood and people are virtually unanimous about the desirability or undesirability of the intervention. A *guideline* is a statement for which outcomes are reasonably well understood and are preferred (or not preferred) by a solid but not unanimous majority. If outcomes are not known or if preferences are unknown, indifferent, or split, then an intervention may be described as an *option* without being recommended. Although this scheme does not directly apply to coverage policies, it is nonetheless a useful way to think about the strength of the case for coverage changes.

For the interventions and outcomes examined here, the committee found little or no systematic evidence about either individual or societal preferences for different outcomes. As a result, the committee had to rely on its own experience and expertise in suggesting how people might value different outcomes for themselves or others. For example, the committee judged that the scarring produced by most biopsies for false negative results for skin cancer screening examinations was not likely to be viewed by most people as an important risk of screening, whereas the disfigurement that might result from late diagnosis and surgical treatment of squamous cell carcinoma was likely to be viewed as important. As explained in Chapter 3, the evidence did not warrant further steps such as efforts to assign utilities or numerical weights for the value of different outcomes.

ESTIMATING COSTS TO MEDICARE OF EXTENDING COVERAGE

A next analytic step was to estimate the costs to Medicare of covering the interventions analyzed in this report. At the outset, the committee decided that it would present cost estimates for each intervention even if analysis suggested that the evidence did not support the extension of coverage. The rationale is, first, that the charge to the committee called for estimates of costs and, second, that the estimates might be useful if Congress continued to consider extending coverage despite the weakness of the evidence base for coverage.

As explained in Appendix E, the method for estimating Medicare costs generally followed the generic approach of the Congressional Budget Office (CBO), which was determined from past cost estimates and in discussions with CBO staff. This decision reflected the committee's wish to provide Congress with estimates that were based on familiar procedures. Unlike cost-effectiveness analyses intended to inform broad public policy decisions, the CBO approach does *not* take a societal perspective, nor does it recognize costs to beneficiaries, families, or others affected by coverage policies. Other differences are that the estimates do not discount future costs to present value,[5] and they consider future benefits only in the form of any direct cost offsets (e.g., avoided hospitalizations but not avoided absences from work) projected to result from covering a service.

Although specific procedures, assumptions, and data sources vary for each service examined as explained in later chapters and Appendix E, the basics of the committee's approach to estimating costs to Medicare are as follows. The estimates:

- cover the five-year period, from 2000 to 2004;
- apply assumptions about the numbers of beneficiaries experiencing the intervention (including initial and referral visits), complications, and other relevant events based on the epidemiological and other literature and guidance from the committee and consultants;
- specify the type and number of physician visits or other services and procedures (e.g., biopsies) that constitute the intervention based on Health Care Financing Administration (HCFA) data, research literature, and guidance from the committee and consultants;
- adjust future costs for inflation but do *not* discount them to present value;
- subtract the amounts beneficiaries would pay in coinsurance (generally 20 percent of the Medicare-approved payment); and

---

[5]Economists typically discount future dollars because individuals tend to favor present over future consumption. A discount rate is an assumption about what a dollar invested today would earn if invested rather than spent. The cost estimation approach used here inflates rather than discounts future dollars. In addition, to the extent that the estimates involve costs that occur in one year and savings that occur in later years, the lack of discounting to present value could be particularly misleading. Further, when offsets are expected to occur beyond the five-year period (as is likely for many preventive services), they are ignored. For more a detailed discussion, see Gold et al., 1996.

• subtract the proportion of the total cost increase that would be transferred to beneficiaries through higher Part B premiums, which are set at 25 percent of Part B spending for elderly Medicare beneficiaries and which flow to the Part B Trust Fund.

The committee's estimates of Medicare costs are based on a series of assumptions, some of which have supporting evidence or data but others of which are best guesses based on committee judgment in the absence of such information. For each condition or service, the estimates are intended to suggest the order of magnitude of the costs to Medicare of extending coverage, but they could be considerably higher or lower than what Medicare might actually spend were coverage policies changed. The tables in Appendix E allow readers to vary some of the committee's assumptions and calculate alternative estimates.

Both Chapter 1 and Appendix E note that the rules now governing Congress generally require that decisions to increase federal government spending in one area be offset with reduced spending in other areas or increases in tax or other revenues. The committee did not explicitly factor these budget rules into its conclusions. Nonetheless, it was aware that, for example, higher net spending for skin cancer screening or dental services would probably have to be matched by increased taxes or by spending reductions elsewhere.

Coverage determinations by HCFA do not entail such explicit "neutrality" criteria. Thus, the services examined in this report—which require decisions by Congress—face a higher hurdle to achieve coverage than do services that fit within already established coverage categories.

The committee was not asked to estimate costs to the federal-state Medicaid program that might be added or reduced if Medicare extended coverage to the services examined in this report. For example, if the three-year limit on Medicare coverage of immunosuppressive drugs were eliminated, federal and state Medicaid costs should decrease because that program would be spending less for these drugs for beneficiaries who were eligible for both Medicare and Medicaid. In this case, the net cost to the federal budget of extending coverage would be less than the cost to Medicare.

Considering Health Outcomes and Costs Together

The possible combinations of overall health and cost outcomes can be set out in simplified terms as shown in Table 2-1. In this table, the rows labeled "better," "same," and "worse" refer to the overall health outcome of using the intervention compared to not using it. Similarly, the columns labeled "lower," "same," and "higher" describe the net cost to Medicare of covering the intervention relative to the cost of not covering it (i.e., the status quo). The pluses in the table's cells indicate support for a positive decision about an intervention,

TABLE 2-1 Expanding Coverage to a New Intervention: Possible Outcomes and Directions for Decisionmakers

Health Outcome of the Intervention	Cost to Medicare for the Intervention		
	Lower	Same	Higher
Better	++	+	?
Same	+	?	–
Worse	?	–	– –

SOURCE: Adapted from Pauker and Col, 1999.

the minuses indicate support for a negative decision, and the question marks indicate more mixed situations.

Thus, the combination of better outcomes and lower costs (upper left corner of Table 2-1) points toward a positive coverage decision whereas the combination of worse outcomes and higher costs (lower right corner) points to a negative decision. The diagonal row of question marks indicates the less clear-cut decision situations, for example, the not uncommon circumstance that an intervention produces better results but at a higher cost. Cost pressures can focus attention on options that might produce worse outcomes but reduce Medicare costs.

A more formal and comprehensive way of considering outcomes and costs together is cost-effectiveness analysis. Cost-effectiveness analyses relate the estimated costs of an intervention to its expected outcomes.[6] They also allow comparisons of different interventions to be made in similar units. For example, the cost per year of life gained from implementing an effective screening test can be compared to the results for other screening tests or other interventions already covered by Medicare. Although such comparisons provide some context for assessing the projected consequences of different interventions, they do not in themselves indicate what is a "reasonable" cost-effectiveness ratio. Some have suggested the use of $100,000 per life year gained as a dividing point (Laupacis et al., 1992), whereas others have cautioned against using such a criterion (Siegel et al., 1996).

Increasingly, cost-effectiveness analyses incorporate measures that reflect an intervention's effect on both the quantity of life achieved (reduced mortality) and the health-related quality of that life (e.g., see Gold et al., 1996; IOM, 1998). Such measures include quality-adjusted life years (QALYs), disability-adjusted life years (DALYs), and years of healthy life (YHLs).

---

[6]In contrast to a cost-effectiveness analysis, a cost-benefit analysis would express both the outcomes (e.g., lives saved) and the costs in monetary terms. For technical, philosophical, and political reasons, health technology assessments rarely include cost-benefit analyses.

The additional dimensions captured in assessments of health-related quality of life could be particularly useful in evaluating services for the Medicare population in which chronic disease is so prevalent. For example, two interventions might be equally effective in extending survival, but they might differ in the extent to which the extra years of life were lived with or without pain or serious limitations in physical or mental functioning. A number of methods and tools have been developed to assess health-related quality of life including methods for assessing people's preferences for different health states (e.g., a year of life lived in severe pain versus nine months lived pain free).

Although formal cost-effectiveness analyses are useful in trying to understand the "value for money" of particular interventions, the committee's charge called only for estimates of the costs to Medicare of extending coverage. Even if the committee had gone further, it would have encountered difficulties given the limited evidence of effectiveness and the lack of quality-of-life or patient preference data for the interventions examined. Studies have compared health-related quality of life for patients on renal dialysis with posttransplant patients taking immunosuppressive drugs, but the committee did not find comparable data on the other conditions considered here. Nonetheless, the approach used here—estimating only the costs to Medicare—provides an incomplete picture of the value for money of covering a service.

3

Screening for Skin Cancer

Today, most Americans are probably familiar with advice to limit sun exposure—actually, exposure to sunlight and other sources of ultraviolet radiation such as sunlamps—to reduce their risk of skin cancer. They are also likely to have heard or seen messages sponsored by the American Cancer Society (ACS), the American Academy of Dermatology (AAD), or other groups explaining how to check their skin for warning signs of skin cancer, especially melanoma.[1]

From a public health perspective, the advice to limit sun exposure—especially during the first two decades of life—is a form of *primary prevention*, which includes counseling and educational interventions that aim to keep people from developing health problems in the first place. Another primary prevention strategy that has been widely advised, sunscreen use, was recently reported to have helped prevent one type of skin cancer in a controlled clinical trial (Green et al., 1999).

The advice about skin self-examination is a form of *secondary prevention*, which promotes early identification of risk factors or subclinical disease in people who have not developed symptoms. Skin self-examination for suspicious moles or other skin features is a form of secondary prevention. Clinical screening—examination by a physician or other trained individual of the skin of an

---

[1]For melanoma, warning symptoms include new or changing pigmented spots that are asymmetrical, larger than 6 mm, irregular in border, or varied in color including blue, black, or gray. For nonmelanoma skin cancer, warning symptoms include the appearance of a new spot, bump, or sore that does not heal or go away in about two weeks, and may or may not bleed or crust. See AAD (1994b) and ACS (1999b).

asymptomatic person—is also a form of secondary prevention, and it is the focus of this chapter. Because primary prevention of skin cancer emphasizes actions to be taken by children and young adults, secondary prevention is the main issue for those over 65.

For people who already have a medical problem, usual clinical management may include measures to prevent additional problems or complications. These measures, sometimes described as *tertiary prevention*, include such steps as identification and elimination of oral infections before organ transplants and treatment with immunosuppressive drugs afterwards. Medicare coverage for diabetes outpatient self-management training and supplies, which was approved by Congress in 1997 as a preventive service, is another example of tertiary prevention.

The primary, secondary, and tertiary labels for preventive services are not rigidly applied. For example, much tertiary prevention is viewed as treatment and thus not subject to Medicare's preventive services exclusion. The exclusion for outpatient drugs would, however, still apply to most of the medications used for tertiary prevention.

The premise underlying both self-examination and clinical screening programs is that detecting a disease earlier than would happen in usual health care will result in earlier treatment that saves lives and reduces the physical and emotional burden of illness. In addition, screening is often promoted as a way of reducing the overall costs associated with treating disease, especially late-stage disease. Nonetheless, when claims about the benefits of particular screening programs are subjected to systematic evaluation, the evidence supports some but is negative, mixed, limited, or otherwise inadequate to support others (see, e.g., Eddy, 1991; Russell, 1994; USPSTF, 1996).[2] As controversies over assessments of breast cancer screening for women ages 40 to 49 demonstrate, conclusions that the evidence does not clearly support screening for a particular disease can generate considerable controversy, given the understandable hopes that screening will prevent or reduce the mortality, disability, and other suffering caused by the disease (see, e.g., Eddy, 1997; Ransohoff and Harris, 1997; Taubes, 1997a,b).

Medicare does not cover screening for skin cancer in asymptomatic people. It does, however, cover a physician visit initiated by a concerned patient who has noticed, for example, a change in the color of a mole (clinically described as a pigmented nevus or, more generally, skin lesion), or a new skin growth. Simi-

---

[2]Claims about other prevention strategies become similarly complex when rigorously investigated. Proponents of evidence-based medicine will note that the results of the controlled trial of sunscreen use that was mentioned on the previous page supported—for squamous cell carcinoma—a prevention strategy that has long been promoted on the basis of biological plausibility without direct evidence (Hill, 1999). For basal cell carcinoma, the trial did not find a significant effect of sunscreen use. The trial also tested the use of beta-carotene supplements to prevent skin cancer. This strategy received some attention based on animal studies but was not confirmed in this trial.

larly, if a physician notices such a suspicious sign during a visit for another purpose and extends the visit to investigate further, Medicare may pay more for the visit if it meets certain criteria for a higher level "evaluation and management service" (which is Medicare payment terminology for a physician visit). In either situation, if the patient is referred to a dermatologist for further assessment, that referral visit is also covered.

Appendix B, which was prepared by researchers at the Oregon Health Sciences University Evidence-Based Practice Center presents the review of the scientific literature on skin cancer screening that was commissioned for this study. Consistent with provisions of the legislation authorizing this study, the review was developed in conjunction with both the IOM committee and the U.S. Preventive Services Task Force (USPSTF). It also follows the general strategy used by an earlier IOM committee evaluating thyroid cancer screening in people exposed to radioactive iodine from atomic weapons testing (IOM/NRC, 1999).[3] The rest of this chapter discusses the committee's analytic approach; the burden of illness associated with different forms of skin cancer; the procedures used for screening and evidence about their effectiveness; estimated five-year costs to Medicare of three alternative screening approaches; statements on skin cancer screening from other groups; and the committee findings and conclusions.

ASSESSMENT APPROACH: INTERVENTION, POPULATION, AND OUTCOMES

Following the general approach set forth in Chapter 2, the committee began by defining the specific procedures or activities that constitute skin cancer screening. As described in Appendix B, skin cancer screening may rely on a case-finding strategy, when a person seeing a health care professional for another reason is offered a total skin examination (or a partial skin examination with referral to a specialist depending on the findings). Such screening may focus on all people or only those identified as high-risk. Another strategy involves mass screening in which people are invited and self-select to undergo a total skin examination by a health care professional and then are referred to their primary care physician or a specialist for follow-up.

The committee considered two case-finding approaches to screening for skin cancer in addition to the mass screening approach just described. The first case-finding approach involves a visual examination of the entire skin (including scalp and nails as well as the mouth) and a patient history to identify risk factors such as family history of skin cancer, level and frequency of sun exposure, or recent change in a mole. The other case-finding strategy separates the process

---

[3]Reflecting differences in IOM and Task Force objectives and presentation needs, the Appendix in this report will differ slightly from the Task Force document expected early in 2000.

into two phases, so that a total skin examination is offered only for those identified by their history as being at high risk of skin cancer. The committee also considered a mass screening approach as a third approach. In all approaches, those with lesions identified as suspicious for skin cancer are offered biopsies.

Because skin cancer screening searches for disease in people who have not noticed symptoms of the disease, the committee defined it as *excluding* several services already covered by Medicare. These covered services include a skin examination and history undertaken by a physician (a) in response to a patient's concern about a skin abnormality, including both new and changing skin features, (b) after the incidental discovery of a suspicious skin lesion during an examination for another purpose, or (c) during a subsequent referral visit to a specialist. Also excluded from the definition of screening are Medicare-covered follow-up visits and skin examinations for patients previously diagnosed and treated for skin cancer or other conditions that put them at higher risk for skin cancer. In contrast to a new program of clinical skin cancer screening, all these services are considered part of usual patient care.

In this analysis the population of primary interest is Medicare beneficiaries age 65 and over. Nonetheless, evidence related to all age groups was reviewed.[4]

The major health benefits sought from skin cancer screening are reduced mortality and associated suffering, lower rates of recurrence and subsequent treatment, and less treatment-related discomfort or disfigurement. Another potential benefit of screening is improved patient knowledge, self-examination skills, and risk reduction behaviors.

Harms from skin cancer screening are also possible, for example, when false positive or inconclusive results lead to unnecessary treatment, pain, scarring, and anxiety, although any pain or scarring is likely to be modest for such false positives. In addition, false negatives may induce complacency and disregard for subsequent skin changes possibly indicative of cancer. Most people have some moles, differently pigmented areas of skin, and other skin features, and the number of skin changes and growths tends to increase with age. Although most of these skin features will not be or become malignant, some may prompt suspicion and further testing.[5] For younger people, possible harms of

---

[4]The benefit would also, presumably, apply to Medicare beneficiaries who are under age 65, for instance those who qualify as disabled. The younger group of beneficiaries is a relatively small part of Medicare, and skin cancer is associated with age, so this discussion emphasizes older beneficiaries.

[5]For example, actinic keratoses (scaly or crusty patches that may be flat or elevated and are associated with cumulative sun exposure) are relatively common and do develop into squamous cell carcinoma in a small percentage of cases. Because they can cause itching and other discomfort, some patients would likely seek evaluation and treatment independent of a screening program. In addition, some actinic keratoses would—like cancerous lesions—be identified incidentally during the course of a physician visit for another purpose.

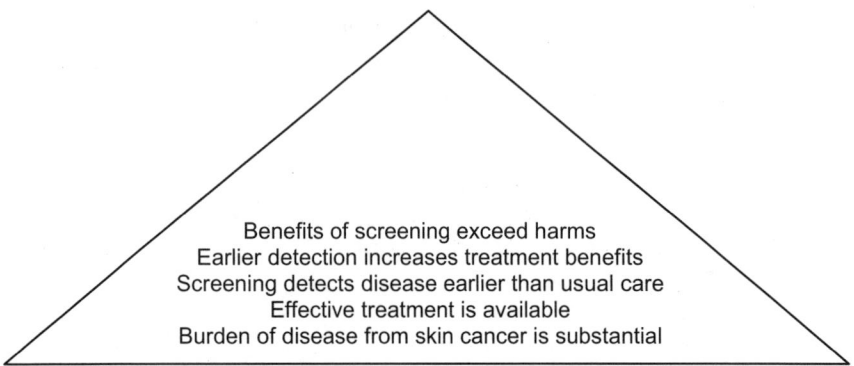

FIGURE 3-1 Evidence pyramid for assessing a screening intervention. SOURCE: Adapted from IOM/NRC 1999, p. 89.

screening and false positives include labeling and denial of health coverage by insurance companies, employers, or others. The committee viewed these possible harms of skin cancer screening as relatively minor.

To guide this assessment of a screening intervention, the committee used Figure 3-1, which is adapted from the simpler, three-tier figure introduced in Chapter 2. Thus, the committee sought evidence that skin cancer is important in terms of prevalence, incidence, and mortality or morbidity (disease burden) for the population 65 and over; amenable to effective treatment; detectable by a screening test that is reliable, accurate, and safe and that detects the disease at an earlier stage than in usual care; and more effectively treated when detected at an earlier stage with overall benefits of treatment outweighing any harms. Appendix B describes the evidence search strategy more specifically.

A test that met all the criteria in Figure 3-1 would clearly have benefits compared to usual care, but the extent of the benefit relative to the cost to Medicare, a health plan, or society generally would still need to be considered. As explained earlier, this report provides only estimates of costs to Medicare and not others, and it does not include formal assessment of the cost-effectiveness of skin cancer screening compared to other interventions (e.g., promotion of skin self-examination). In addition, this chapter covers only a subset of feasibility issues that might arise in implementing a new program of skin cancer screening.

Although not considered in depth here, certain ethical considerations relevant to screening recommendations should also be noted (see, e.g., Malm, 1999). Screening—even when targeted to higher-risk groups—typically involves examination or testing of a large number of healthy people who will turn out not to have the disease or who may have subclinical disease that will never progress to cause problems. For this reason, those making recommendations about screening interventions may want the margin of benefits over harms to be greater or clearer than they would for interventions intended to cure or improve the well-being of those who are ill. The general enthusiasm for screening may lead to screening promotions that do not adequately inform the public and the professions about the potential for harm (e.g., see Woloshin and Schwartz, 1999b).

POPULATION BURDEN OF DISEASE

The skin cancers considered here are melanoma, basal cell carcinoma, and squamous cell carcinoma.[6] The latter two are often lumped together as nonmelanoma skin cancers, which also include other, far less common skin malignancies such Kaposi's sarcoma and cutaneous T-cell lymphoma. These uncommon conditions are not the focus of general skin cancer screening programs.

Melanomas originate in cells that can produce melanin, a pigment found in the skin, hair, eyes, and sometimes elsewhere. Basal cell carcinoma and squamous cell carcinoma originate in the epidermis, the outermost layer of the skin.

Melanoma

Melanoma is the least common but most deadly of the three skin cancers considered here. It accounts for less than 5 percent of reported cases but about 80 percent of skin cancer deaths (ACS, 1999a).

Although melanoma occurs most commonly in the skin, it may be found in the eye and, rarely, elsewhere. It may arise either de novo or from an existing mole and can spread through the lymph system or blood.

Risk factors for melanoma include light skin color, older age, large numbers of common moles, atypical moles, history of severe sunburns (especially at younger ages), and family history of the disease. Unlike basal cell and squamous cell carcinomas, a majority of melanomas occur on skin surfaces not normally exposed to the sun.[7]

Melanoma of the skin is primarily a disease of fair-skinned people. It is also more common in white men than in white women with an incidence in 1996 of 19.3 per 100,000 for the former and 13.2 per 100,000 for the latter (SEER, 1999).[8] (The corresponding rates for black men and women are 1.3 per 100,000 and 0.6 per 100,000.) The disease is also much more common in older age

---

[6]This discussion draws on AAD, 1994a; ACS, 1999b,c; Albert et al., 1990; NCI, 1999b–e; USPSTF, 1996; Whited and Grichnik, 1998).

[7]There are four types of melanoma: superficial spreading melanoma (the most common form of melanoma), acral lentiginous melanoma, nodular melanoma and lentigo maligna. Lentigo maligna melanoma is most often found among the elderly, and usually on areas with high cumulative sun exposure.

[8]Unless otherwise indicated, data come from the Surveillence, Epidemiology and End Results (SEER) program of the National Cancer Institute.

groups; the 1992–1996 age-adjusted incidence rate for those age 65 and over was 72.3 per 100,000 for white men and 31.8 per 100,000 for white women. In 1999, approximately 44,000 cases of melanoma are expected to be diagnosed (ACS, 1999a). Based on 1994–1996 data, the lifetime risk of being diagnosed with invasive melanoma is 1.84 percent in white men and 1.34 percent in white women, which ranks it 6th among common cancers for white men and 11th for white women.

The age-adjusted incidence of the disease has been increasing, from 5.7 per 100,000 population in the 1973 to 13.8 per 100,000 in 1996 with higher rates of increase occurring during the earlier part of this period (SEER, 1999). As noted in Appendix B, changes in record-keeping procedures, diagnostic criteria, and preventive practices may be contributing to increased detection and reporting. Some suggest that more melanomas of a relatively nonaggressive and clinically unimportant kind are being detected, but no studies have established this (Burton and Armstrong, 1995; Swerlick and Chen, 1996, 1997).

The age-adjusted mortality from melanoma has, however, also been increasing, rising from 1.6 per 100,000 in 1973 to 2.3 per 100,000 in 1996. This trend suggests that the increasing incidence of the disease is not just an artifact of increased detection or changing criteria for diagnosis. Again, older white men are most at risk. For 1994–1996, their age-adjusted mortality rate was 17.4 per 100,000 compared to 7.5 for older white women. Most of the increase in overall mortality since 1973 has been among white men. White men have a 0.38 percent lifetime risk of dying from melanoma, which ranks it 13th among major kinds of cancers; for white women the comparable risk of dying is 0.28 and 18th in rank. In comparison, the lifetime risks for white men of dying from lung or prostate cancer are 6.94 percent and 3.09 percent, respectively; for white women, the lifetime risks of dying from lung cancer or invasive breast cancer are 4.77 percent and 3.47 percent, respectively. In 1999, about 7,300 deaths are expected from melanoma (ACS, 1999a).

When melanomas of the skin are diagnosed in their early stages while thin and localized (i.e., no spread beyond the development site), prospects for long-term survival are very good. Data from the Surveillance, Epidemiology and End Results (SEER) program of the National Cancer Institute show a five-year relative survival rate (1989–1995) for localized disease of over 95 percent; for regional disease that involves nearby lymph nodes, the rate drops to 58 percent; and for distant metastatic disease, it is only 13 percent. SEER data also show that more than 80 percent of melanomas are diagnosed while still local.

Nonmelanoma Skin Cancers

Basal cell carcinoma and squamous cell carcinoma are the most common skin cancers, accounting for about one million new cases a year and about 1,900 deaths (ACS, 1999a). Risk factors include older age, sun exposure (primarily childhood exposure for basal cell carcinoma and both early and recent exposure for squamous cell carcinoma), and fair hair, eyes, or skin. For squamous cell carcinoma, immunosuppression and cigarette smoking are an additional risk factors. European and U.S. data suggest that people who have been diagnosed with these cancers are at higher risk of subsequent skin cancers (including melanoma) and other noncutaneous cancers (Kahn et al., 1998; Karagas, 1994; Karagas et al., 1992; 1998). Because of their relatively low lethality, neither cancer is included in the major reports issued by the SEER program.

Basal cell carcinoma accounts for about three-quarters of all skin cancers. This cancer is slow growing and usually does not spread to other parts of the body. It is highly curable by surgical removal but may, if neglected, cause death, functional impairment, or disfigurement. Because basal carcinomas often appear on the face, scarring or coloration changes associated with even minor surgical treatment may cause distress.

Squamous cell carcinoma occurs primarily in the skin but may also occur elsewhere, including the mouth and genitals. Another skin condition, actinic keratosis, is a concern because a small proportion may develop into squamous cell carcinomas (Mittelbronn et al., 1998; NCI, 1999e; Schwartz, 1997). Like basal cell carcinoma, squamous cell carcinoma usually is slow growing, but it is more likely to be lethal. It is usually curable if detected early but may cause death, functional impairment, or severe disfigurement if neglected. Squamous cell carcinoma of the skin accounts for about one-fifth of all skin cancers and most of the deaths from nonmelanoma skin cancer (ACS, 1999a).

AVAILABILITY OF EFFECTIVE TREATMENT

Melanoma

Surgical treatment is widely accepted as effective in achieving long-term survival for patients with localized melanoma (Holmstrom, 1992; Kelly et al., 1984; NCI, 1999b,c; NIH, 1992). Recent research has focused on identifying the effect on survival of more limited surgical excisions that remove smaller margins of skin surrounding the tumor. Results suggest that smaller margins are acceptable for early-stage disease and reduce the need for skin grafts (Karakousis et al., 1996).

Other research has examined the effectiveness of routine lymph node resection when there is no clinical indication of spread to the lymph nodes, but trials to date have not established its value for most patients (Hochwald and Coit, 1998). A more focused approach for identifying and treating people with subclinical spread of the disease, the sentinel lymph node biopsy (which targets the lymph nodes that first drain a primary tumor site), is being tested (Gershenwald et al., 1998; Glass et al., 1998).

The thinner the melanoma, the higher the survival rate (Halpern and Schuchter, 1997; Sabin et al., 1997; Straume and Akslen, 1996). For patients with thicker melanomas or melanomas that have spread, effective treatments are still being sought. For example, the NCI recommends that physicians discuss with such patients the possible benefits and harms of enrolling in clinical trials that are testing various interventions such as chemotherapy, biological therapy, or therapy with immunologically active agents such as interferons (NCI, 1999b). If cancer has spread to regional lymph nodes, surgery to remove the tumor and affected lymph nodes can be successful, but survival rates are lower than for less advanced disease (Karakousis et al., 1998). For melanoma that has spread beyond the skin and lymph nodes, treatment is primarily palliative, aimed at relieving pain and other symptoms rather than at improving long-term survival.

Nonmelanoma Skin Cancers

Most nonmelanoma skin cancers can be successfully treated with one of several kinds of surgical procedures including surgical excision, cryosurgery (which uses liquid nitrogen to kill cancer cells), and electrodessication and curettage (drying the lesion with electric current and then scraping the debris away) (NCI, 1999d; Preston and Stern, 1992). These procedures are also commonly used to remove premalignant actinic keratoses. Radiation therapy, chemotherapy, and other nonsurgical approaches are also used in certain situations.

The choice of procedure depends on the type of tumor, its location, and patient history (e.g., past nonmelanoma skin cancers). For small excisions, surrounding skin may be stretched over the wound and stitched; large excisions may require grafts of skin from elsewhere on the body. Microsurgical techniques have been developed to check tissue as it is removed to minimize the removal of healthy tissue and subsequent scarring. In general, the smaller the lesion is, the easier the procedure (Thomas and Amonette, 1988). An important benefit of early detection and treatment of these cancers is reduced scarring and a better cosmetic appearance.

SCREENING AND DIAGNOSTIC PROCEDURES

Screening

As described earlier, the committee reviewed evidence for a mass screening strategy and two case-finding approaches to screening. One case finding approach used a history and total skin examination for all patients, and the second used the patient history to identify high-risk people to undergo total skin examination. This examination takes approximately three to five minutes for an experienced clinician if nothing suspicious is detected that requires further in-vestigation.[9]

In examining the skin for possible melanoma, American clinicians are ad-vised to remember the "ABCDs" (and sometimes E) of pigmented lesions sug-gestive of melanoma: *A*symmetry (a lesion not regularly round or oval), *B*order irregularity (poorly defined edges, scalloping, notching), *C*olor variegation, and *D*iameter greater than 6 millimeters (Friedman, et al., 1985; Harris et al., 1999). The fifth item sometimes suggested is *E*levation of the lesion (Thomas et al., 1998). Public awareness and education programs promoting skin self-examination describe the same or similar warning signs (AAD, 1994b), and about half of all melanomas are initially found by patients (Koh et al., 1992). Physicians, however, are more likely to detect thin, early-stage melanomas (Ep-stein et al., 1999).

If nothing suspicious is found during the skin examination, the result of the screening examination is described as negative. If a clinician identifies a mole or other lesion suspicious for melanoma or nonmelanoma skin cancer, the exami-nation is considered positive. The next step—and the "gold standard" for identi-fication of any skin cancer—is a skin biopsy, usually a simple and easily toler-ated outpatient procedure.

Diagnosis

If examination of the skin detects something suspicious for melanoma or nonmelanoma skin cancer, a diagnostic biopsy and microscopic examination of the removed tissue is used to confirm or rule out the presence of skin cancer. If melanoma or other cancerous tumor is identified, the tissue analysis also identi-fies characteristics useful for "staging" the cancer (judging how advanced it is) and assessing a patient's prognosis. An excisional biopsy removes the suspi-cious lesion with a narrow margin of normal-appearing skin as well as a portion of underlying subcutaneous fat (Arndt et al., 1995; Geisse, 1994). Such an exci-sional biopsy may also serve as effective treatment for early-stage lesions. For large lesions, an incisional biopsy may be used to remove enough tissue for a diagnosis to guide subsequent treatment decisions. Either kind of biopsy usually requires local anesthetic; scarring is likely but the extent will depend on the type, size, and location of the biopsy.

As part of the diagnosis, cancer staging systems are intended to classify characteristics of the disease related to prognosis. The most common staging system for melanoma uses information about the tumor's size; the extent to which it has invaded the skin or nearby tissue; involvement of the lymph nodes; and spread or metastasis to more distant sites (NCI, 1999b). Appendix B pro-

---

[9]Dermatologists may also use in vivo epiluminescence microscopy, a noninvasive test that is still being assessed for accuracy (Kittler et al., 1999; USPSTF, 1996).

vides more information on diagnosis and staging of melanoma and nonmelanoma skin cancers.

Accuracy of Screening Tests

The literature review in Appendix B identified four recent studies of screening by total skin examination for both melanoma and nonmelanoma skin cancers (De Rooij et al., 1995, 1997; Jonna et al., 1998; Limpert, 1995; Rampen et al., 1995).[10] As summarized in Table B-1, these studies found suspicious lesions in from 4 to 28 percent of those screened. Between 30 and 58 percent of those found to have a suspicious lesion who then followed up and had a biopsy were diagnosed with some form of skin cancer, mostly basal cell carcinomas.[11] It is important to distinguish between the number who were referred for biopsy on the basis of a positive screen and the usually smaller number who actually followed up and had a biopsy. When analyses of the outcome of the screening program also included those who were referred for a biopsy but did not have one, the percentages of those with a positive screening result who were diagnosed with skin cancer dropped considerably for two studies. This latter kind of analysis—including all those referred for further testing—better reflects the reality that people do not always follow up as advised.

In a study focused on the much less common melanoma, one very large, free mass-screening project (over 280,000 participants) reported 0.3 percent (or 763) of the participants had lesions suspicious for melanoma (Koh et al., 1996). An additional 1.3 percent had lesions for which "rule-out melanoma" biopsies were recommended. The diagnosis of melanoma was confirmed by biopsy in 130 of the 763 patients with a suspected melanoma. Thus, of those with a lesion suspicious for melanoma, about 19 percent of those who had a biopsy were diagnosed with the disease. Not all of the participants (especially those in the "rule-out" melanoma category) followed up by having a biopsy as advised. Among those in the rule-out category who had a biopsy, an additional 234 cases of melanoma were identified, but finding those cases required biopsies for additional 2,316 disease-free individuals.

Two commonly used measures of screening test accuracy—specificity and sensitivity—cannot usually be computed for skin cancer screening studies because only the suspicious lesions that are detected are biopsied, and people with negative screening result are not followed. *Sensitivity* (the proportion of people who have the disease and who also have positive test results) is relevant in assessing screening tests because the lower the sensitivity, the more likely a test is

---

[10]Earlier studies reviewed in USPSTF, 1996, and Elwood, 1994, and 1996, were consistent with these studies.

[11]As discussed further in Appendix B, the proportion of people with a positive test result who are found to have the disease is referred to as the positive predictive value of a screening test.

to miss people who actually have the disease (i.e., show false negative test results). [12] *Specificity* (the proportion of people who do not have the disease and who also have negative test results)[13] is useful to know because the lower the number for specificity, the more people who do not have the disease (i.e., show false positive results) will be told they do have it—and may, as a result, undergo further testing and treatment unnecessarily.

One study did follow patients with negative screening results (1551 of a total of 1961) for 42 months (Rampen et al., 1995). Of the 15 patients diagnosed with skin cancer by the end of that period, a review of their records showed three lesions (no melanomas) that had been misdiagnosed during the earlier screening (i.e., were false negatives). (The other 12 patients were determined to have developed new lesions since the screening.) Thus, those with an initial negative result had a 99.8 percent chance that the initial negative result was accurate.

A few studies have compared biopsy results with results of visual examinations identifying the ABCD(E) signs described above and similar checklists (reviewed in Whited and Grichnik, 1998). In these studies, the percentage of those diagnosed with melanoma who had been identified by visual examination ranged from 79 percent to 100 percent, and the percentage of those with negative biopsies who had negative results by visual examination ranged from 32 percent to 37 percent. The reviewers concluded that, at present, the data suggest that clinicians would be unlikely to miss a melanoma, based on application of the checklist criteria. It is not clear how often a benign lesion might be classified as melanoma using the same criteria.

If a new program of skin cancer screening were to be adopted, a number of practical questions would arise. One is how accurate primary care clinicians—who form the front-line in most screening programs—are likely to be in identifying skin cancers or skin cancer risk factors. Most studies comparing dermatologists with other examiners involve relatively weak research designs and rely on examinations of color photographs or slides rather than patients. As might be expected, studies generally indicate that dermatologists are more likely to accurately identify skin cancers than primary care physicians or trained nonprofessionals (Burton et al., 1998; Byles et al., 1994; Cassileth et al., 1986; Federman et al., 1997; Gerbert et al., 1998, but see also McGee et al., 1994a,b). Although some studies suggest that training can improve accuracy in identifying photo-

---

[12]To compute sensitivity requires some way of identifying those who have the disease who have negative test results. For example, studies of screening for thyroid nodules using palpation of the neck have been compared to ultrasound examinations, which can detect nonpalpable lesions. Only a biopsy, however, can distinguish between cancerous and noncancerous thyroid nodules.

[13]To compute specificity also requires some way of determining that those who have negative test results really do not have the disease.

graphs of lesions, performance in everyday clinical practice may not improve (Burton et al., 1998; Weinstock et al., 1996). One recent survey of skin cancer screening practices by primary care physicians found that only half of those surveyed were confident that they could detect skin cancer (Kirsner et al., 1999).

In an effort to improve the yield and reduce the cost of skin cancer screening, some studies have examined screening targeted to high-risk individuals identified by a patient history or self-administered questionnaire. These studies tend to show that individuals are more accurate in reporting some risk factors (hair color, freckles, number of moles) than others (number of raised moles or sunburn history) (Jackson et al., 1998; Westerdahl et al., 1996). One study found that not quite 10 percent of those administered a risk-factor questionnaire reported responses that would classify them as high risk (Jackson et al., 1998). No studies have assessed the accuracy of primary care physicians in accurately identifying risk factors for skin cancer.

In sum, although data are limited, they suggest that clinical screening by dermatologists is moderately accurate. They also suggest reason for some concern about the accuracy of screening by primary care physicians and the need to develop and test strategies to assure reasonable accuracy in this group's performance in practice.

Accuracy of Diagnostic Tests

Assuming a positive screening result, the accuracy of diagnostic tests also needs to be considered. Histopathological examinations are not perfect, which puts those with false positive screening results at risk of unnecessary further surgery or other treatment as well as anxiety, possible insurability problems, and other harms.

Studies have found varying levels of agreement among pathologists in diagnosis and classification of tissue samples (see, e.g., Cook et al., 1996; Corona et al., 1996; Heenan et al., 1984). Agreement is higher for basic distinctions between benign and malignant lesions than for more specific characterizations or for borderline conditions (Cook et al., 1996). To improve diagnostic accuracy and consistency, recommendations include efforts to achieve agreement among pathologists on the use of standardized terminology, diagnostic criteria, and definitions as well as better education about the appearance and behavior of certain lesions (CRC, 1997).

BENEFITS AND HARMS OF SKIN CANCER
SCREENING
General Issues

The major benefit desired from any screening program is early detection of disease followed by early treatment that permits better outcomes including longer life (not just a longer period between diagnosis and death), reduced morbidity, and better quality of life. A negative screening result may also bring benefits in the form of relief from anxiety, particularly for those who consider themselves to be at high risk.

Although discussions of screening generally emphasize expected benefits, potential harms to those screened should also be examined and weighed. Those who test positive during screening but actually have no disease can suffer harms including anxiety, inconvenience, explicit or covert discrimination by insurers or employers, and unnecessary further testing and treatment. Thus, one factor cited in recommendations against prostate cancer screening is the high rate of false positives and the significant risks of impotence, incontinence, and other harms associated with surgical treatment (USPSTF, 1996). In addition, some cancers including many prostate and thyroid cancers will never progress to do harm, which means that a screening program that identifies large numbers of such cancers may cause many people to suffer needless anxiety and unnecessary treatment. Further, people who have false-negative screening results as determined by follow-up biopsy may be less alert to symptoms of their disease and seek treatment later than if they had not been screened.

Assessing benefits and harms from screening typically involves a subjective as well as an objective component. Although research and analysis can generate estimates of the probabilities and magnitudes of different outcomes, individual decisions about the relative importance of these possible outcomes will reflect personal circumstances, preferences, and priorities.

As stated in a recent IOM report, "when the evidence of screening benefits or harms is limited or weak, when patient perceptions of benefits and harms are variable or not well understood, or when patient preferences about outcomes are crucial to good decision making, then the strong involvement of the patient in a process of shared decision making . . . becomes particularly important (IOM/NRC, 1999, p. 103; see also Emanuel and Emanuel, 1992; Flood et al., 1996; Woolf, 1997). For toss-up or close-call situations, decision theory emphasizes patient views about possible benefits and harms as the key variable in determining a course of action (Kassirer and Pauker, 1981; Pauker and Kassirer, 1997).

Few studies have examined the possible harms of various cancer screening interventions or how such harms are viewed by potential screenees. Likewise, few researchers have attempted to assess how people weigh potential harms against potential benefits.

EVIDENCE OF BENEFITS FROM EARLY DETECTION OF SKIN CANCER THROUGH SCREENING

The best evidence of benefit from skin cancer screening would come from a prospective randomized clinical trial that randomly selected people to be screened or not screened (i.e., to continue "usual" care) and then followed both groups long enough for differential outcomes (e.g., five-year mortality rates) to be evident. Because cancer screening trials typically require very large study populations, long follow-up periods, and significant administrative complexities, they usually have been undertaken only for cancers that affect many people and cause major mortality and morbidity.

The committee identified no randomized trials of clinical skin cancer screening. Discussions during the committee's June 1999 workshop indicated that such a clinical trial would require from one-half million to one million participants and would not likely be funded in the United States. The committee heard that a trial is underway in Australia (where skin cancer rates are much higher than in the United States) involving at least 500,000 people in 60 communities that have been randomly assigned to have a screening program established or to continue with current care. Current care includes intensive education and awareness campaigns for both the general population and the health professions. The study was reported to be in its first year of a 10-year follow-up period.

The committee also found no case-control studies of the effectiveness of clinical skin cancer screening in reducing mortality or morbidity. Lacking direct evidence of a link between skin cancer screening and better outcomes, the committee searched for indirect evidence. Because the underlying assumption is that screening will lead to earlier detection of disease, the committee considered evidence for this link in the pathway from screening to better outcomes (see arc 3 in the diagram in Figure B-3 of Appendix B). Appendix B summarizes eight screening studies (none of which included an unscreened comparison group) that measured thickness of detected melanomas. Four found no melanomas over 1.0 mm, and another study found only 8 percent in this category. Three studies reported 67 to 87 percent of melanomas were 1.5mm or less. Data from SEER indicate that more melanomas are being discovered at a thinner stage than in the past but are still diagnosed more often at thicker stages than reported in the screening studies (Dennis, 1999). One recently reported French study suggested that delay in diagnosis of melanomas was less important to prognosis than aggressive tumor growth, a finding consistent with other retrospective studies trying to identify reasons for delay in diagnosis and its impact (Richard et al., 1999). In general, however, the evidence suggests that screening can identify melanomas at a thinner stage than usual care.[14]

---

[14]The committee notes that "usual" care is not precisely defined (compared to a studied intervention) and that such care may change over time. For example, on the one hand, participation in or competition from managed care may prompt shorter office visits and less direct patient access to specialists; on the other hand, HMOs may encourage more patients to have a periodic preventive care visit. The committee found no specific evidence to document changes in usual primary or specialist care related to identification

Studies of survival following excision indicate that greater thickness is associated with poorer survival. These data, although suggestive, are not definitive evidence that detecting thinner melanomas *through screening*, as opposed to detection through usual care by alert health care professionals, will improve survival. One reason is that screening of asymptomatic people might just lengthen the time between diagnosis and death (*lead-time bias*). A second possibility is that screening may mostly discover more nonaggressive tumors that exist for long periods of time while missing many faster growing, more lethal tumors (*length bias*) that arise between screenings. Randomized clinical trials are the best strategy for assessing the effects of screening programs on mortality and morbidity.

The committee identified one case-control study of skin self-examination, which reported suggestive evidence that such examination might reduce the risk of lethal melanoma (Berwick et al., 1996). However, the study also found that older men—those most at risk of melanoma—were less likely than women to examine their own skin, although they were much more likely to have a melanoma identified by a spouse. It is reasonable to expect that patients who examine their own skin for skin cancer will do so more frequently than a physician would for any class of patients, so the generalizability of this study to clinical screening is not clear. Conversely, the extent to which effective self-examination could occur in the absence of initial education by a clinician is also uncertain.

If Congress was persuaded to extend coverage for a new program of skin cancer screening in asymptomatic people, the statute or implementing regulations would have to address the question of screening frequency. No evidence is available to guide such a policy decision. The most limited option would be to pay for a single screening examination in combination with education about skin self-examination. Whatever the frequency of screening, skin cancer screening could be incorporated in a periodic preventive services visit that also included other recommended preventive services. Again, regardless of how skin cancers or suspicious lesions are identified, current Medicare policy covers follow-up services.

ESTIMATED COSTS TO MEDICARE OF EXTENDING COVERAGE

As discussed in Chapter 2, the cost estimation approach used by the committee follows the generic practices (e.g., not discounting estimates to present value) employed by the Congressional Budget Office (CBO) in making estimates for Congress. A more detailed presentation of the committee's cost estimates appears in Appendix E, which was prepared by the Lewin Group in con-

---

of skin cancers. One analysis indicated that patients in managed care plans were less likely to have skin care provided by a dermatologist than those in fee-for-service plans (Feldman et al., 1996). Most Medicare beneficiaries are not enrolled in HMOs, but their care may still be influenced by managed care depending on their community and the composition of an individual physician's practice.

sultation with the committee and background paper authors. To illustrate how Medicare costs would be affected by different skin cancer screening strategies and behaviors, the committee developed estimates for the three models of screening described earlier. As summarized in Box 3-1 and explained below, for the five-year period 2000 to 2004, net estimated costs to Medicare range from about $150 million for the most limited screening scenario to about $900 million dollars for the most expansive.

The committee's estimates of Medicare costs are based on a series of assumptions, some of which have supporting evidence or data but others of which

---

BOX 3-1 Summary of Estimated Costs to Medicare for Covering a New Program of Screening Asymptomatic Beneficiaries for Skin Cancer

Screening Strategy Assumptions

• *Case Finding Approach 1.* 30% of beneficiaries are screened each year by total skin examination during a physician visit that includes other covered services; those with skin lesions identified as positive (suspicious for melanoma or nonmelanoma skin cancers) are referred to a dermatologist, who may order a biopsy. Estimate assumes 5% of those screened would be referred to and visit a dermatologist; 50% of this group would have a biopsy.

• *Case Finding Approach 2.* Same as above except that beneficiaries would first be assessed for skin cancer risk; only those identified as high risk would be examined. Estimate assumes that physicians would identify 10% of beneficiaries as high risk and then examine them; 20% of those examined would be referred to and visit a dermatologist; 50% of this group would have a biopsy.

• *Mass Screening Campaign.* Public information campaign encourages beneficiaries to assess their own risk for skin cancer and then see a dermatologist if they conclude they are at high risk. Estimate assumes that 10% of beneficiaries are at high risk and that 20% of that group visit a dermatologist, who biopsies 20% of this group.

Cost Estimate Assumptions for Years 2000 to 2004 (see also Appendix E)

• In 2000, Medicare pays $20 for screening added to a physician visit, $50 for a separate visit, and $90 for a biopsy.
• Medicare payments increase at 2% per year.
• Costs are not discounted to present value.
• Costs are subject to 20% cost sharing.

Continued

BOX 3-1 *Continued*

Cost Estimate Assumptions for Years 2000 to 2004 (*continued*)

- No cost offsets for program savings are attributed to screening.
- Net costs are total estimated gross costs offset by 25% for premium increase borne by Medicare beneficiaries.

Data Sources (see Appendix E for specifics)

- Beneficiary population data from HCFA Office of the Actuary.
- Assumptions about use of screening visits, referrals, and biopsies and cost of biopsy based on advice of IOM committee and its consultants.
- Payment per visit data (before adjustments) from 1998 Medicare Physician Fee Schedule.

Estimated Costs (in millions) to Medicare Summed Over 2000–2004

	Screening Model		
	Case Finding 1	Case Finding 2	Mass Screening
Gross 5-Year Cost to Medicare	$1,199.4	$510.8	$199.5
25% Medicare Premium Offset	299.9	127.7	49.9
Net 5-Year Cost to Medicare	899.5	383.1	149.6

are best guesses based on committee judgment in the absence of such information. The estimates are intended to suggest the order of magnitude of the costs to Medicare of extending coverage, but they could be considerably higher or lower than what Medicare might actually spend were coverage policies changed. The tables in Appendix E allow readers to vary some of the committee's assumptions and calculate alternative estimates.[15]

The unit cost of skin cancer screening services (physician visits and diagnostic biopsies) is not high, which means that the cost estimates are driven primarily by the number of individuals who would be screened. Some 39 million beneficiaries are expected to be enrolled in Medicare in 2000. A majority visit a primary care physician each year, so the number of persons who could be offered screening is quite large. Even if all beneficiaries were entitled to screening, however, not all would seek or accept screening nor would all physicians advise or conduct screening for their patients. A recent survey of primary care physi-

---

[15]The CBO and HCFA actuaries would undoubtedly be asked to develop their own estimates for any specific proposals under active consideration by Congress.

cians in Dade County, Florida, and New Haven, Connecticut, reported that about 30 percent said they routinely performed a full-body skin examination on all their patients, and about 30 percent of the remainder say they did so for high-risk patients (Kirsner et al., 1999). A retrospective analysis of patient records at two Veterans Affairs Medical Centers found skin cancer screening documented for only 28 percent of 200 patients and only 18 percent when those without a skin-related complaint were excluded (Federman et al., 1997). Reports on use of other preventive services likewise show considerably less than complete adherance to recommendations by both physicians and consumers (HCFA, 1998a, and USPSTF, 1996; see also Chapter 6).[16]

For the single-step case-finding approach, the estimates below assume that of 30 percent of Medicare beneficiaries, 5 percent would then be referred to a dermatologist who would do biopsies on half of those referred. For the two-step strategy involving an initial risk assessment, the estimates assume that primary care physicians would identify 10 percent of beneficiaries as high risk and refer them to a dermatologist for further evaluation. Both estimates assume that other beneficiaries would have skin examinations (and referrals and biopsies) prompted by a physician's incidental discovery of a skin abnormality or patient concern about a skin abnormality. These services are already covered by Medicare.

Consistent with the CBO approach, estimates are not discounted to present value, and total direct costs for screening are offset by 25 percent to reflect the increase in the Medicare premium that would be paid by beneficiaries based on the projected increase in expenditures resulting from extended coverage. The screening models assume that the costs listed for visits and biopsies are actual Medicare reimbursements with nothing subtracted for cost sharing by patients. Absent relevant evidence, the models assume no offsetting savings to Medicare during the period.

The committee did not attempt to assess the cost-effectiveness of skin cancer screening. During its workshop, however, the committee was presented with an analysis that modeled the cost-effectiveness of a single occurrence of skin cancer screening among high-risk individuals, compared to no screening (see Freedberg et al., in press). This analysis assumed that the screening was performed by a dermatologist. More important, the analysis also assumed (1) that the screening would result in melanomas being detected at earlier, thinner stages; (2) that these screening-detected melanomas would be more effectively

---

[16]Skin cancer screening is less demanding than some other screening services because it is not invasive, nor does it involve expensive, specialized equipment that is not available in the office of a primary care physician (thus requiring the patient to go elsewhere). Still, the patient or physician would have to be motivated to request or recommend the skin examination. For a physician, discussing skin cancer screening and doing a risk assessment or skin examination could add several minutes to office visits that are often scheduled for less than 15 minutes.

treated than if they had been detected in the course of usual care; and (3) that the result would be reduced Medicare costs for treating skin cancer. Analysts then estimated the cost of screening a population of one million and the quantity of life saved (mortality avoided) due to the screening. The result was an estimated $29,170 expended per year of life saved, a figure not greatly different from several other cancer screening strategies. It is important to note that the assumptions of the analysis are significantly different than those used here, namely, that screening would in fact detect melanomas at earlier stages leading to earlier and less costly treatment. The analysis did not assess the costs or benefits of screening for nonmelanoma skin cancers.

In developing its estimates, the committee took into account past experience with cost estimates that have assumed that more people would take advantage of screening benefits than actually do. Underuse and underprovision of effective screening services are important public health issues. Chapter 6 discusses the challenge of "putting prevention into practice," that is, turning clinical recommendations and coverage into actual delivery of preventive services to those likely to benefit from them.

STATEMENTS OF OTHERS ABOUT SKIN CANCER SCREENING

A number of organizations have made statements and recommendations about clinical screening for skin cancer. The organizations vary in the extent to which they explicitly link their conclusions to systematic assessments of the evidence.

The U.S. Preventive Services Task Force (USPSTF, 1996) stated that "there is insufficient evidence for or against routine screening for skin cancer by primary care physicians using total body skin examination. . . . Clinicians should remain alert for skin lesions with malignant features . . . when examining patients for other reasons" especially those with established risk factors (p. 148). "A recommendation to consider referring [patients with melanocytic precursor or marker lesions] to skin cancer specialists for evaluation and surveillance may be made on the grounds of patient preference or anxiety . . . although evidence of benefit from such referral is lacking." The USPSTF is again reviewing the evidence related to skin cancer screening and could reaffirm or change its 1996 recommendation, but an announcement is not expected before the release of this report.

Since 1985, the American Academy of Dermatologists has sponsored free skin cancer examinations as part of a public education program (Koh et al., 1996). The Academy's materials for the public stress sun avoidance and skin self-examination rather than routine clinical skin examinations for asymptomatic individuals.

Statements from the National Institutes of Health (NIH) are not fully consistent. The National Cancer Institute's on-line PDQ information system for physicians states "there is insufficient evidence to establish whether a decrease in mortality occurs from routine examination of the skin" (NCI, 1999f). In contrast, a 1992 NIH consensus conference stated that "there is sufficient evidence to warrant screening programs for melanoma in the United States. . . . The public should be encouraged to ask their primary care physicians and nurses for periodic skin examinations when seeing them for other purposes, for example, a physical examination . . . [and] should be made aware of (1) the increased risk of melanoma related to excessive sun exposure, particularly in childhood; (2) the clinical appearance of early melanoma; (3) the excellent prognosis associated with detection and treatment of early melanoma; and (4) the need for regular skin examinations by themselves and by their health professionals." A specific screening interval is not cited. The consensus statement does not link its recommendations to specific citations of the literature or evaluate the strength or quality of the evidence but does note that no randomized clinical trials are available.

The American College of Preventive Medicine (ACPM) recommends "periodic total cutaneous examinations be performed, targeting populations at high risk for malignant melanoma." The ACPM, however, finds insufficient evidence to set a screening interval more precisely and recommends well-conducted observational or case-controlled studies or randomized clinical trials to better identify the screening interval and the risk-benefit ratio for different groups.

The strongest and most comprehensive screening recommendation comes from the American Cancer Society. It recommends a cancer-related screening— including a skin examination—every year for those over 40 (ACS, 1999b).

COMMITTEE FINDINGS AND CONCLUSIONS

In developing its findings and recommendations, the committee recognized that the pathway from adoption of a new program of skin cancer screening to improved health outcomes for Medicare beneficiaries would have many uncertainties. Figure 3-2 illustrates a simple pathway and indicates some of the uncertainties associated with each element of the pathway. This figure does not include every possible step or uncertainty but rather summarizes some major variables that would likely affect the success of a screening program. These are the sort of potential issues to be weighed in the formulation of any final policy. Most of these uncertainties would affect the cost of covering screening.

Findings

After reviewing the literature, considering the discussion at its workshop, and drawing on its members' judgment, the committee reached several findings relevant to decisions about coverage of a new program for skin cancer screening for Medicare beneficiaries. The first findings listed below relate to the assessment criteria depicted in Figure 3-1. The last relate to directions for further research.

Population for Screening

  Definition of higher-risk subpopulations
  Public and professional education about risk factors, benefits/risks of
    screening
  Recognizability of candidates to themselves or medical personnel
  Noncoverage barriers to screening (e.g., patient interest, location,
    bureaucracy)

Screening Examination

  Skill, training, and experience of examiner
  Extent of exam (full body or partial)
  Frequency of exams
  Accuracy of exam
  Characteristics of lesions (e.g., location, stage)
  Cooperation of patient

Positive Result and Referral to Dermatologist

  Patient follow-up on referral
  Skill, training, experience of examiner
  Extent of exam (full body or partial)
  Accuracy of exam
  Characteristics of lesion

Biopsy Ordered

  Cooperation of patient
  Skill of biopsy preparation and pathology interpretation
  Characteristics of lesion

Positive Biopsy, Treatment

  Cooperation of patient
  Characteristics of lesion (size, depth, location)
  Skill of surgeon
  Health of patient (ability to heal)

Outcome for Patient (positive: improved survival, reduced morbidity;
  negative: scarring if any, anxiety, insurability problems)

FIGURE 3-2 Causal Pathway: Skin cancer screening, with examples of uncertainty that could affect outcome at several key points. Note: Events are in **bold** and in the main path; examples of variables that increase uncertainty of outcomes are offset to the right.

Disease Burden. Basal cell and squamous cell carcinoma are relatively common among older people. Squamous cell carcinoma is sometimes lethal and both can cause disfigurement or functional impairment. Melanoma is much less common but more often lethal. Older white males appear to be at particular risk of developing and dying from melanoma.

Treatment Effectiveness. Basal and squamous cell carcinomas are effectively treated by excision or other therapies. Earlier diagnosis and treatment is likely to result in less scarring. Excision is also effective for early-stage melanoma, but effective treatments have not been found for late-stage melanoma.

Accuracy of Screening Tests. Although studies are limited and show somewhat mixed results for total skin examination, the test appears acceptably accurate when performed by a dermatologist. Diagnostic biopsy is also not perfectly accurate but has good results in making the basic distinction between benign and malignant lesions.

Effect of Screening on Outcomes. Because basal cell carcinoma and squamous cell carcinoma are highly treatable and rarely lethal, it is unlikely that a new program of screening asymptomatic people could appreciably improve survival rates. Direct evidence is not available on the effect of screening on morbidity and disfigurement from these conditions. Direct evidence is not available to support conclusions about the effect of clinical screening on mortality or other health outcomes related to melanoma. Physicians identify a substantial proportion of the melanomas and tend to detect them at a thinner stage than do patients, and thinner melanomas have a better prognosis. This indirect evidence is only suggestive about the possible benefits of a new program of skin cancer screening for those without symptoms, in part because of inadequate knowledge about the rate of growth of melanomas, especially thin melanomas in older people. Another uncertainty involves the degree to which beneficiaries, particularly those at greatest risk, would avail themselves of a screening benefit and pursue recommended follow-up care.

Benefits Versus Harms. No controlled studies provide direct evidence about the benefits or harms of skin cancer screening. Patient perspectives on possible harms have not been explicitly assessed. Unlike breast, prostate, and certain other cancers, unnecessary surgery for a lesion misdiagnosed as skin cancer is unlikely to be life- or function-altering, disfiguring, or very painful. Scarring and anxiety may be expected from unnecessary diagnostic and treatment services if screening falsely identifies someone as having skin cancer, but such scarring usually will be minimal.

Possible Directions for Future Research

The committee identified several areas where further research would be helpful, although it did not attempt to set priorities. As noted above, a randomized controlled trial of skin cancer screening is underway in Australia, although substantial results are years away. Also, the much higher incidence of skin cancer in Australia would have to be taken into account in assessing the study's relevance to this country.

In the absence of evidence from controlled trials, it would be useful to have more research on the early stages of cancerous and precancerous lesions and their progression to more advanced states. Such research would help answer questions about how quickly different kinds of melanomas progress in different risk groups and about how likely it is that earlier detection of disease through a new program of clinical screening would make a difference in outcomes. More research would also be useful to understand how frequently and how quickly actinic keratoses develop into squamous cell carcinoma and what factors predict such progression.

Key issues in arguments against screening involve the effect of the intervention on healthy participants, which both exposes many individuals to unnecessary harm including inconvenience, discomfort, and anxiety, and drives up the cost of the program relative to any benefit. These concerns would be reduced if those most likely to benefit from the program could be accurately and efficiently identified, for example, during a preventive care office visit. To this end, further research on the effect of training primary care physicians in the accurate assessment of skin features should examine change in actual clinical practice (not just identification of photographs).

Accurately identifying those most at risk of skin cancer is part of the problem, but reaching the members of that group in the community is a different problem. One question is what kinds of communication strategies will encourage people at higher risk to limit sun exposure, to be alert to the warning signs of cancer (especially melanoma), to visit a physician when something suspicious is found, and to follow up on referrals for further assessment or treatment. Except for communication of sun exposure, a particular focus should be identifying ways of communicating more effectively with older white males.

Continued work to develop and assess educational programs and skin self-examination initiatives makes sense. For example, although outcome data are limited, research suggests that women are more likely to self-identify melanoma than men and that men are more likely than women to have a melanoma identified by a family member. This may suggest investigating whether self-examination education programs might also emphasize the role of family members and close friends in being alert for, and telling one another about, abnormal-appearing areas of skin, which should then be professionally evaluated.

More generally, in addition to research that could clarify the benefits, harms, and cost-effectiveness of clinical skin cancer screening and primary prevention programs, other interesting lines of investigation exist in the area of treatment. These include more effective chemotherapy for nonlocalized melanoma and vaccination or immunotherapy for melanoma.

Conclusions

In summary, **the committee concluded that evidence for the effectiveness of skin cancer screening is insufficient to support positive or negative conclusions about the adoption of a new program of clinical screening of asymptomatic Medicare beneficiaries.** Direct evidence that detection of skin cancer through clinical screening leads to better health outcomes is lacking rather than negative, inconsistent, or ambiguous. The indirect evidence for screening is suggestive but not compelling. The committee is aware that Medicare coverage has been extended for other services (e.g., prostate-specific antigen testing and bone densitometry testing) for which direct and indirect evidence of benefit is inconclusive or disputed. Those precedents are not sufficient grounds for covering a new program of clinical screening for skin cancer.

Because evidence does support benefits of early detection and treatment as part of usual medical care, clinicians and patients should continue to be alert to the common signs of skin cancer—with a particular emphasis on older white males and on melanoma—and should investigate suspicious signs further. Medicare already covers skin examination and testing by primary care physicians and dermatologists prompted by patient concern about a skin abnormality or by incidental physician discovery of an abnormality during a visit for other purposes.

Further, **dermatological and other organizations should continue skin cancer educational programs for people of all ages, including programs that encourage people to limit sun exposure and inform themselves about skin cancer risk factors and warning signs, especially those for melanoma.** Perhaps the major challenge related to the Medicare population is identifying and implementing better ways of reaching the group at highest risk of death from skin cancer—older, fair-skinned males.

4

Medically Necessary
Dental Services

From the outset, the Medicare program has excluded coverage "for services in connection with the care, treatment, filling, removal, or replacement of teeth or structures directly supporting the teeth" (Section 1862(a)(12) of the Social Security Act). The 1965 legislation authorizing the program provided a narrow exception that payment could be made "in the case of inpatient hospital services in connection with the provision of dental services if the individual, because of his/her underlying medical condition and clinical status, or because of the severity of the dental procedure, requires hospitalization in connection with the provision of such services."

As described in regulations and the program manuals used by the intermediaries and carriers who administer Medicare claims, the Health Care Financing Administration (HCFA) has interpreted the statutory exceptions language to permit payments for professional dental services when they are performed as an "integral part" of covered inpatient procedures (*Carriers Manual,* section 2136 [HCFA, 1999b]). For example, if the extraction of a tooth in the line of a jaw fracture is integral to treatment of the jaw injury, then dental treatment (i.e., the extraction) is covered. If a beneficiary has to be hospitalized for a dental procedure (e.g., an extraction not integral to a covered medical service) to be safely performed given his or her clinical status, Medicare covers the hospital services but not the dental procedure itself. In general, Medicare-covered services that are within the scope of practice (as defined by states) for a physician as well as a dentist are covered when provided by a dentist. Examples include management of mucositis and treatment of oral infections using antibiotics.

TABLE 4-1 Medicare Coverage of Dental Services as Specified in
Statute or by the Health Care Financing Administration

Clinical Condition	Medicare-Covered Service
Underlying medical condition and clinical status requires hospitalization for dental care	Inpatient hospital services only (Medicare Part A)
Severity of dental procedure requires hospitalization for dental care	Inpatient hospital services only (Medicare Part A)
Any oral condition for which nondental services are covered	All dental services if incident to and an integral part of a covered procedure or service performed by the same person (Medicare Part B)
Neoplastic jaw disease	Extractions prior to radiation and prior to oral examination if extractions occur (Medicare Part B)
Renal transplant surgery	Oral or dental examination on an inpatient basis (Medicare Part A if performed by hospital-based dentist; Part B if performed by a physician)

Table 4-1 summarizes Medicare's limited coverage of dental services. The summary is based on HCFA policy statements rather than on sometimes conflicting carrier policies.

HCFA has explicitly approved coverage exceptions for the extraction of teeth to prepare the jaw for radiation treatment of cancer (*Carriers Manual,* section 2136 [HCFA, 1999b]) and for an oral examination performed as part of a comprehensive inpatient work up prior to kidney—but not other organ—transplantation (*Coverage Issues Manual,* section 50.26 [HCFA, 1999b]). HCFA has proposed additional exceptions based on arguments that the services would reduce the risk of infection and other complications, but its Technology Advisory Committee suggested that such exceptions (which would include some approved earlier) went further than the Medicare statute allowed and that Congress needed to indicate its approval of coverage based on such an argument (TAC, 1996).

Neither the statutory nor the regulatory language related to coverage exceptions for dental services is straightforward to interpret.[1] Moreover, carrier inter-

---

[1]For example, HCFA's *Carriers Manual* (section 2136 [HCFA, 1999b]) instructs carriers to pay "for a covered dental procedure no matter where the service is performed. The hospitalization or nonhospitalization of a patient has no direct bearing on the coverage or exclusion." In HCFA's *Coverage Issues Manual* (section 50-26), however, oral examinations by a dentist prior to a kidney transplant are covered under Part A of the program if performed by a dentist on the hospital's staff but under Part B only when per-

pretation is not always consistent. For example, at least one carrier's policies appear to approve coverage for an oral examination not only for kidney transplant patients but also for heart, liver, and other covered organ transplants, whether performed on an outpatient or an inpatient basis (e.g., see Conway, 1995; WPSIC, 1996).

DEFINING MEDICALLY NECESSARY DENTAL SERVICES

The 1997 Balanced Budget Act, which provided for this study, included no definition of "medically necessary dental services." One definition of such services is found in a bill submitted earlier in 1997 (but not passed). It called for coverage of "dental services that are medically necessary as a direct result of, or will have a direct impact on, an underlying medical condition if the coverage of such services is cost-effective" (H.R. 1288, introduced April 10, 1997). It also included explicit provisions for Medicare to cover dental care related to several specific illnesses. The bill's language—minus the wording about cost-effectiveness—is similar to that used three years earlier in a bill that included "medically necessary oral health care" in a proposed set of "basic benefits" to be covered as part of broad health care reform (H.R. 3600, introduced May 1994). This earlier proposal also included oral care intended to control pain and infection and to restore function. The committee understands these definitions of medically necessary services—particularly the one proposed in 1997—to be narrowly constructed (1) to continue the general exclusion of Medicare coverage for dental care[2] but (2) to broaden the scope of the exceptions to include dental care needed to prevent or effectively manage systemic conditions including the oral complications of specific illnesses or their medical treatment.

Certainly, the prevention and management of oral infection have significant health implications when such infection has the potential to increase systemic morbidity in patients who are immunocompromised or otherwise at greater risk of adverse medical outcomes because of their underlying health problems. The importance of immunosuppression as a medical problem reflects scientific and

---

formed by a physician. This manual (unlike the *Carriers Manual*) also says that a dentist is not recognized as a physician when performing such an examination.

[2]As defined in HCFA's *Carriers Manual* (section 2136), dental care involves care limited to the teeth and the structures directly supporting the teeth. These structures are the periodontium (connective tissue surrounding the tooth root and attaching it to its socket), which includes the gingivae (gums), dentogingival junction, periodontal membrane, cementum of the teeth (layer of bone-like mineralized tissue that covers dentin and blends with fibers of the periodontium), and alveolar process (projecting ridge on the upper and lower jaw containing tooth sockets). Thus, dental care is understood as involving not only the teeth but also parts of the oral cavity and the structures therein.

therapeutic developments that have occurred in the three decades since the adoption of Medicare.

From the broader perspective of individual and public health, the coverage-oriented definitions of "medically necessary dental services" are unduly narrow. The concept that such care involves only care related to an "underlying medical condition" could suggest to some for example, that periodontal or other tooth-related infections are somehow different from infections elsewhere. More generally, such narrow definitions could imply that the mouth can be isolated from the rest of the body, a notion neither scientifically based nor constructive for individual or public health.[3] Thus, the remainder of this chapter refers to "medically necessary dental services," using quotation marks as a reminder of the term's specialized and restricted meaning in this discussion of Medicare coverage policy and, more generally, of the difficulty of precisely defining such care in most contexts.[4] (Appendix C includes further examination of the concept of "medically necessary dental services.")

Given the limited time and resources available, the committee could provide an evidence-based consideration of "medically necessary dental services" only for a subset of services that might qualify for this designation. The next section of this chapter reviews the approach the committee took to selecting and assessing specific medical conditions and associated dental services. The rest of the chapter reviews the evidence for each condition and presents the estimated costs to Medicare of covering the dental services examined. The final section summarizes the committee's findings and its conclusions about Medicare coverage for the general category of dental care needed to prevent or effectively manage nondental illnesses or injury including oral complications of other therapies. The background paper commissioned by the committee is found in Appendix C.

ASSESSMENT APPROACH: INTERVENTION, POPULATION, AND OUTCOMES

The selection of conditions and services for assessment was guided in part by historical context. A few months before the passage of the 1997 Balanced Budget Act, legislation had been introduced, first, to cover a specific set of "medically necessary dental services" that were described as "cost-effective" and, more generally, to provide for future coverage of other services subsequently determined to "result in reductions in expenditures . . . that exceed expenditures resulting from such coverage" (H.R. 1288, April 1997). This latter

---

[3]For a discussion of the inadequate integration of oral health care with other health care, see IOM (1995a).

[4]The committee retained the term "dental" services rather than using a term that might perhaps seem more inclusive such as "oral health care" to maintain consistency with its charge and the language of the BBA.

requirement is quite stringent; generally, services are considered to be cost-effective (i.e., to have net benefits worth the costs) whether or not they produce cost savings that fully offset direct service costs. The more restrictive language reflects the rules that Congress has adopted requiring increases in spending in one area to be offset by cuts elsewhere or by increased taxes.

The five conditions listed in the 1997 bill had been presented in prior analyses of health conditions that sought to identify those for which the cost of covering inpatient dental services would likely be offset by savings related to complications avoided, especially additional hospitalization (Cameron et al., 1995; Rutkauskas, 1995). The five conditions were

1. head and neck cancer,
2. leukemia,
3. lymphoma,
4. organ transplantation, and
5. valvular heart disease.

Although the Balanced Budget Act provisions calling for this study did not mention any particular conditions, the committee decided that those identified in the prior 1997 legislative proposal were a reasonable focus for its analyses. Table 4-2 summarizes current Medicare coverage (as specified by HCFA) of dental services for these conditions.

Following the general approach set forth in Chapter 2, the committee began by defining the specific dental services that would be investigated for the five identified conditions. It assumed that these services follow referral from a physician caring for a patient with one of the designated medical conditions. The dental care normally provided for these conditions includes a mix of preventive services (e.g., oral examinations to detect infections that might compromise transplant outcomes, cleaning of the teeth to eliminate potential sources of infection) and treatment services (e.g., extraction of abscessed teeth or treatment of gingival or gum enlargement associated with use of cyclosporin). The specific services examined for each condition are described in Appendix C and later sections of this chapter.

The population of interest includes Medicare beneficiaries age 65 and over as well as younger people qualified for Medicare on grounds of disability or diagnosis of end-stage renal disease (ESRD). Evidence related to all age groups was reviewed.

The potential beneficial outcomes investigated include reduced mortality and morbidity due to more effective prevention or management of oral problems related to the five medical conditions or to complications of their treatment. More generally, dental care may improve patient knowledge of good oral health habits. In addition, dental care may bring quality-of-life benefits related to appearance and self-esteem and enjoyment or comfort in eating. Preservation of teeth is clearly valued by many, although data on the value that people place on teeth—having most of their teeth, a few teeth, or no teeth, or having good versus bad teeth—indicate that the value varies in different cultural subgroups (Hollister and Weintraub, 1993; Slade et al., 1996; Strauss and Hunt, 1993). Potential harms of dental care include the possibility that such care may exacerbate infection or infection risks; cause pain, disfigurement, or functional impairment; or delay other treatment. The literature identified by the committee focused on morbidity (including pain and other discomfort) rather than on quality-of-life outcomes.

TABLE 4-2 Summary of Dental Services Currently Covered and not Covered Under Medicare for Selected Diseases or Conditions

Disease or Condition	Dental Services Currently Covered Under Medicare	Dental Services not Currently Covered Under Medicare
Head and neck cancer	Extraction of teeth prior to radiation Oral examination if extractions are to be performed	Oral examination if no extractions are to be done prior to radiation Preventive care to reduce risk of radiation caries (e.g., fluoride trays, supplemental topical fluoride) Treatment of radiation caries
Lymphoma and leukemia	Management of mucositis, hemorrhage, and related side effects of underlying disease	Oral examination prior to treatment Dental treatment to reduce risk of infection or eliminate infection prior to or following treatment
Organ transplantation	Management of infection following transplantation Oral examination prior to renal transplant surgery on an inpatient basis	Oral examination for transplants other than kidney Outpatient oral examination performed by a dentist prior to kidney transplant Dental treatment to reduce risk of infection or eliminate infection for any transplantation prior to or following transplant
Heart valve repair or replacement	None	Oral examination prior to repair or replacement Dental treatment to reduce risk of infection or eliminate infection prior to or following repair or replacement of valve

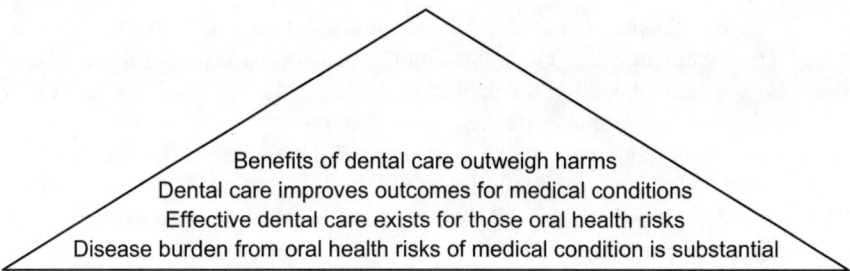

Benefits of dental care outweigh harms
Dental care improves outcomes for medical conditions
Effective dental care exists for those oral health risks
Disease burden from oral health risks of medical condition is substantial

FIGURE 4-1 Evidence pyramid for assessing "medically necessary dental services." SOURCE: Adapted from IOM/NRC, 1999, p. 89.

To guide its assessment of the evidence about dental care for these five conditions, the committee adapted the evidence pyramid introduced in Chapter 2 as shown in Figure 4-1. One distinguishing feature of Figure 4-1 compared to the generic pyramid is that it requires a link between a nondental condition or treatment and either dental services or dental complications. The first tier of the pyramid refers accordingly to the relationship between the medical conditions listed earlier and oral health conditions. The relationship could be manifest either as an increased risk to oral health caused by the medical condition (or its treatment) or as an increased risk to systemic health related to poor oral health. The tiers above refer to the effectiveness of dental care in treating oral problems and improving outcomes for the medical condition.

A test that met all of the criteria in Figure 4-1 would clearly have benefits compared to usual care, but the extent of benefit relative to the cost to Medicare, a health plan, or society generally would still have to be considered. The committee did not formally assess the cost-effectiveness of the dental services considered here. As called for by its charge, it did estimate the cost to Medicare of covering these services. Part of this analysis included identifying any offsetting savings to Medicare that might occur as a result, for example, of shorter or avoided hospital stays or reduced use of hyperbaric oxygen therapy for complications associated with treatment for head and neck cancer.

HEAD AND NECK CANCER

Burden of Disease

Cancers of the head and neck are commonly defined to include primary or metastatic cancers involving the oral cavity, pharynx, and larynx[5] but to exclude

---

[5]The oral cavity includes the lips, the front two-thirds of the tongue, the lining of the cheeks and lips (buccal mucosa), the floor of the mouth, the gums (lower and upper gingiva), the hard palate, and the area behind the last molar. The pharynx or throat is the part

cancers invoving other parts of the head, notably the eyes, skin, thyroid, and brain. The treatments, as well as head and neck cancer itself, can have serious implications for the health of the patient.

Cancers of the head and neck are more common among persons age 65 and older than among younger persons. Statistics often track invasive cancers of the oral cavity and pharynx and cancers of the larynx separately (SEER, 1999).[6] These two categories of head and neck cancers account for approximately 2.6 and 1.6 percent, respectively, of all cancers.

An estimated 29,800 new cases of cancer of the oral cavity and pharynx are expected to be diagnosed in 1999, more than 48 percent (or nearly 14,400) in people age 65 or older (ACS, 1999a). The age-adjusted incidence rate (1992–1996) in those diagnosed at age 65 or older is 45.0 per year per 100,000 population, compared to 6.5 per 100,000 in younger persons. Five-year relative survival rates (1989–1995) do not differ greatly by age—52.3 percent for those age 65 or older and 54.1 percent for younger persons. The lifetime risk of being diagnosed with cancers of the oral cavity or pharynx is 1.47 percent for men and 0.73 percent for women, while the lifetime risk of dying of this cancer is 0.41 percent for men and 0.23 for women.

For cancer of the larynx, an estimated 10,600 new cases are expected in 1999, nearly 55 percent (or about 5,800) in patients age 65 or older. The five-year age-adjusted incidence rate in those age 65 or older is 19.7 per 100,000, compared to 2.3 per 100,000 in younger persons. Five-year relative survival rates again do not differ greatly by age—63.2 percent for those age 65 or older and 65.7 percent for younger persons. The lifetime risk of being diagnosed with cancer of the larynx is 0.72 percent for men and 0.18 percent for women, while the lifetime risk of dying of this cancer is 0.22 percent for men and 0.06 for women.

Most cancers of the oral cavity, pharynx, and larynx are squamous cell carcinomas (affecting the outer layers of the tissue covering the cavity and structures). Epidemiological studies have repeatedly shown head and neck cancers to be positively associated with use of tobacco and alcohol, with both independent and interactive effects. Viral exposures and nutritional deficiencies also are associated with these cancers (reviewed in Carroll et al., 1998).

A dentist or physician may detect cancers of the oral cavity and upper pharynx while the lesions are still asymptomatic. This is more likely for people undergoing regular oral examinations, although evidence has been described as

---

of the digestive tube lying between the esophagus and the mouth and nasal cavities. The larynx, which includes the vocal cords, lies below the pharynx and connects to the trachea or windpipe.

[6]Unless otherwise indicated, data are from the most recent report of the National Cancer Institute's Surveillance Epidemiology and End-Results Program (SEER), which is available at www-SEER.ims.nci.nih.gov/publications.

"insufficient" to justify recommendations for or against routine screening for oral cancer (USPSTF, 1996, p. 175). In general, however, patients with cancer of the head and neck tend not to be identified until the disease is fairly advanced.[7] The exception is cancer of the vocal cords, where even a very tiny tumor will result in notable hoarseness and thus is likely to be noticed sooner (reviewed in Carroll et al., 1998).

Treatment of Cancers of the Head and Neck

Treatment for most cancers of the head and neck involves radiation, surgery, or a combination, although some chemotherapy is also used (see Appendix C, and Carroll et al., 1998). Treatment is a team effort, involving the head and neck medical oncologist, radiation oncologist, head and neck surgeon, dentist, and other personnel. Surgery to excise cancerous tumors can impair function and appearance. Dental services may be an integral part of treatments to reduce or correct such damage.

Surgery can be especially difficult and risky around the fine structures of the larynx. As a result, clinicians have pressed ahead with the development of chemotherapy (often with radiation) for laryngeal cancers.[8] Anticancer drugs in general work by inhibiting cell division in active tissues, which has the side effect of inhibiting healing and growth in the healthy tissue lining the mouth. The resulting irritation and inflammation of the oral mucosa is called mucositis, which can be treated by both physicians and dentists and is discussed further below.

Radiation therapy is used with surgery for most cancers of the oral cavity and pharynx. Radiation, like chemotherapy, can affect both tumor cells and healthy cells. The damage to healthy tissue depends on the size and number of radiation doses and on the location of the tumor and the therapy. Radiation therapy can be from either an external source or an implant; in some cases, both are necessary (Carroll et al., 1998).

The oral side effects of cancer treatment that result from drugs, radiation, and surgery will often be managed by the physicians or surgeons overseeing treatment. For instance, they may modify the dose of anticancer drugs, take a "break" in the course of radiation therapy, or prescribe therapeutic mouthwashes

---

[7]Less regular care and later detection of cancers may partly explain the difference between black and white subpopulations in overall five-year survival rates for oral cavity and pharyngeal cancer (32 percent and 55 percent, respectively) (reported in Landis et al., 1999). Men are also somewhat less likely than women to have regular dental examinations (CDC, 1997) and tend to have more advanced disease at the time of diagnosis.

[8]Some success with chemotherapy in combination with radiation—and without surgery—has been reported for some cancers of the larynx. Surgical removal of the larynx means loss of normal speaking ability. Chemotherapy has not been shown to be as effective in other head and neck cancer sites as radiation and surgery.

to allow serious mucositis to heal. In any case, such management would generally fall under the scope of practice for a physician and would therefore be covered even if delivered by a dentist. Radiation therapy has additional, and specifically dental, implications that are examined next.

Oral Health Problems Associated with Radiation Treatment of Cancers of the Head and Neck

Because radiation therapy disrupts cell division in healthy tissue as well as in tumor(s), it also affects the function and structure of the oral mucosa (lining of the mouth) and underlying organs and tissues such as salivary glands and bone. If directed at the lymph nodes in the jaw area, radiation may impinge in varying degrees on the salivary glands, which are very sensitive to radiation effects. Radiation can irreversibly damage these glands, resulting in insufficient production of saliva, known technically as xerostomia (dry mouth). Saliva is important to keep the oral tissues moist and to buffer the acidity of the oral environment, which is critical both to reducing bacterial growth and infection and to laying down new mineral deposits that keep the teeth strong and dense. After radiation, the teeth tend to become demineralized (more porous) and to develop cavities easily, a tendency so marked that it has the special name radiation caries.

Radiation for head and neck cancer is also an important contributing factor in less common but very serious adverse consequences to the underlying bone. Especially in high or multiple doses, radiation affects bone by injuring the small vessels that supply blood to the cells in the bone, so that these cells die. The death of bone cells means that remodeling, which occurs continuously in healthy living bone tissue, proceeds very slowly, as does healing, with the result that the bone becomes susceptible to infection. The bone cell death resulting from radiation is called osteoradionecrosis (ORN). In head and neck radiation, the lower jaw or mandible is the most susceptible because it is a very dense bone, having a relatively low proportion of cells and blood supply to start with. ORN can require surgery to excise the dead tissue, which can in turn leave the jaw and face badly disfigured as well as functionally impaired—with serious consequences for the patient's quality of life.

The likelihood of ORN is increased by trauma to the bone, including the trauma to the jawbone caused by a tooth extraction (Murray et al., 1980a,b, reviewed in Appendix C). The effect of such trauma on the risk of ORN is especially marked when the extraction or other trauma occurs near (before or after) the time of the radiation (Epstein et al., 1987, reviewed in Appendix C). This occurs presumably because the radiation damage to blood vessels makes healing a recent extraction wound more difficult.

Dental Care for Patients Undergoing Radiation Therapy for Cancer of the Head and Neck

Thirty years ago, the standard of care for patients with head and neck cancer involved extracting teeth before beginning radiation therapy. HCFA has ruled that this treatment meets the criteria for coverage as an exception to Medicare's general exclusion of dental care, even though extraction is generally carried out as a separate step rather than as an integral part of the radiation therapy. The rationale for covering such extractions was that tooth removal would preclude radiation-related caries and the possible later need for extractions that would increase the risk for ORN.

In the 1970s, however, dentists began to experiment with aggressive tooth-sparing approaches to dental care before, during, and after radiation therapy for head and neck cancer. The new approach to care called for a preradiation program to improve and protect the patient's oral health through an evaluation, careful oral hygiene, fluoride applications, restoration of the teeth that were salvageable, and removal of unrestorable or periodontally diseased teeth with adequate healing time if possible. During and after radiation, this approach called for the patient to continue very thorough oral hygiene and home fluoride treatments. After radiation therapy, the dentist provides further monitoring and restoration as needed (Keys and McCasland, 1976, as reviewed in Appendix C). None of the care involved in this tooth-preserving approach is covered by Medicare unless an extraction occurs prior to radiation, in which case the oral examination may also be covered.

Absent unexpected negative research findings, the role of tooth-preserving therapy should continue to increase. Surveys of the population ages 65 to 74 taken in 1971–1974 and in 1985–1986 show that the percentage of older persons who have lost all their teeth dropped from 45 to 41.1 percent, a trend that has continued (Bloom et al., 1992; Marcus et al., 1996; MMWR, 1999; NIDR, 1987). In recent years, approximately 33 to 43 percent of patients diagnosed with head or neck cancers have already lost all their teeth (Appendix C; Lockhart and Clark, 1994; Niewald et al., 1996, Roos et al., 1996). Of those retaining some teeth, the average patient still possesses only about a third of the full complement of 32 adult teeth, and most have accumulations of plaque and some tooth decay (Lockhart and Clark, 1994; Niewald et al., 1996). The challenge is how best to manage such patients to minimize further dental and medical problems—including loss of additional teeth, bone destruction, surgical treatment, functional impairment, and disfigurement—associated with radiation therapy for patients with head and neck cancer.

Effectiveness of Dental Care in Improving
Health Outcomes for Head and Neck Cancer Patients
Treated with Radiation

No randomized controlled trials have compared the effectiveness of tooth-preserving protocols and protocols that emphasize tooth extraction without preventive care for head and neck cancer patients undergoing radiation therapy. One of the earliest retrospective studies comparing tooth-preserving and aggressive tooth extraction protocols was carried out at Walter Reed Army Medical Center (Keys and McCasland, 1976). It showed that patients in the tooth-preserving protocol lost fewer teeth than their predecessors treated under an aggressive tooth extraction protocol. (Other key patient care procedures, including the radiation techniques and doses, remained stable during the time periods compared.) Patients in the tooth-preserving protocol also required fewer dental visits both before and after radiation therapy (Keys and McCasland, 1976). ORN rates were historically low before and after the change in protocol, so the study did not demonstrate an effect on ORN.

Another retrospective analysis during the same period, however, demonstrated the potential for dental conservation to reduce ORN (Bedwinek et al., 1976). Researchers at M.D. Anderson compared two periods of dental management for patients treated with radiation to the jaws. Among those treated when extractions were the favored treatment, 19.7 percent developed ORN, with the precipitating factors assigned to dental extraction (11.8 percent), denture irritation (2.5 percent), and spontaneous or unknown causes (5.4 percent). During the period that tooth-preserving protocols were in place, 7.9 percent developed ORN, with the precipitating factors assigned to dental extraction (2.3 percent), denture irritation (1.1 percent), and spontaneous or unknown causes (4.5 percent). Other research indicates that the highest incidence of ORN occurs when extractions immediately precede or follow radiation therapy (Epstein et al., 1987).

Studies to identify causes of ORN have repeatedly identified extractions and lack of preventive dental care as major contributing factors (Beumer et al., 1984; Curi and Dib, 1997; Kluth et al., 1988; Murray et al., 1980a,b). As tooth-preserving treatments have become more common and the rate of ORN has dropped, unknown causes of ORN are proportionately more likely to be identified as causes than are extractions.

Evidence from a randomized, placebo-controlled trial suggested that fluoride treatments following radiation were responsible for much of the effectiveness of the tooth-preserving protocols in reducing postradiation caries in patients with xerostomia (Driezen et al., 1977). Patient compliance with daily fluoride application on an indefinite basis is a challenge, just as patient compliance is challenging in other areas; compliance may likewise be increased by contact with clinicians (see Epstein et al., 1995, 1996; see also Chapter 5).

Because ORN is associated with injury to blood vessels and failure to heal, several centers have investigated the use of hyperbaric oxygen (HBO) therapy to prevent ORN resulting from extractions after radiation therapy. HBO, which supplies oxygen at a higher concentration than in normal air, may facilitate healing by promoting blood vessel formation and supporting tissues that are poorly supplied with oxygen. HBO therapy has been used prophylactically to help avoid ORN and to treat patients who have developed ORN. Although the treatment has been reported to be effective, the equipment required is not currently available in many places and is expensive even when available (Marx et al., 1985; Myers and Marx, 1990).

HBO prevention of ORN can be less expensive than treatment of serious ORN, but both are considerably more costly per patient than tooth-preserving dental care and self-care. Although tooth-preserving dental interventions for those with head and neck cancer are not covered by Medicare, HCFA has approved coverage of HBO therapy for osteoradionecrosis (*Coverage Issues Manual,* section 35.10 [HCFA, 1999b]). As noted earlier, the extraction of teeth to prepare the jaw for radiation treatment of neoplastic disease such as head and neck cancer is covered by Medicare. The costs to Medicare of adding coverage for certain tooth-preserving dental services for head and neck cancer patients and the possible offsetting savings are discussed later in this chapter.

LEUKEMIA AND LYMPHOMA

The first parts of this section discuss the general burden of disease and the oral health problems associated with leukemia and lymphoma and the treatment of these cancers. The later parts present a combined discussion of the management of oral health problems associated with these conditions or their treatment.

Leukemia

Burden of Disease

Leukemias are malignancies of the blood cells and blood-forming organs. They account for about 1.7 percent of all cancer cases (ACS, 1999a). Of the four major kinds of leukemia, the incidence of three—chronic lymphocytic leukemia, acute myeloid leukemia, and chronic myeloid leukemia—is higher in those age 65 and over than in those younger than 65 (SEER, 1999).[9] The incidence is only slightly lower for the fourth kind, acute lymphocytic leukemia. All leukemias taken together are predicted to cause 30,200 new cases in 1999. Of these cases, 56.4 percent (or about 17,000) are expected to be diagnosed in patients age 65 or older. The incidence rate in those age 65 or older is 51.4 per 100,000, compared

---

[9]Unless otherwise indicated, all data are from SEER, 1999.

to 5.8 per 100,000 in younger persons. Five-year survival rates also vary by age, 33.9 percent for those age 65 or older and 51.2 percent for younger persons. For specific types of leukemia, five-year survival rates for the older age group are less than 6 percent for the acute leukemias and do not exceed 25 percent for chronic myeloid leukemia. For chronic lymphocytic leukemia, the five-year survival rate is 65.9 percent for those age 65 or older, compared to 78.8 percent for younger persons.

Leukemia is typically diagnosed by blood and bone marrow tests. The lifetime risk of being diagnosed with any leukemia is 1.38 percent for men and 1.06 percent for women, and the lifetime risk of dying from leukemia is 0.94 percent for men and 0.77 percent for women.

Oral Health Problems and Leukemias

Oral symptoms are a common reason for patients to seek care that leads to a diagnosis of leukemia. The majority of those found to have acute or chronic leukemia have such symptoms early in the course of the disease. Symptoms include bleeding or infected gingiva (gums), gingival overgrowth, hemorrhagic points (petechiae) or spots (ecchymoses) resulting from reduced platelet levels (thrombocytopenia), ulcers, and other inflammations. Because those with leukemia often have suppressed immune systems due to the disease (and may become more immunosuppressed as a result of chemotherapy), they are at higher than usual risk of oral and other infections. Septicemia is a major cause of death in leukemia patients (Bodey et al., 1978; Rintala, 1994; as discussed in Appendix C).

Treatment for Leukemias

Medical treatment for acute leukemias typically involves single- or multiple-agent chemotherapy with supportive red blood cell or platelet transfusions to manage the anemia and thrombocytopenia often associated with the disease. Because chronic lymphocytic leukemia often progresses slowly and is not curable with current treatments (which generally have unpleasant side effects), it is often managed conservatively by observation and treatment of associated infections, anemia, hemorrhage due to platelet deficiency, and other complications of the disease. For chronic myeloid leukemia, the only cure is bone marrow transplant, which is generally not recommended for older patients. Chemotherapy, radiation, or biologic therapy may lengthen survival for some patients with this type of leukemia.

Lymphoma

Burden of Disease

Lymphomas are malignancies of the lymph system. One type, Hodgkin's disease, is most common in two age groups—young adults and those over 55 (NCI, 1999a). The incidence of Hodgkin's disease is declining, however, especially among those 65 and over. In 1999, 7,200 new cases of Hodgkin's disease are predicted to cause 7,200 new cases, less than 0.6 percent of all new cancer cases. The disease still accounts for about 1.9 percent of all cancer cases (ACS, 1999a). Of the new cases, only 15 percent (about 1,100) are expected to be diagnosed in patients age 65 or older. The incidence rate in those age 65 or older is 3.6 per 100,000, compared to 2.6 per 100,000 in younger persons (SEER, 1999).[10] Five-year survival rates are 45.3 percent for those age 65 or older and 86.6 percent for younger persons. The lifetime risk of being diagnosed with Hodgkin's disease is 0.24 percent for men and 0.20 percent for women, whereas the lifetime risk of dying from it is 0.06 percent for men and 0.04 percent for women.

Non-Hodgkin's lymphoma, which actually includes nearly 30 types of cancers, presents a very different epidemiological picture. The same data and estimate sources predict 56,800 new cases in 1999, 4.6 percent of all new cancer cases and 3.6 percent of all cancer cases taken together. Of the new cases, 51.6 percent (or 29,300) are expected to be diagnosed in patients age 65 or older. The incidence rate in those age 65 or older is 75.5 per 100,000, compared to 9.2 per 100,000 in younger persons. Five-year survival rates differ less by age, 46.7 percent for those age 65 or older and 54.4 percent for younger persons. The lifetime risk of being diagnosed with non-Hodgkin's lymphoma is 2.08 percent for men and 1.71 percent for women, while the lifetime risk of dying from it is 0.96 percent for men and 0.92 percent for women.

Oral Health Problems and Lymphomas

Lymphoma patients, particularly Hodgkin's disease patients, are at increased risk for infections of all sorts. Non-Hodgkin's lymphoma patients can develop mouth ulcers. As discussed below, other oral problems may follow the treatment of either disease.

Treatment for Lymphomas

Depending on the type of lymphoma, treatment may include radiation, chemotherapy, or both. Early stages of non-Hodgkin's lymphoma may be treatable by radiation alone, but later-stage disease often requires both treatment modalities. Chemotherapy and radiation may be used alone or in combination for

---

[10]Unless otherwise indicated, data are from SEER, 1999.

patients with Hodgkin's disease, depending on the stage and other characteristics of the disease (NCI, 1999a).

Oral Health Problems Related to Treatment for
Leukemia and Lymphoma

In addition to oral symptoms arising from the disease (leukemia or lymphoma) itself, chemotherapeutic treatment (including high-dose chemotherapy with bone marrow transplant) frequently induces oral health problems, in particular, mucositis and stomatitis (an inflammatory condition of the mouth). These problems arise both from immunosuppression, which results from damage to the blood-forming cells in the bone marrow, and from direct drug toxicity to the oral mucosal cells lining the mouth.

Severe mucositis and stomatitis can involve extensive ulceration, intense pain, and disfiguring destruction of tissue. These problems may interfere sufficiently with chewing or swallowing to cause malnutrition or dehydration. In addition, while patients are severely immunosuppressed from chemotherapy, they may experience acute exacerbations of asymptomatic periodontal disease (Overholser et al., 1982). In general, the more extensive the chemotherapy, the more serious and widespread these adverse oral conditions are likely to be. For some patients, adjustment of the chemotherapy regimen (types and amounts of drugs) may reduce the severity of mucositis or stomatitis.

When patients with lymphoma are treated with radiation that includes the jaw area (where many lymph nodes are located), these patients—like those with head and neck cancer—may suffer injury to the salivary glands and resulting xerostomia. Xerostomia, as described earlier, promotes infection, demineralization of the teeth, and dental caries. Systemic infection is also a threat when patients have preexisting oral infections and when oral tissue damaged by chemotherapy becomes secondarily infected. Researchers have documented oral lesions colonized by one or more types of organisms in 34 percent of patients undergoing chemotherapy for leukemia (Dreizen et al., 1986). One cohort study that tracked bacteremia (presence of viable bacteria in the circulating blood) and bacterial cultures from saliva in high-dose chemotherapy patients suggests that the oral mucosa likely was the point of entry for the infecting organism but could not demonstrate that oral sources were exclusively responsible (Richard et al., 1995). Research also suggests that acute oral infections may contribute to fevers and septicemia in these immunocompromised patients, but the specific contribution of oral organisms remains unclear (Bergmann, 1988, 1989; Greenberg, 1990; Greenberg et al., 1982). Older age, type of cancer, and oral health status prior to chemotherapy have been identified as risk factors for the subsequent development of chemotherapy complications (Sonis and Clark, 1991).

Dental Care for Patients with Leukemia or Lymphoma

As described in Appendix C, the standard evaluation for patients diagnosed with leukemia or lymphoma includes a careful oral examination and full-mouth radiographs to identify both existing infection and potential sources of infection. In addition to cleaning of the teeth, indicated periodontal or extraction procedures, and instruction in oral hygiene, mouth rinses may be prescribed to prevent or control microorganisms associated with oral infection and reduce the probability and severity of mucositis and stomatitis and systemic infection. Other patient management goals for leukemia and lymphoma patients are to relieve symptoms and encourage adequate nutrition and hydration. Topical anesthetics, saline rinses, and other strategies, which may be prescribed by both physicians and dentists, may provide some relief of symptoms.

Because bacteria in the mouth may enter the bloodstream through oral ulcers and areas of mouth tissue breakdown, the goals of dental care for patients who have developed treatment-related stomatitis or mucositis include reducing the level of organisms in the mouth and preventing any breach of its epithelial lining that provides an avenue for infection. Histopathological or microbiological analysis to identify the infectious organisms involved may be useful in guiding antimicrobial therapy (Dreizen et al., 1983; Ostchega, 1980; Schimpff 1990).

Effectiveness of Dental Care in Improving Health Outcomes for Leukemia and Lymphoma Patients

No large, multicenter, randomized clinical trials have assessed the effectiveness of dental interventions to prevent or manage oral or systemic complications of chemotherapy for leukemia or lymphoma patients. A few controlled studies suggest that dental care (examination, periodontal treatment, and extractions for unrestorable teeth) for leukemia patients prior to chemotherapy may prevent or reduce subsequent episodes of septicemia and prevent or reduce the severity of common oral complications of chemotherapy that are associated with the prior burden of oral disease (Borowski, 1994; Levy-Polack et al., 1996; Peterson, 1982, 1990). Unfortunately, these studies involve few elderly patients.

A recent study with no control group that tested the effect of not treating chronic dental disease prior to chemotherapy concluded that treatment for chronic problems could be safely postponed with little effect on the subsequent risk of acute dental disease (Toljanic et al., 1999). It also concluded that a prechemotherapy oral examination was still needed to identify acute dental disease for treatment to prevent local exacerbations or systemic spread of infection

These few studies of prechemotherapy dental treatment have involved mostly or entirely leukemia patients, who tend to receive aggressive, combination chemotherapy that is associated with more severe immunosuppression. Additional studies would be needed to determine the effects of prechemotherapy dental treatment on lymphoma (and other cancer) patients.

For prevention and treatment of oral infections, research has produced inconsistent findings about the effectiveness of different mouth rinses, notably chlorhexidine (a standard broad-spectrum antimicrobial that can bind to oral surface tissue but is not readily absorbed in the gastrointestinal tract) (e.g., see Epstein et al., 1992; Ferretti et al., 1988; Wahlin, 1989; Weisdorf et al., 1989; as discussed in Appendix C). Some other prescription drugs have also been studied for their effectiveness in the management of specific oral infections, but the committee did not further review prescription rinses and other outpatient drugs that are not now covered by Medicare.

SOLID ORGAN TRANSPLANTS

Burden of Disease

As briefly reviewed in Chapter 4 and Appendix D, many medical conditions can lead to the failure of major organs including the kidney, heart, liver and lung, and thus to consideration for transplantation. Immunosuppressive drugs are essential to reduce the chance of graft rejection in transplant recipients. Renal failure accounts for the great majority of transplants among Medicare beneficiaries.[11] Many younger patients receiving other kinds of transplants qualify for Medicare at some point before or after the transplant due to disability. As described further in Chapter 5, more than 20,000 solid organ transplantations were performed in the United States in 1998 (UNOS, 1999a). According to regional data from 1997, more than 12,000 kidney transplants and several hundred heart and liver transplants were performed in Medicare-eligible patients age 65 and over (UNOS, 1999a; see Table 5 of Appendix C).

Oral Health Problems and Organ Transplantation

The primary oral health issues for recipients of solid organ transplants are related to the drug therapy they must take to control graft rejection. This immunosuppressive therapy limits their ability to fight infections. Posttransplant infections can lead to very serious consequences including hospitalization, loss of the grafted organ, return to dialysis, retransplantation, or death. Thus, as people are evaluated before, during, and after transplantation, a central goal is to identify and eliminate existing infections and obvious potential sources of infection. These include infections associated with the mouth, although there is no direct evidence of serious infections linked specifically to oral sources (see Appendix

---

[11]Since the end-stage renal disease (ESRD) provisions of Medicare define ESRD patients as a category of beneficiaries, ESRD patients covered by Medicare may be of any age.

C). Some transplant centers will not operate on a patient with an active oral infection.

People with suppressed immunological function are vulnerable to several kinds of bacterial, viral, and fungal infectious agents that may be harbored in the mouth and elsewhere in the body. Many organisms that do not normally create problems in healthy people are a threat to those with suppressed immune systems. For example, a transient, typically asymptomatic bacteremia often occurs following various dental treatments, especially those involving the gums. This condition is of no concern in the patient with a fully functioning immune system but may be dangerous in the severely immunosuppressed transplant recipient.

Cytomegalovirus (CMV) and herpes simplex virus (HSV) are common in humans (found in 40–80 percent of adults who are asymptomatic), and most transplant patients test positive for CMV (Berry et al., 1988; Rubin and Tolkoff-Rubin, 1988; reviewed in Appendix C). In transplant patients the viruses are frequently found in oral ulcers during the six months immediately following surgery, but they may occur elsewhere along the gastrointestinal tract.

Some of the immunosuppressive drugs so necessary to the transplant recipient have the unfortunate side effect of gingival overgrowth. Gingival overgrowth, a condition of gum enlargement, makes removal of bacteria through brushing and flossing of teeth more difficult. It can also be disfiguring and can interfere with eating and maintenance of adequate nutrition. CMV has been found in areas of gingival overgrowth.

In addition to the risks associated with posttransplant immunosuppressive therapy, certain common causes of organ failure (or their treatment) may put people at higher risk of oral problems. Diabetes is a common cause of renal failure and is associated with periodontal disease in its own right, and untreated oral disease may complicate effective diabetic management (Grossi and Genco, 1998). Hypertension is another common cause of organ failure, and its treatment with certain calcium channel blockers is associated with gingival overgrowth (in addition to any overgrowth caused by certain immunosuppressants).

The overall rate of periodontal disease, caries, and abscesses is not documented specifically for transplant candidates, but it is reasonable to expect that these conditions are at least as common in these populations as in adults generally. In the most recent National Health and Nutrition Examination Survey, approximately 20–30 percent of older adults were found to have moderate periodontal disease (which would not necessarily indicate active disease that poses a risk of self-infection), and serious disease was found in approximately 5 percent (with higher percentages for men and lower for women) (Albandar and Kingman, 1999). Although some studies have linked posttransplant infections to organisms ubiquitous in the oral cavity (e.g., lactobacillus, as well as several fungi) (Suresh et al., 1996; reviewed in Appendix C), the rate of posttransplant infection associated with oral sources specifically is not documented. Similarly, the extent to which oral problems associated with diabetes or the use of certain calcium channel blockers contributes to poor outcomes for transplant patients is not known.

Dental Care for Patients Before or After
Organ Transplantation

As noted above, the standard of care for transplant candidates includes the prevention and elimination of oral infection. Such care involves an oral examination that includes visual and tactile inspection of the mouth and is usually accompanied by x-rays. An oral examination also typically includes instruction in personal oral hygiene (brushing, flossing, use of antiseptic mouth rinses) intended to help patients avoid posttransplant gingivitis and other oral problems. At least one controlled study has found less gingivitis, plaque, or gingival overgrowth in transplant patients who received hygiene instruction compared to those who did not (Somacarrera et al., 1996; reviewed in Appendix C).

Dental prophylaxis (not currently covered by Medicare for any patient group) removes plaque, a tenacious film of germs that adheres to the teeth, and calculus (tartar) that can build up to cause periodontal disease. When periodontal disease is diagnosed, treatment—which can be limited or quite extensive—removes hardened plaque, calculus, and infected tissue under the gum and smoothes the root surfaces of teeth so that damaged tissue can heal and reattach to the teeth. If damage to teeth or gums is serious enough, teeth may have to be extracted. If the base of the tooth root is infected, a root canal may be performed.

As noted earlier, HCFA has ruled that an inpatient oral examination prior to renal transplant is covered but the ruling does not mention beneficiaries receiving other kinds of transplants. Some carriers, however, provide for such coverage in their local medical policies. Dental care prescribed following an oral examination is not covered. In addition to services normally provided by dentists, both dentists and physicians may manage oral infections with drugs. These drugs are not covered by Medicare if provided on an outpatient basis.

Effectiveness of Dental Care in Improving
Health Outcomes for Organ Transplant Recipients

As described in Appendix C, no direct evidence is available regarding the effect on survival of prevention, early detection, or treatment of oral health problems in transplant patients. As noted above, people with oral infections may be ruled out for transplants at some transplant centers, but the committee found no research comparing patient outcomes in centers with and without this policy. It also found no studies comparing transplant patients who had received periodic oral prophylactic services with those who had not. For those with identified oral infections, no trials have compared different treatment strategies. One controlled study, as mentioned above, did suggest that oral hygiene instruction reduced subsequent oral problems, but the study did not examine more important outcomes such as acute or chronic graft rejection.

More generally, controlled studies have not evaluated the overall strategy of identifying and eliminating infection prior to transplantation. The approach is based on biological principles, experience, and concern about the significant mortality and morbidity risks that infection poses to transplant recipients taking immunosuppressive drugs.

HEART VALVE REPAIR OR REPLACEMENT

Burden of Disease

Heart valve disease may arise congenitally or develop later in life. The diseased valve is functionally impaired so that it cannot open properly, close sharply, or both. This causes irregularities in blood flow through the heart, which are often first heard with a stethoscope. Some valve disease can be treated with medication, but other cases require surgical repair or even replacement with synthetic or transplanted tissue.

Those with valve disease are at risk of endocarditis, a serious and often fatal inflammation of the tissue lining the chambers of the heart. Any sort of uneven or rough surface, which may be present with a diseased, abnormal, repaired, or replaced valve, creates a niche where bacteria can lodge and multiply to cause endocarditis. Such infections can be difficult and costly to treat. Those at high or moderate risk of endocarditis include people with a prosthetic heart valve or past episodes of endocarditis and those with certain other cardiac problems including a number of congenital cardiac conditions (AHA, 1999). Although mitral valve prolapse has frequently been cited as a risk factor, only those meeting certain criteria (e.g., mitral regurgitation demonstrated by Doppler examination) appear to be at higher-than-normal risk for endocarditis.

Data on the incidence and prevalence of heart conditions are less extensive than data for common cancers. Population-based studies in limited geographic areas in the United States have reported an overall incidence of 1.7 to 4.0 cases per 100,000 (Berlin et al., 1995). According to Medicare records, the number of Medicare-paid hospital stays involving heart valve disease has been increasing (from 42,700 in 1990 to 58,800 in 1995), and the number of stays for which endocarditis was specifically reported has also increased (from 3,900 in 1990 to 4,950 in 1995) (HCFA data discussed in Appendix C). The American Heart Association (AHA, 1999) reported more than 16,000 hospital discharges for bacterial endocarditis in all age groups in 1995. In 1996, valvular heart disease was listed as the cause of death in more than 17,000 cases in the population overall and was mentioned as a factor in almost 36,000. In 1995, the latest year for which information was available, bacterial endocarditis was specified in 2,100 reports of death in the population overall (AHA, 1999). Among other heart conditions, diseases of the arteries and congestive heart failure each accounted for more than 43,000 deaths in 1995.

Many studies of risk factors and other aspects of endocarditis are based on data from major medical centers that treat many patients referred from other communities. A study undertaken by investigators at the Mayo Clinic that compared incidence cases for Olmstead County, Minnesota, with referral cases seen at the clinic reported that age was a much more significant factor in the community cohort than in the hospital cohort. For the former, the incidence rate was nearly 9 times higher for those age 65 and over than for younger age groups (Steckelberg et al., 1990). The population-based incidence rate for those age 70–79 was 18 per 100,000; it was 40 per 100,000 for those age 80 or older.

Oral Health Problems and Heart Valve Disease

The oral cavity in general, and common oral infections in particular, can provide sources of organisms that may lead to heart valve infection, which in turn can lead to endocarditis. Clinicians have observed an association between oral disease and endocarditis, and Appendix C describes a causal model offering a possible explanation (after Drangsholt, 1998).

The oral cavity harbors a lot of bacteria, most commonly in the form of plaque, but also associated with gingivitis, periodontitis, and periapical disease (infection around the base of the tooth root). Oral flora, particularly streptococcus, are implicated in approximately 40 percent of cases of infective endocarditis (Roberts, 1999; Strom et al., 1998; van der Meer et al., 1992a). Bacteremia can arise from dental procedures but also from such routine activities as tooth brushing and chewing, especially if extensive oral infection and inflammation are present. Patients with dentures may develop bacteremias associated with poorly fitting dentures.

Although dental procedures for hygiene, restoration, or extraction of diseased teeth can cause breaks in the epithelium lining the mouth that allow bacteria to spill into the bloodstream causing bacteremia, most cases of orally related endocarditis are not attributed to dental procedures (Bonow et al., 1998; Pallasch and Slots, 1996). The burden of oral disease of itself is a concern for the patient at high risk of endocarditis (Strom, 1998; van der Meer, 1992b).

Dental Care for Patients Undergoing Surgery for Heart Valve Disease

Standard clinical practice is to eliminate as many potential sources of oral infection as possible before a patient undergoes a surgical procedure to repair or replace a defective heart valve. This typically involves an oral examination and x-rays, thorough cleaning, and treatment for any gingival, periodontal, or periapical disease identified. None of these services are covered by Medicare. Standard practice also includes prophylactic use of antibiotics prior to bacteremia-producing dental procedures (Bonow et al., 1998).

Effectiveness of Dental Care in Promoting Better Health Outcomes for Patients with Heart Valve Disease

The committee and the authors of the background paper were unable to locate any published controlled studies on the effectiveness of dental care prior to heart valve repair or replacement. Further, they found no such studies documenting the effectiveness of antibiotic prophylaxis during dental or other bacteremia-inducing procedures involving people at risk of endocarditis. A randomized controlled trial, especially one assessing treatment and outcomes in elderly patients, would be difficult to organize in part because the main outcome of concern—infective endocarditis—is relatively uncommon. Less rigorous comparative studies might be possible for some topics, for example, the value of a preoperative dental examination before cardiac surgery.

The committee and the background paper authors managed to find one 1997 paper describing the dental health of 156 patients with valve disease requiring a prosthetic valve implant (Terezhalmy et al., 1997). Nearly all of the patients had some level of significant periodontal disease, suggesting that they would be at increased risk if untreated prior to surgery. This study did not include a comparison group and provided no information on the patients regarding either their dental care prior to surgery or the prevalence of endocarditis subsequent to surgery.

Bacteremia can cause local pockets of infection wherever the bacteria get caught and accumulate—for example, on the irregular surface of a diseased or surgically repaired heart valve. One case control study found that patients who have undergone valve surgery or have other valve abnormalities remain indefinitely at increased risk of endocarditis (Drangsholt, 1998).

In summary, the committee was unable to find any published clinical trial data bearing on whether dental care prior to heart valve repair or replacement affects the outcome of valve surgery. The explanatory model addressing the observed association between oral disease and endocarditis is intellectually attractive but not supported by direct evidence at this time.

ESTIMATED COSTS TO MEDICARE OF EXTENDING COVERAGE

The committee considered the likely costs of extending limited Medicare coverage for dental services provided in conjunction with surgery, chemotherapy, radiation, or pharmacological treatment for beneficiaries with the serious medical conditions reviewed above. Box 4-1 summarizes the assumptions and data on which the estimates are based. As explained in Chapter 2, the cost estimation approach follows the generic practices (e.g., not discounting estimates to present value) used by the Congressional Budget Office (CBO) in making estimates for Congress. A more detailed presentation of the committee's cost estimates and the associated assumptions and data sources appears in Appendix E, which was prepared in consultation with the committee and background paper authors.

BOX 4-1 Summary of Estimated Costs to Medicare for "Medically Necessary Dental Care" Associated with Certain Medical Conditions

Coverage Model Assumptions

• The demand for the dental services will be determined by the number of Medicare-eligible patients who have the medical condition in question (with no significant induced demand).
• Services are provided only during the year of the medical procedure.
• Each condition calls for similar dental services (oral examination and x-rays; dental cleaning, scaling, or root planing; restoration or extraction of teeth; treatment of soft-tissue disease).

Cost Estimate Assumptions for Years 2000–2004 (see also Appendix E)

• Cost per visit is assumed the same for all patients and data from 1987 are adjusted for inflation through 2000–2004 using the dental services Consumer Price Index (CPI).
• Cost per visit is reduced by 20% for the Medicare Part B copayment and then by 30% for an assumed Medicare "discount" from provider charges.
• Average visits per patient were estimated by committee members and consultants and, except for head and neck cancer patients, include only patients with teeth.

Medical Condition	Dentate (patient still has teeth)		Edentulous (patient has no teeth)	
	Average No. of Visits	% Medicare Population	Average No. of Visits	% Medicare Population
Head and neck cancer	2	65	1	35
Leukemia	2	65	0	35
Lymphoma	2	65	0	35
Organ transplant	2	80	0	20
Heart valve	2	65	0	35

Continued

BOX 4-1 *Continued*

Cost Estimate Assumptions for Years 2000–2004 (*continued*)

• Spending offsets occur only for head and neck cancer from reduced ORN treatment costs.
• Net costs are total estimated gross costs offset by 25% to reflect premium increase borne by Medicare beneficiaries as a result of increased Part B expenditures.

Data Sources

• Cost per visit is from National Medical Expenditure Survey 1987(before adjustment).
• Inflation adjustment is from CPI, dental.
• Expected prevalence of the cancers is from SEER and Medicare data. Expected prevalence of transplants was from UNOS. Expected prevalence of heart valve disease is from Medicare data on relevant diagnosis-related groups.

Estimated Costs (in millions) to MEDICARE, 2000–2004

Medical Condition	Costs
Head and neck cancer	$18.6
Leukemia	20.9
Lymphoma	32.3
Organ transplant	24.2
Heart valve	117.5
Total gross cost to Medicare	213.3
Head and neck cancer savings offset	−5.6
25% Medicare premium offset	−51.9
Net cost to Medicare	155.8

The committee's estimates of Medicare costs are based on a series of assumptions, some of which have supporting evidence or data but others of which are best guesses based on committee judgment in the absence of such information. The estimates are intended to suggest the order of magnitude of the costs to Medicare of extending coverage, but they could considerably higher or lower than what Medicare might actually spend were coverage policies changed. The tables in Appendix E allow readers to vary some of the committee's assumptions and calculate alternative estimates

The total net cost to Medicare of covering services for the five conditions examined for the five-year period from 2000 to 2004 is estimated to be $155.8

million. This estimate takes into account $5.6 in offsetting savings from reduced medical care costs and $51.9 million in offsets related to increases in the Medicare premium that would result from increased Medicare spending for the elderly.

The main procedures likely to be needed by patients with the five medical conditions are similar: examination and diagnostic radiographs; restorations where possible; extractions where restoration is not an option; and treatment of periodontal, gingival, and periapical disease. The overall cost per patient is driven primarily by the number of visits that each patient would be likely to need. The average number of dental visits per patient is based on the judgment of committee members and background paper authors. Except for head and neck cancer patients undergoing radiation therapy, visits were assumed only for patients with teeth. Head and neck cancer patients are typically examined to identify any retained tooth roots, impacted teeth not detected by visual inspection, and any residual bone pathology warranting treatment prior to radiation therapy. The proportion of older people with no teeth appears to have been declining (Bloom et al., 1992; Marcus et al., 1996; MMWR, 1999) and could reach lower levels for the period 2000–2004. This would mean more dental examinations and higher costs.

The number of Medicare beneficiaries likely to experience one of the conditions mentioned was estimated using Medicare or Surveillance Epidemiology and End-Results (SEER) incidence data for the conditions applied separately to the aged and disabled Medicare Part B beneficiaries. The cost estimates assume coverage only for the year of the transplant procedure or other surgery, radiation therapy, or chemotherapy, although some patients (e.g., transplant recipients taking immunosuppressive drugs) will be at risk indefinitely. Longer periods of coverage would raise the estimates.

Payments were calculated on a per-visit basis, based on 1987 data from the National Medical Expenditure Survey. Figures were adjusted to reflect the increased intensity of service likely for the treatment population compared to the general population. The figures were also adjusted for inflation since 1987 and for expected Medicare discounts, copayments, and Medicare premium offsets (see Appendix E). The cost per visit was then multiplied by the expected average number of visits per patient.

Based on the research described earlier in this chapter and in Appendix C, offsetting savings due to the dental services (as opposed to increases in Medicare premiums) were applied only for head and neck cancer. As discussed in Appendix E, previous HCFA and CBO estimates of the cost to Medicare of extending coverage of medically necessary dental treatments have included a broader range of conditions and services than the committee's estimates.

STATEMENTS OF OTHERS ON "MEDICALLY NECESSARY DENTAL SERVICES"

The U.S. Preventive Services Task Force did not examine the narrowly focused kinds of services examined in this chapter. It has examined counseling to prevent dental and periodontal disease and stated that "counseling patients to visit a dental care provider on a regular basis, floss daily, brush their teeth daily with a fluoride containing toothpaste, and appropriately use fluoride for caries prevention and chemotherapeutic mouth rinses for plaque prevention is recommended based on evidence for risk reduction from these interventions" (USPSTF, 1996, p. 711).[12] It also stated that "while examining the oral cavity, clinicians should be alert for obvious signs of oral disease" (p. 711), but it concluded that there was "insufficient evidence to recommend for or against routine screening of asymptomatic persons for oral cancer by primary care clinicians." (p. 175).

The House of Delegates of the American Dental Association (ADA) has defined "medically necessary dental care" to include care to control or eliminate infection, pain, and disease and has resolved that the ADA "make every effort on behalf of patients to see that the language specifying treatment coverage in health plans be clarified so that medical necessary adjunctive care, essential to the successful treatment of a medical condition being treated by a multidisciplinary health care team, is available to the patient" (Conway, 1995, p. 188). The ADA endorsed the AHA recommendations related to endocarditis (see below). It also recommended more research on specific heart conditions and dental procedures, following the publication of a recent study in *Annals of Internal Medicine* (Strom et al., 1998) that concluded that dental treatment did not appear linked to infective endocarditis and that antibiotic prophylaxis should be reconsidered. An accompanying editorial encouraged the AHA, the Infectious Diseases Society of America, and others to rise to the challenge of crafting appropriate new recommendations (Durack, 1998).

To prevent bacterial endocarditis, the American Heart Association has recommended prophylactic regimens for high- and moderate-risk patients undergoing dental, oral, respiratory tract, or esophageal procedures (Bonow et al., 1998). The recommendations related to dental practice were, as noted above, endorsed by the ADA's Council on Scientific Affairs. The recommendations were based on retrospective studies, animal studies, and in vitro susceptibility data. The AHA noted, however, that no randomized and carefully controlled human trials had established the effectiveness of antibiotic prophylaxis in protecting against endo-

---

[12]For a population with additional health problems who would presumably be more motivated, counseling about dental hygiene would be presumed to be equally or more effective. For example, interviews with 60 liver transplant patients transplanted between 1992 and 1996 found that 75 percent reported having sought a yearly dental examination, one of the higher levels of preventive behavior reported (Zeldin et al., 1998).

carditis in patients with underlying structural heart disease. It also noted that most cases of endocarditis are not attributed to invasive procedures.

In addition to recommendations relating to antibiotic prophylaxis, the AHA has recommended that those at risk for bacterial endocarditis should establish and maintain the best possible oral health to reduce the potential for bacteremia. They should seek regular professional care and undertake thorough self-care, including brushing of teeth, use of dental floss, and other plaque-removal techniques. For patients undergoing cardiac surgery (e.g., heart valve repair), the AHA recommended a careful preoperative evaluation and the completion of required dental treatment before cardiac surgery whenever possible to reduce the potential for late postoperative endocarditis.

The American Society of Transplantation (formerly the American Society of Transplant Physicians) developed guidelines for evaluating renal transplant candidates. These include recommendations to identify and treat overt infections and assess patients for possible occult infections including dental caries (Kasiske et al., 1995).

The National Institutes of Health held a Consensus Development Conference on Oral Complications of Cancer Therapies: Diagnosis, Prevention, and Treatment in 1989 (NIH, 1989). Conclusions included that (1) all cancer patients should have an oral examination before initiation of cancer therapy; (2) treatment of preexisting oral disease is essential to minimize oral complications in all cancer patients; (3) prophylactic acyclovir is beneficial in selected patients to prevent HIV reactivation. (4) precise diagnosis of mucosal lesions and specific treatment of fungal, viral, and bacterial infections are essential; (5) mucosal ulcerations should alert the cancer team to the risk of systemic infection; (6) the best current treatments for chronic xerostomia include fluorides, attention to oral hygiene, and sialagogues (agents that promote the production of saliva); (7) osteoradionecrosis can be prevented and, when present, is best managed with hyperbaric oxygen alone or with surgery; and (8) in the pediatric population, it is important to recognize the long-term consequences of radiation therapy, which include dental and developmental abnormalities and secondary malignancies. Given the limited research base, the conference also recommended that studies of oral complications be incorporated into ongoing and future cooperative clinical oncology group protocols.

In 1999, the National Institute of Dental and Craniofacial Research (NIDCR), one of the National Institutes of Health, launched a health awareness campaign: Oral Health, Cancer Care, and You: Fitting the Pieces Together. Partners in this campaign include the National Institute of Nursing Research (NINR), the Centers for Disease Control and Prevention (CDC), the National Cancer Institute (NCI), and the Friends of the NIDCR. Materials are available through the National Oral Health Information Clearinghouse, an information dissemination service of NIDCR. The campaign promotes medically necessary oral care prior to, during, and after cancer treatment to prevent or reduce the incidence and severity of oral complications, enhancing both patient survival and quality of life (NIDCR, 1999).

COMMITTEE FINDINGS AND CONCLUSIONS

The committee utilized the extensive review of literature provided by the panel of background paper authors, four experts in dental research. The committee also benefited from a two-day public workshop featuring many guest speakers and attended by members of the public with expertise in dental research and hospital-based dental practice (see Appendix A). Unfortunately, little systematic research is available to assess the prevention and management of the oral–medical problems examined in this chapter.[13] Standards of practice for these problems have been developed, often on the basis of plausible biological reasoning but without much evidence from well-controlled clinical trials. The committee's findings, as discussed in this chapter, are summarized briefly below. Its conclusions about Medicare coverage follow.

Findings

Cancers of the Head and Neck

Disease Burden. The committee found that cancers of the head and neck are relatively common, accounting for approximately 3.3 percent of the total estimated new cancers for 1999 and about 4 percent of overall cancer prevalence. Of the estimated 40,000 new cases reported each year, almost half are diagnosed in patients age 65 or older. Treatment is associated with serious oral health risks including damage to the salivary glands, radiation-related caries, and osteoradionecrosis.

Dental Care Effectiveness. The committee found that standard clinical practice for head and neck cancer patients anticipating radiation to the jaw includes reliable identification of active and potential oral health problems for which effective management exists. Evidence is limited but supports the effectiveness of tooth-preserving regimens—especially the role of topical fluoride applications—for head and neck cancer patients prior to and after radiation therapy. Evidence suggests the tooth-preserving approach (not covered by Medicare) is associated with lower rates of ORN and, thus, overall better patient outcomes than the older strategy that emphasized tooth extractions (covered by Medicare).

---

[13]An earlier IOM report found a relatively weak base of systematic oral health research, including in university settings that are strong contributors to medical research (IOM, 1995a).

Benefits Versus Harms.   The committee found evidence suggesting that tooth-preserving therapies are preferable to full mouth extraction not only in limiting ORN but also in avoiding some of the functional and quality of life problems associated with tooth loss. Not all patients, however, are able to adhere to the rigorous hygiene and fluoride treatment programs required by this strategy. To the extent that such patients can be identified prior to therapy, these individuals may benefit more from full mouth extraction to avoid the greater risk of extractions after radiation. Both classes of patients, however, benefit from oral examination and assessment. The committee found no types of patients that would be more likely to suffer harm from oral examination and appropriate treatment compared to no oral care.

Leukemia

Disease Burden.   The committee found that leukemia is a relatively common form of cancer, with approximately 30,000 new cases reported annually. The incidence rate in the population age 65 or older is much greater than that in the under age 65 group, and survival rates are lower than for younger people. Leukemia patients, who are often immunosuppressed from their disease, are especially susceptible to septicemia, which is a leading cause of death. Oral health problems are common from both the disease and its treatment. Chemotherapy can cause mucositis, which can lead to serious secondary and systemic infections. Another treatment, bone marrow transplantation, also can result in oral health problems such as xerostomia, oral lesions, and oral infections, which may contribute to systemic infection.

Dental Care Effectiveness.   The committee found that standard clinical practice includes reliable identification of active and potential oral health problems for which effective dental and medical management exists. The committee found clinical experience to be suggestive that dental cleaning and restoration or extraction services are effective in reducing oral infection in leukemia patients as in other patients. Limited direct evidence from small studies suggests that dental treatments for leukemia patients prior to chemotherapy that is focused on the elimination of acute oral infection and prevention of bacteremia may (a) prevent or reduce subsequent episodes of septicemia and (b) prevent or reduce the severity of the common oral complications of chemotherapy associated with a prior burden of oral disease.

Benefits Versus Harms.   In addition to the scarcity of direct evidence about the systemic benefits of dental treatment, patient perspectives on possible benefits and harms of dental treatments related to the overall management of leukemia have not been explicitly assessed. To the extent that dental care helps to eliminate oral sources of infection and reduce patient discomfort and dysfunction, the committee finds it biologically plausible that dental care promotes a better overall health outcome. An experienced oncologist is in the best position to judge whether a particular leukemia patient should be referred to a dentist for further examination and treatment, taking into account the risk of any delay in the initiation of chemotherapy.

Lymphoma

Disease Burden. Lymphoma is more common than cancers of the head and neck or leukemia, with approximately 64,000 new cases of lymphoma reported in a year, approximately 57,000 of which are non-Hodgkin's lymphoma. The incidence rate in the population age 65 or older is almost eight times higher for non-Hodgkin's lymphoma and is somewhat higher for Hodgkin's disease, compared to the population under age 65. Survival rates are lower in older people. Both non-Hodgkin's lymphoma and Hodgkin's disease are treated with radiation and often chemotherapy as well (especially Hodgkin's disease), so the treatment can result in increased oral health problems such as mucositis and dental caries due to xerostomia.

Dental Care Effectiveness. The committee found that standard clinical practice includes reliable identification of active and potential oral health problems for which effective dental and medical management exists. The committee located no published clinical trials providing direct evidence that dental care improves health outcomes of treatment for non-Hodgkin's lymphoma or Hodgkin's disease or prevents or reduces the severity of treatment-related oral problems. The committee found clinical experience to be suggestive that reduction of oral sources of infection by extraction of abscessed teeth and periodontal cleaning prior to chemotherapy may prevent some septicemias in patients with non-Hodgkin's lymphoma or Hodgkin's disease.

Benefits Versus Harms. In addition to the lack of direct evidence about health benefits, patient perspectives on possible benefits and harms of dental treatments related to the overall management of lymphoma patients have not been explicitly assessed. To the extent that dental care helps to reduce oral infection and patient discomfort, the committee finds it biologically plausible that dental care promotes a better overall health outcome.

Organ Transplantation

Disease Burden. The committee found that organ transplants occur less frequently than the cancers mentioned earlier, but they have become much more common in the last 15 years, with about 20,000 organ transplants performed in the United States annually. All organ transplant recipients require some level of immunosuppressive therapy, especially at the time of and just after the transplant operation, and they are therefore more susceptible to infection. The committee found no data, however, documenting infections from specifically oral sources in immunosuppressed transplant patients. Regarding the treatment following a transplant, the committee noted that gingival overgrowth is a well-known adverse effect of some immunosuppressive drugs, although it is less severe with newer products and must be managed by a physician or dentist along with other adverse drug effects.

Dental Care Effectiveness.   The committee found that the standard clinical practice of preparing a patient to receive a transplant includes reliable identification of active and potential oral health problems for which effective dental and medical treatments exist. The committee located no published clinical trials providing direct evidence that dental care improves health outcomes for transplant recipients. Clinical experience suggests that dental cleaning and restoration or extraction services are effective in reducing oral infection in transplant candidates, as in other patients. In general, however, controlled studies have not evaluated the overall strategy of identifying and eliminating infection prior to transplantation. The approach is based on biological principles and experience.

Benefits Versus Harms.   In addition to lack of direct evidence of systemic benefits, patient perspectives on possible benefits and harms of dental treatments related to the overall management of transplant surgery and maintenance have not been explicitly assessed. To the extent that it helps to reduce oral infection, the committee finds it biologically plausible that dental care promotes a better overall health outcome.

Heart Valve Repair and Replacement

Disease Burden.   The committee found that the number of hospital stays involving heart disease paid for by Medicare has been increasing and had reached 58,800 by 1995. Endocarditis was specifically reported in 4,950 of these cases. The committee found that valvular disease causes a substantial disease burden in the Medicare population and that endocarditis, although relatively uncommon, is associated with significant mortality and morbidity. Clinicians have observed an association between oral disease (gingivitis, periodontitis, periapical disease) and endocarditis.

Dental Care Effectiveness.   The committee found that the standard clinical practice for preparing a patient for valve surgery includes reliable identification of active and potential oral health problems for which dental and medical treatments exist. Clinical experience is suggestive that cleaning and restoration or extraction services are effective in reducing infection in patients preparing to undergo valve surgery, as in other patients. The committee located no published clinical trials providing evidence that dental care improves the overall health outcome of patients undergoing valve surgery.

In addition, the committee found no controlled studies demonstrating that dental procedures increase the incidence of endocarditis by introducing oral bacteria into the bloodstream, although the committee did find the model to be biologically plausible. Poor oral health may, however, produce bacteremia in the course of routine activities such as tooth brushing or chewing.

Benefits Versus Harms.   In addition to the lack of direct evidence of systemic benefit or harm, patient perspectives on possible benefits and harms of dental treatments related to the overall management of patients undergoing valve surgery have not been explicitly assessed. To the extent that dental care helps to reduce oral infection, the committee finds it biologically plausible that dental care promotes a better overall health outcome.

Possible Directions for Future Research

The committee identified several areas in which further research would be helpful, although it did not attempt to set priorities. In general, it was disappointed to find so little evidence documenting the effectiveness of accepted clinical practices in the oral health care of patients with leukemias, lymphomas, cardiac valvular disease planned for valve replacement or repair, and organ transplants. Lack of evidence is not itself evidence that the current standards of care are inappropriate, but it does point to the desirability of studies that could help assess the benefits and harms of that care. [14]

Widespread acceptance of such standards, coupled with the biological plausibility of the clinical protocols for identifying and eliminating infections, may however make controlled studies difficult to design and carry out. Nonetheless, the recent retrospective case-control study of antibiotic prophylaxis to prevent endocarditis in patients with various heart conditions suggests that some trials could in fact be devised to clarify practice within standards of appropriate scientific and ethical rigor (Strom et al., 1998). Given the risk of infection and grave outcomes for such patients, the committee encourages efforts to devise and implement such studies. For example, a prospective study designed to control for differences in patient populations and other factors could compare hospitals that

---

[14]As this report was being completed, under an Intra-Agency Agreement between the NIDCR and the AHCPR, AHCPR awarded a three-year contract to the Evidence-Based Practice Center from the Research Triangle Institute/University of North Carolina at Chapel Hill (RTI-UNC) to produce both comprehensive evidence reports and/or limited reviews on topics identified by the NIDCR. The aim is to strength the scientific basis for the diagnosis and management of dental, oral, and craniofacial conditions.

include a dental examination and indicated treatment as part of standard preoperative care for cardiac surgery patients with those that rely on physicians to identify patients with dental problems needing further evaluation and treatment. Controlled research is also feasible to test the effectiveness of different dental care protocols for leukemia and lymphoma patients prior to or during chemotherapy.

Research on education and other strategies to encourage patient adherence to self-care regimens is important in dental care as in other areas. For example, even at the risk of tooth loss and bone damage, some patients who have undergone radiation therapy for cancers of the head and neck do not follow the recommended but very rigorous self-care routines, which may result not only in worse health outcomes but also in higher Medicare costs.

The committee was interested in emerging reports linking improved oral health to improved health outcomes for people with systemic conditions not evaluated in this study. A primary example is diabetic patients for whom treatment of periodontal infection is associated with better blood glucose control (Grossi et al., 1997; Grossi and Genco, 1998; Westfelt et al., 1996). Given the prevalence of diabetes and its significance as a problem among older adults, further study of the implications of oral health status and the effect of dental care should be encouraged.

In addition, the link between oral health and coronary artery disease and stroke remains an important area for further research (Beck et al., 1996). With new research suggesting a relationship between oral health status and pneumonia (an important cause of mortality and morbidity in older people), further investigation of this link and of the effectiveness of dental care and oral hygiene in preventing pneumonia also is warranted (Limeback, 1998; Scannapieco, 1999; Yonayama et al., 1999).

Finally, although AIDS patients constitute a relatively small proportion of Medicare beneficiaries, the burden of suffering associated with oral problems is significant. The contribution of dental care to better health status and quality of life has so far been little studied (Capilouto et al., 1991; Migliorati et al., 1994). The results of new research on the relationships between oral and systemic diseases for these and other medical conditions not studied in this report could inform both clinical practice and future coverage policies.

Conclusions

The committee concluded that the direct evidence to support coverage for "medically necessary dental services" varies depending on the medical condition to which dental services are related. Such evidence is, in general, lacking rather than negative or ambiguous. More and better research is needed on the systemic implications of dental problems and dental interventions to guide clinicians in caring for people with serious health problems and policymakers in supporting financial access to effective care.

Although no large randomized clinical trials have investigated outcomes of dental care for head and neck cancer patients receiving radiation therapy to the jaws, the committee concluded that small retrospective studies of patients treated before and after implementation of tooth-preserving protocols provide limited direct evidence that the replacement of tooth extraction protocols with tooth-preserving protocols prior to radiation can reduce xerostomia-induced radiation caries and associated postradiation tooth extractions that place patients at high risk for osteoradionecrosis. Other retrospective analyses show higher rates of ORN for patients with inadequate dental care and preradiation extractions. HCFA has approved coverage of extractions but not of tooth-preserving strategies. **Given this limited evidence, the severe consequences of radiation-induced osteoradionecrosis, and Medicare's investment in treating patients with head and neck cancer, it is reasonable for Medicare to cover both tooth-preserving care and extractions, which may be medically appropriate for certain patients.** Patients should be referred for dental examinations by their oncologist.

The committee also concluded that weak direct evidence suggests that the provision of dental care targeted to prevent or eliminate acute oral infection for leukemia patients prior to chemotherapy can prevent or reduce subsequent episodes of septicemia and prevent or reduce the oral complications of treatment. **Given this limited evidence, the severe consequences of septicemia and other complications of chemotherapy, and Medicare's investment in treating leukemia patients, it is reasonable for Medicare to cover a dental examination, cleaning of teeth, and treatment of acute infections of the teeth or gums for a leukemia patient prior to chemotherapy.** Again, patients would be referred to a dentist by their physician.

The committee concluded that **the evidence is insufficient to support positive or negative conclusions about dental services for patients with lymphoma, organ transplants, and heart valve repair or replacement.** Direct evidence through controlled clinical trials is lacking rather than negative or ambiguous. Indirect evidence and biological plausibility are suggestive that health outcomes may be improved by the elimination of oral sources of infection that may cause septicemia in the immunosuppressed lymphoma or organ transplant patient or endocarditis in the patient with a diseased, abnormal, or surgically repaired or replaced heart valve. Dental services for persons with these life-threatening illnesses do not differ from currently covered medical services that are considered prudent care but for which no controlled clinical studies exist. Widely accepted clinical protocols for identifying and eliminating all infections and potential sources of infection before transplantation are based largely on biological principles, animal studies, and clinical experience, not controlled trials. The committee's conclusion does not negate the value of clinical judgment in selecting appropriate individual patients for such interventions.

Although the evidence base for "medically necessary dental services" is mixed and frequently based on weak research designs, the committee is concerned about interpretations of the current law that could preclude HCFA from approving further coverage exceptions for dental services to identify and eliminate oral infections or potential sources of infection for immunocompromised high-risk patients. As noted earlier, widely accepted clinical protocols for identifying and eliminating all infections and potential sources of infection before transplantation are based on biological principles and clinical experience, not controlled trials. The committee is also concerned about legislative proposals requiring that "medically necessary dental services" produce savings that exceed the direct costs of care. As described in Chapter 5, even elimination of the three-year limit on coverage of immunosuppressive drugs—drugs that clearly improve outcomes for transplant recipients—is unlikely to meet this standard.

Given the scientific and therapeutic advances since the creation of Medicare in 1965 and the concerns about current coverage interpretations, the committee concludes that it is reasonable for Congress to update the statutory language relating to coverage of dental services so that it would clearly cover dental care that is effective in preventing or reducing oral and systemic complications associated with serious medical conditions and their treatment. Specifically, the committee suggests that **Congress should direct the Health Care Financing Administration (with assistance as appropriate from the Agency for Health Care Policy and Research and the National Institutes of Health) to develop recommendations—on a condition-by-condition basis—for coverage of dental services needed in conjunction with surgery, chemotherapy, radiation, or pharmacological treatment for a life-threatening medical condition.** The phrase "in conjunction with" would allow HCFA to limit the window of coverage to a specified period before or after surgery or other treatment but would not require that the services be provided at the same time as or as an immediate part of a surgical or other procedure. This minimal revision in the 1965 exclusion of coverage for dental services would not alter Medicare's basic focus on treatment of acute illness or injury.

If Medicare were to cover "medically necessary dental services" for some or all of the medical conditions reported here, it is uncertain how many beneficiaries in each category would avail themselves of this benefit. The referral for "medically necessary dental care" would likely come from the treating physician at the time of diagnosis or planning of the medical therapy. The patient's physician would in this way serve as a gatekeeper for this benefit, especially among patients who are not under regular dental care. In addition, physicians would continue to manage many oral problems themselves, for example, by prescribing antibiotics and therapeutic rinses.

5

Immunosuppressive Drugs for Transplant Patients

Successful transplantation of human organs is one of the most dramatic achievements of modern medicine. The first successful kidney transplant was performed in 1954 between identical twins, and the first transplants of other organs such as pancreas, liver, and heart followed in the 1960s. Organ transplantation was, however, restricted by the limited effectiveness of the treatment then available to control the body's rejection of grafted organs. With the development of more effective immunosuppressive drugs in the 1980s, transplants have become an accepted treatment for an increasing number of deadly diseases (described in detail in Appendix D, Part 1). More than 20,000 transplants were performed in 1998. With the increasing survival of recipients with functioning grafts, estimates of the number of people now living with a graft range up to 125,000, but a precise figure is not available.

Today, a major limit on transplantation is the shortage of organs available. Nearly 65,000 people were registered on waiting lists for organ transplantation in 1998, and more than 4,500 were removed from waiting lists due to death (UNOS, 1999b). Maintaining the health of transplanted organs not only protects the recipients of transplants from death, retransplantation, or other trauma; it also protects a scarce resource. Immunosuppressive drugs are essential for these dual protections, but their high cost means that most transplant recipients need financial assistance to pay for them.

Immunosuppressive drugs prescribed to recipients of solid organ transplants represent one of the few exceptions to the statutory exclusion of Medicare coverage for outpatient drugs. Even so, coverage is limited to three years following a transplant, which is an increase from the initial single year of coverage authorized in 1986.[1] Consistent with the provisions in the 1997 Balanced Budget Act calling for the present report, this chapter investigates the benefits of eliminating the three-year coverage limit on immunosuppressive drugs and the costs to Medicare of that step. The analysis here differs from that in Chapters 3 and 4 because the emphasis is less on the effectiveness of the drugs themselves than on the effects of the coverage limitation on patient outcomes. As this chapter and Appendix D describe, the former is well documented but the latter is not.

The special status of immunosuppressive drugs for transplant recipients has evolved through a complex series of incremental exceptions to the basic framework of Medicare coverage established in 1965. The next section reviews this evolution as context for the analysis of coverage issues that follows. Appendix D, Part 2 provides more detailed background.

EVOLUTION OF IMMUNOSUPPRESSIVE DRUG COVERAGE BY MEDICARE

When the Medicare program was created, outpatient drugs (and drugs in general) played a markedly smaller role in the treatment of people with serious medical problems. Many people died from conditions that now can be either cured or managed effectively for years by drugs that were not available in 1965. With the growing supply of effective drugs have come higher costs in this as in many other areas of medicine. What was once seen as a minor part of the financial burden of illness is now a major worry for many Medicare beneficiaries and an increasing concern for policymakers.

Nonetheless, coverage for immunosuppressive drugs arose less from concerns about high-cost outpatient drugs in general than from a historical anomaly, the creation by Congress of a special entitlement to Medicare for those diagnosed with permanent kidney failure (end-stage renal disease, or ESRD). For a condition that meant near-certain death, the emerging technologies of dialysis and renal transplantation could be lifesaving. Medicare coverage made these treatments financially accessible and promoted the development of dialysis services around the country (IOM, 1991).

Because transplantation was both rare and risky in 1972, the Medicare amendments mainly affected dialysis, a more developed but still relatively early-stage technology that had been introduced to clinical practice on a limited basis in the early 1960s. As long as ESRD patients were treated with dialysis, they were assured of Medicare benefits—and this remains true today. If, however,

---

[1] As this report was being completed, Congress passed the Balanced Budget Act Refinements of 1999 (P.L. 106-113), which included a provision extending the coverage of immunosuppressive drugs for eight months (subject to expenditure limitations).

patients received a transplant, their eligibility lapsed after one year and did not, in any case, include outpatient medications. The assumption at the time was that a renal graft cured ESRD. As it became evident the transplantation created its own set of continuing medical needs for those who survived past one year, in 1978, the one-year limit on Medicare benefits for renal transplant recipients was extended to three years. This three-year limit remains in place for people who cannot qualify for Medicare by virtue of age or disability.

Although the need for immunosuppressive drugs was recognized when the ESRD benefit was created and then extended for transplant patients, the drugs available were neither effective nor expensive enough to prompt an exception to Medicare's general exclusion of coverage for outpatient drugs. After the introduction of much more effective immunosuppressive drugs, starting with cyclosporine in 1983, transplantation became much more successful. Likewise, immunosuppressive therapy became much more expensive, in part because the new drug regimens were very costly to patients and in part because the drugs would be used for many years as survival times lengthened.

As the combination of the longer survival of transplant recipients and the heavy financial burden for immunosuppressive drugs became increasingly understood, Congress in 1986 authorized Medicare coverage of immunosuppressive drugs for one year following a Medicare-covered transplant.[2] This coverage was extended to three years (on a phased-in basis) beginning in 1995.

People with ESRD have a special entitlement to Medicare that other transplant recipients lack. Regardless of age or eligibility for disability benefits, they become Medicare eligible by virtue of being diagnosed with ESRD, and they remain eligible for benefits for three years following the transplant. If, however, someone with ESRD has employer-sponsored or other group health insurance, the group plan has primary payment responsibility for 30 months following the diagnosis, with Medicare serving as secondary payer to cover certain costs not covered by the group plan.

Recipients of other solid organ grafts establish and retain eligibility for Medicare coverage in the same way as other non-ESRD patients, namely, by reason of age or disability. Many establish eligibility through disability demonstrated prior to or while recovering from transplant surgery. Nonetheless, if they remain eligible for Medicare for a three-year period following their transplant, these other transplant recipients also have the special benefit of immunosuppressive drug coverage for three years.

---

[2]Kidney is the most common solid organ transplant, followed by liver, heart, lung, and pancreas. Medicare covers such transplants for beneficiaries under specified circumstances. For example, pancreas transplant is covered only when performed simultaneously with a kidney transplants or after such a transplant (*Coverage Issues Manual*, section 35.82 [HCFA, 1999b]).

Table 5-1 summarizes current Medicare policy (prior to the changes noted in footnote 1) for covered transplant recipients. Some proposals to eliminate the three-year limit on Medicare coverage of immunosuppressive drugs would extend coverage indefinitely only for transplant recipients who remained eligible for Medicare by virtue of age or disability (H.R. 1115). Another bill would also include those who are no longer eligible for general Medicare benefits, primarily renal transplant recipients (S. 631). The latter bill would also extend indefinitely legislation that makes Medicare the secondary payer for beneficiaries covered under a group health plan. This would limit Medicare costs but continue to discourage employment and provide an incentive for transplant recipients to establish and maintain eligibility for coverage by reason of disability.

ASSESSMENT APPROACH

Following the approach described in Chapter 2, the committee explored the evidence base related to the effectiveness of immunosuppressive drugs and the effect of current time limits on Medicare's coverage of these drugs. It adapted the evidence pyramid discussed in Chapter 2. Figure 5-1 shows two pyramids, the lower one relating to immunosuppressive drug therapy and the upper one to the coverage extension. For both "interventions," the desired outcomes are patient survival, graft survival, minimal complications or side effects, and good health-related quality of life. Health-related quality of life has additional dimensions for the "coverage intervention" related to the stress that people may experience in trying to arrange alternative financial access to care when Medicare coverage ends.

In contrast to the interventions discussed in Chapters 3 and 4, the evidence base for the lower pyramid is strong and is only briefly reviewed below. The real question for the committee involved coverage, that is, whether there is an additional burden of disease stemming from the loss of Medicare coverage related to people not following their prescribed immunosuppressive regimen *and* whether this behavior is related to lack of financial access. Here the committee sought evidence that coverage could result in enhanced adherence by patients to drug regimens and improved outcomes, taking possible harms into account.

Even if all the criteria in Figure 5-1 were met, the extent of benefit relative to the cost to Medicare or society generally would still have to be considered. As explained earlier, this report provides estimates of costs to Medicare only and does not include formal assessments of cost-effectiveness. It does explore briefly (in Chapter 6) the various ethical questions arising from special Medicare entitlements or exceptions to the outpatient drug exclusion for a few categories of expensive drugs that leave other needed drug therapies still uncovered.

TABLE 5-1 Summary of Current Medicare Coverage Policy on Transplants

Patient Characteristics	Pretransplant		Up to 3 Years Posttransplant[a]		More than 3 Years Posttransplant	
	Immuno Drugs	Standard Services[b]	Immuno Drugs	Standard Services	Immuno Drugs	Standard Services
Renal Transplant						
Patient disabled or ≥ 65	NA	Y	Y	Y	N	Y
Patient not disabled or ≥ 65	NA	Y	Y	Y	N	N
Other Covered Organ Transplant						
Patient disabled or ≥ 65	NA	Y	Y	Y	N	Y
Patient not disabled or ≥ 65	NA	N	N	N	N	N

NOTE: NA = not applicable; N = not covered; Y = yes, covered.

[a]Reference for coverage of immunosuppressive drugs: Social Security Act (SSA), Title XVIII, section 1861(s)(2)(J); reference for other eligibility for renal transplant recipients: SSA, Title II, section 226A.
[b]Standard services are those normally covered under Medicare (e.g., dialysis services, physician care prior to or following transplantation).

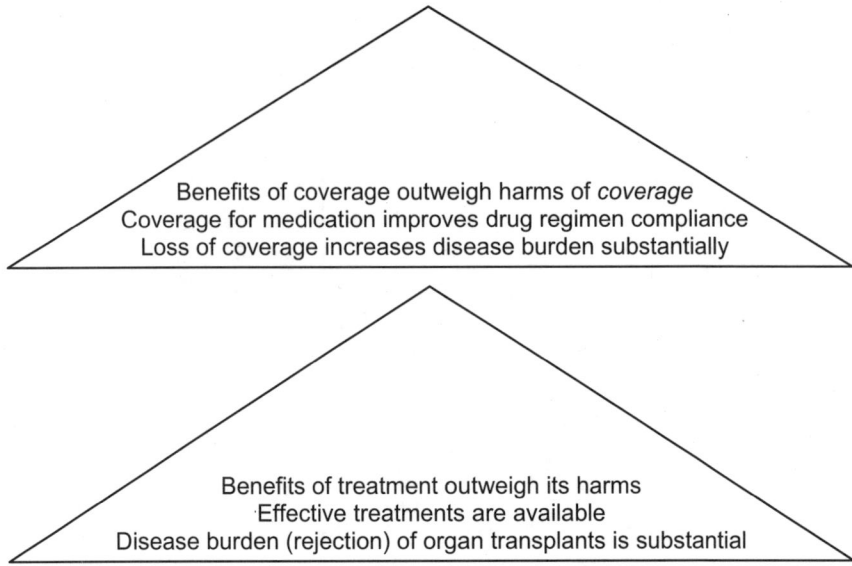

FIGURE 5-1 Evidence pyramids for extending coverage of immunosuppressive drugs.

BURDEN OF DISEASE

Organ transplantation has become the treatment of choice for a number of advanced life-threatening conditions. In 1997, the latest year for which data on primary diagnoses were available (UNOS, 1999a), nearly two-thirds of those receiving kidney transplants had glomerular diseases (diseases of the basic filtering unit of the kidney), diabetes, or hypertensive nephrosclerosis. The majority of liver transplants resulted from noncholestatic cirrhosis (59 percent), with another 14 percent due to cholestatic liver disease or cirrhosis. The great majority of heart transplants were due to either coronary artery disease (45 percent) or cardiomyopathy (42 percent). The much less common lung transplants are most often the result of emphysema or chronic obstructive pulmonary disease (37 percent), cystic fibrosis (19 percent), or idiopathic pulmonary fibrosis (14 percent).

In 1998 alone, the United Network for Organ Sharing (UNOS) reported that well over 20,000 solid organ transplants were performed in the United States. Table 5-2 shows their distribution.

For some conditions such as congenital malformation of an organ, transplantation cures the condition that made the operation necessary. In other cases such as viral hepatitis or diabetes, the condition persists and may ultimately destroy the transplanted organ, which can result in death, retransplantation, or—for patients with renal transplants—a return to dialysis.

TABLE 5-2 Number and Types of
Transplants Performed in 1998

Type	Number
Kidney–pancreas	965
Kidney alone	11,990
Pancreas alone	253
Liver	4,450
Heart	2,340
Heart–lung	45
Lung	849
Intestine	69
Total	**20,961**

SOURCE: UNOS Scientific Registry data as of
April 14, 1999. Double kidney, double lung,
and heart–lung transplants are each counted as
one transplant.

In 1995 there were more than 70,000 persons in the United States living with a functioning transplanted kidney. With roughly 12,000 kidney transplants performed per year and more than 80 percent of patients surviving five years with a functioning graft, this number is now estimated at over 80,000, but the exact figure is not known. Numbers of liver, heart, and other transplants are smaller, but the long-term survival of both grafts and recipients is growing rapidly—the total number of all living transplant recipients has been estimated, as previously mentioned, at up to 125,000.

The increasing success of transplantation has brought great benefits to many people. It has also created a new—but almost always more tolerable—type of burden, the continued need for immunosuppression to manage the continued risk of graft rejection.

Need for Immunosuppression

As described in more detail in Appendix D, Part 1, it quickly became apparent based on observations from animal research and early organ transplants in humans that the survival and functioning of grafted organs required suppression of the recipient's natural immune response to the graft. The immune system reacts to the presence in the body of proteins that do not belong to the individual, whether these proteins are from ragweed pollen, infecting bacteria, blood of another blood type, or an organ from the body of another individual. For a transplanted organ, this reaction leads to organ rejection and eventual destruction. Absent successful intervention, the death of the "host" follows.

In the early days of transplantation, physicians and researchers hoped that the patient would accommodate the graft completely and thus render pharmacological immunosuppression unnecessary. Although a degree of accommodation does occur in most patients, allowing the dosages of immunosuppressive drugs to be reduced, accommodation is not so complete as to allow drug-free graft survival in any but rare cases involving particularly tolerant organs. The liver, for instance, needs less immunosuppressive support than other types of grafts, and a few liver transplant recipients (less than 1 percent) have been able eventually to cease immunosuppressive therapy. Most patients, however, cannot cease immunosuppressive therapy without serious risk of graft rejection.[3]

Although research has demonstrated the effectiveness of immunosuppressive drugs, they are not 100 percent effective. Some patients still experience acute rejection of their graft despite immunosuppressive therapy, and others suffer chronic rejection that may eventually lead to graft failure.[4] Acute rejection is most common in the first few months after the transplant. In 1995, graft loss during the first year after a kidney transplant was reported as about 12 percent (USRDS, 1998; discussed in Appendix D, Part 1), but more recently, various centers have reported lower rates of early graft loss due to acute rejection: 7 to 8 percent (Gaston, 1998). Chronic rejection, the gradual failure of an organ due to immunologic rejection, is a more complex phenomenon, or at least more difficult to measure, and it varies by organ. In the more immunologically tolerant liver, for instance, chronic rejection has been reported to account for only 9 to 10 percent of late graft loss (Abbasoglu et al., 1997). In the kidney, on the other hand, chronic rejection has been considered a major cause of late graft loss, but this is now being reexamined. One center had reported chronic rejection as the primary cause of graft loss in 44 percent of cases of loss between six months and approximately four to five years after transplantation. When the cases attributed to chronic rejection were critically reevaluated, however, more than half appeared to have involved lack of patient adherence to demanding medication regimens rather than ineffectiveness of the drugs themselves (Gaston, 1998). It is therefore difficult to tell how many cases of graft loss that have

---

[3]One very unusual exception was recently reported (Spitzer et al., 1999) in which the patient received a kidney and bone marrow transplant following failure of her own kidneys due to multiple myeloma and has survived without immunosuppression.

[4]Different types of rejection are mediated by different immunologic mechanisms but are named according to the rate at which rejection occurs. One type, acute rejection, occurs over days to weeks. Another type, chronic rejection, occurs over months or years. Although acute rejection is most common just after surgery, it can also occur on one or repeated occasions long afterward. Thus, "acute" and "chronic" are not synonyms for early and late rejection. The terms "early" and "late" are not precise, but early usually means within a year of the operation, sometimes less than six months, whereas "late" means more than a year but often refers to episodes several years after the operation.

been labeled chronic rejection actually represent a failure of therapy rather than patient noncompliance.

In summary, the rate of graft loss due to acute rejection has decreased as more effective drugs have been introduced; the rate of late graft loss due to chronic rejection may be lower than believed; and it could perhaps be reduced by greater attention to factors affecting patients' ability to take their medications as prescribed. Neither form of rejection, however, has been eliminated. The goal of achieving adequate immunosuppression, even with today's more effective drugs, remains a challenge that cannot be met for every patient.

Waiting Lists for Transplantation

The increased transplant success rate has meant that renal transplantation became a better treatment for ESRD than dialysis. For kidneys and other organs as well, increased success has made the supply of donated organs a critical concern.

The relative scarcity of organs is evident in the growing number of patients on the waiting lists for transplantation (Table 5-3). This growth is due in part to the increasing number of people with organ failure and in part to the improved safety and effectiveness of the procedure that allows it to be offered to a wider population of patients including some who have survived the failure of a first grafted organ. Long waits for a transplant—waits that may end in death before an organ becomes available—are a significant part of the burden of the diseases treated by transplantation. The main "treatment" for these waits would be an increase in organ donation or the development of effective, acceptable alternatives to human organs. For the present, however, every transplanted organ that is successfully maintained also helps prevent further increases in the waiting list and waiting times.

Further, patients whose grafts have failed and who have successfully applied for a second graft may have a worse prognosis than the patient who is receiving a graft for the first time, due in part to the likelihood of increased immunologic sensitivity among patients who have already had a graft. This phenomenon has been reported in adult recipients of, for example, regrafts of hearts (Chan and Hunt, 1998), livers (Markmann et al., 1997), and kidneys (Cecka, 1997). It should also be noted, however, that the largest body of data, which involves renal regrafts, indicates that the gap between the outcomes of first and second transplants has been cut in half in recent years (Cecka, 1997). Any retransplantion uses a donated organ from a very small pool and leaves some other patients on the waiting list longer.

TABLE 5-3 Number of Patients on Waiting Lists at Year's End, Selected Years

| | Organ Type | | | | | | | |
Year	Kidney	Liver	Pancreas	Kidney–Pancreas	Heart	Lung	Heart–Lung	Total
1988	13,943	616	163	0	1,030	69	205	16,026
1992	22,376	2,323	126	778	2,690	942	180	29,415
1997	38,270	9,647	361	1,593	3,899	2,672	236	56,678

NOTE: The table shows data for the number of patients on the waiting list by type of organ in 1988 and 1997 (the earliest and latest years for which data were displayed), and the intermediate year 1992 (the first year that there was a kidney–pancreas waiting list).

SOURCE: UNOS, 1999a, Table 6.0.

AVAILABILITY OF EFFECTIVE TREATMENT

Questions that the committee had to grapple with in the previous chapters—whether evidence showed that the clinical intervention proposed for coverage improves outcomes—have largely been settled in the case of immunosuppression after organ transplantation.[5] As shown in Table 5-4, more than 75 percent of kidneys, livers, hearts, and even lungs are now functioning one year after transplantation, and in all categories except lung grafts, more than 60 percent of the grafts are still functioning five years after transplantation. Patients are surviving at somewhat higher rates than grafts. More than two-thirds of transplant recipients now survive at least five years.

Of the four classes of drugs that have contributed to the major improvements in graft and patient survival in recent years, products in one class (antilymphocyte agents) are used on a short-term basis and, thus, are not a Medicare coverage issue. Products in the other three classes (antiproliferative agents, corticosteroids, and calcineurin phosphatase inhibitors) are used on a long-term basis. Physicians generally prescribe a combination regimen for long-term use because the different classes of drugs work in different ways and have different side effects. The combination approach helps achieve high levels of immunosuppression without letting any particular type of side effect become as bad as it might otherwise be.

TABLE 5-4 Graft and Patient Survival Rates at One and Five Years

Organ	Graft Survival (%)		Patient Survival (%)	
	One Year	Five Years	One Year	Five Years
Cadaveric kidney	87.5	61.0	94.8	81.1
Live donor kidney	93.5	76.6	97.7	90.8
Liver	79.2	62.0	86.9	73.2
Heart	85.5	67.7	87.8	69.4
Lung	75.0	40.6	75.8	43.7

NOTE: One-year survival rates refer to transplant recipients in 1995 1996, and five year rates to any transplant recipients between October 1987 and December 1996. Graft survival is survival without loss of the graft or death of the patient; if the patient dies with a functioning graft, the death is counted as a failed graft.

SOURCE: UNOS 1999a.

---

[5]The committee did not re-review evidence showing that the individual drug products indicated for immunosuppression were acceptably safe and effective, but rather assumed that the products that have already been reviewed and approved by the Food and Drug Administration for marketing have been shown in adequate and well-controlled clinical trials to be safe and effective for their intended uses.

The level of immunosuppression needed varies from person to person, depending on the immunologic compatibility of the recipient and the graft. As the time after transplant increases, physicians generally decrease the dose of immunosuppressive agents on an empirical basis, testing small changes to see whether side effects can be reduced without threatening graft rejection.

The major benefits of immunosuppressive drugs for transplant recipients are clear: longer survival and improved quality of life (Wolfe et al., 1999). A functioning renal graft has the great advantage of working all the time, rather than periodically like dialysis, so the transplant patient generally feels healthier and has fewer dietary restrictions. Further, a transplanted kidney works while the patient does other things, but dialysis requires the patient to spend several long periods a week undergoing treatment, which can be very disruptive to work and other activities. Nonetheless, kidney transplant patients do at least have an alternative in the case of graft failure. Patients suffering failure of another vital organ have no options except transplantation.

The major harm that comes from immunosuppressive drugs is the result of a suppressed immune system. That is, the suppressed immune system protects against graft rejection but simultaneously leaves patients at risk from many organisms that normally are present but kept under control by a properly functioning immune system. Many patients take some prophylactic medication, and all require close monitoring for emerging infections.

Each immunosuppressive agent also has its own specific complement of other adverse effects, as does any effective drug. These side effects can include hypertension, decreased kidney function, diabetes, various gastrointestinal complaints, leukopenia or thrombocytopenia, unusual growth of gums or hair, and an increased tendency to develop malignancies. Management of these side effects often requires additional medications.

Although this committee did not systematically address quality of life or cost-effectiveness, one analysis of renal transplantation in Canada compared kidney transplantation to dialysis (starting from the initiation of either procedure) on the basis of several health-related quality measures (Laupacis et al., 1996). Except for the first month following transplantations, all showed higher quality-of-life scores for transplant recipients during both the year of the transplant and the following year (compared to the first two years of dialysis). The quality-adjusted life years (QALYs) for the transplant and subsequent year were 0.65 and 0.62, respectively. The comparable figures for dialysis were 0.53 and 0.51.

Overall, the benefits of immunosuppression for transplant patients are widely accepted as outweighing the harms. Nonetheless, this partial listing of harms makes clear that these patients require continued medical monitoring and often additional therapies to sustain the benefits achieved by transplantation.

BARRIERS TO ADEQUATE THERAPY

For many medical problems including those examined in this report, the existence of effective treatment does not ensure that it will be available to and used by all who could benefit from it. Medicare coverage has helped make transplantation and posttransplantation therapy available to thousands of people, but the cost of continued care, especially immunosuppressive drug therapy, is a problem for many after the three-year coverage period for drugs has passed. Nonetheless, it is not clear to what extent financial problems contribute to people's failure to follow their treatment regimens or to what extent this accounts for graft rejection and failure.

Following Complex Drug Regimens: General Issues

Despite the critical importance of immunosuppressive drugs, a significant proportion of patients—several studies estimate about 22 percent—do not take their drugs as prescribed (Greenstein and Siegal, 1999). This lack of compliance[6] with the treatment regimen puts patients at risk of graft loss. Because patients may be reluctant to admit that they are not taking their drugs as prescribed, the amount and type of noncompliance are difficult to assess, which makes a direct link to graft loss difficult to establish. A study cited earlier from one transplant center suggests that noncompliance is a significantly more important cause of graft loss in patients who have had a successful transplant than has previously been appreciated (Gaston, 1998).

The compliance responsibilities of transplant patients are formidable. A representative kidney transplant medication regimen could very well include an immunosuppressive agent from each of the three classes described earlier, plus a routine prophylactic antibiotic, an antifungal medication, and medications for concomitant conditions including hypertension, angina, hypocalcemia (depletion of calcium and consequently bone disease, which is common among patients who are or have recently been on dialysis), and short- and long-acting antacids for gastrointestinal side effects. A patient on this regimen would have to take at least eight medications in the morning, another four in the evening, plus antacids and antifungal mouth treatments after every meal and before going to bed.

The reasons for lack of full compliance are varied (e.g., see Raiz et al., 1999; Siegal and Greenstein, 1997). With such complex medication regimens, problems may include ordinary forgetfulness, difficult or stressful living ar-

---

[6]The committee recognized that the terms "compliant" and "noncompliant" may suggest a model of authoritarian physicians directing subservient patients rather than the now more commonly advanced model of shared decisionmaking about a course of action. For this reason, the terms "adherent" and "nonadherent" are often more acceptable and commonly used. The transplant literature (e.g., see Cramer, 1995) typically retains the compliance terminology, so the committee followed this pattern.

rangements, or inadequate understanding of the importance of spacing doses throughout the day or in relation to meals. Lack of formal education may contribute to a lack of understanding for some patients. In addition, the side effects of many immunosuppressive drugs are unpleasant and can make compliance difficult. Because noncompliance with immunosuppression can have such serious consequences, transplant professionals have developed various strategies to help patients, for example, assisting them in designing a clear schedule and suggesting various reminder aids. Some transplant centers not only emphasize compliance as part of their pretransplant preparation of patients but also ask patients to sign a written contract agreeing to comply with the prescribed regimen to maintain the donated organ.

One review of studies of patient compliance pointed to greater compliance of patients just prior to physician contact (Cramer, 1995). This suggests that compliance might be increased by more frequent contact with health care workers.[7] Maintaining such contact may be a greater problem for those renal transplant recipients who reach not only the three-year coverage limit for immunosuppressive drugs but also the three-year limit on Medicare coverage overall, including coverage for physician visits.[8]

Patient compliance is a concern in many areas of medicine, not just transplantation. Urquhart (1996) reviewed studies of compliance, concluding that roughly 30 percent or more of patients do not comply with their prescribed therapy regimens, regardless of the severity of the consequences. In one revealing study, researchers introduced medical students to the difficulties that patients face by electronically monitoring the students' compliance with a two- or three-times-a-day drug regimen over a two-week interval (Kastrissios et al., 1996). Although 71 percent of the doses were taken, only 46 percent were taken at the prescribed frequency (doses per day) and 28 percent at the prescribed intervals (hours between doses). The most common explanation given by the students, a hectic schedule, would apply to many patients as well.

In older people, compliance difficulties are associated with a variety of factors, including multiple medications and concern about the cost of the medi-

---

[7]An extreme version of this approach—required observation of medication taking—is already in place for certain patients with tuberculosis and other conditions that pose a significant infectious threat to the community (Davidson, 1998; see also Sbarbaro, 1998, for editorial comment, and see Sbarbaro and Johnson, 1968, discussed in editorial, for study of effectiveness of technique). This measure has not been suggested for transplant recipients.

[8]As explained earlier, those renal transplant recipients who remain eligible for Medicare by virtue of age or disability (not previous ESRD diagnosis alone) lose coverage for immunosuppressive drugs only after the three-year limit is exceeded. The same applies to nonrenal transplant patients who qualify for Medicare by virtue of age or disability. If those qualified by virtue of disability lose this status, they also lose all Medicare coverage regardless of any time limits on drug coverage.

cations (Cool et al., 1990; Coons et al., 1994), both of which are often aspects of the regimen that transplant patients must manage. Nonetheless, studies indicate that elderly patients in general tend to be more compliant with their regimens than younger patients (Bame, 1995; Greenstein and Siegal, 1999).

Cost of Immunosuppressive Drugs

The cost of the combination immunosuppressive drug regimens can vary widely (see Appendix D, Part 1, Table D-1). For example, the least expensive three-part combination regimen might cost roughly $5,900 per year and could be sufficient for many patients. Those who did not do well on this combination might require one or more of the higher-priced drugs, which could bring the cost to more than $16,000 per year.[9]

As noted above, many transplant patients require additional outpatient medications such as antihypertensive agents and antibiotics for infections. Medicare does not cover these outpatient drugs for any beneficiary.

Because immunosuppressive therapy is complex, patients must be monitored for both drug effectiveness and side effects by an experienced physician. As described above, clinical and laboratory services are covered only for long-term transplant survivors who remain eligible for Medicare by virtue of age or disability ("ESRD-only" patients lose coverage after three years).[10] Informal estimates suggest that the visits and laboratory work solely to monitor immunosuppressive drugs could cost such a patient roughly $500 to $700 per year. Any additional problems, infections, or side effects would result in additional costs.

An important question for this study is whether *longer coverage* of immunosuppressive drugs will result in better outcomes for transplant recipients. The answer depends on the degree to which the lack of coverage for the costs of the medication stands as a significant barrier between the patient and adequate immunosuppression. (Cost is not the only factor in noncompliance, as mentioned above; see also Dew et al., 1999.)

Expiration of Medicare Coverage and Alternative Funding

As the committee heard during its workshop on coverage for immunosuppressive drugs (see Appendix A), a number of programs have been created to provide drugs to those without coverage. Still, it may be difficult or impossible

---

[9]Immunosuppressive drugs and other drugs with specific coverage exceptions are not the only costly drugs used by significant numbers of Medicare beneficiaries. For example, Zidovudine (AZT) and other drugs now available to treat people with AIDS (some of whom qualify for Medicare as disabled) cost thousands of dollars a year.

[10]As discussed later in this chapter, the committee's cost estimate includes coverage only for immunosuppressive drugs, not for physician monitoring or other services.

for some patients to assemble sufficient assistance from one or more programs to solve the problem of long-term, stable access to the drugs needed. Some are eligible for Medicaid programs that cover the drugs; others will have coverage under a spouse's insurance; still others may qualify for assistance from companies that manufacture the drugs; and charitable programs may assist more. Some patients may be able to work and find employment that offers health benefits. However, the structure of existing public programs provides incentives for patients to retain their status as disabled to avoid losing Medicare coverage.

Identifying or qualifying for the public or private programs that assist people in paying for or otherwise obtaining needed drugs is a complex undertaking. Programs vary from location to location and also change over time. Patients often need the help of a specialist to locate, apply for, and maintain assistance for their medical expenses (Jacobs, 1998; Sisson et al., 1994). One group documented a substantial increase in compliance with medications when its transplant center provided a specialist to assist patients in assembling coverage (Paris et al., 1998). Several workshop participants reported that patients assist one another and are sometimes forced to resort to seeking compassionate but illegal help to obtain medications. For example, patients may share or lend drugs to help someone through a coverage gap. "Underground" networks have been organized to buy drugs from less expensive foreign sources[11] or to secure donations of unused drugs from the families of deceased patients.[12]

Evidence About the Effects of Providing or Withdrawing Coverage[13]

As noted earlier, if the elimination of time limits on the coverage for immunosuppressive drugs is viewed as an "intervention," the desired results are both improved outcomes in graft survival, and also increased ability of patients to engage in normal activities of living. Although both the effects of immunosuppressive drugs themselves and the effort currently required for maintenance of coverage (e.g., submitting bills or otherwise following Medicare requirements) may have some negative implications, the *loss* of coverage has many more negative aspects, including devoting exorbitant time and energy to the pursuit of

---

[11]The reasons drugs may be less expensive in other countries than in the United States are complex and somewhat controversial, and may range from more regulation in the form of government-negotiated prices, to less regulation of manufacturing and distribution facilities and procedures, to frankly extraregulatory activity such as counterfeit products—and any of these scenarios may be affected by what price the local market can bear.

[12]This phenomenon was also recently described in the popular press (Lagnado, 1999).

[13]This section is concerned with the effects on patients of withdrawal of coverage for cyclosporine A and ought not be confused with studies of the clinical and pharmacological effects of withdrawing cyclosporine A.

alternative ways of getting the needed drugs, and of course, the risk of graft rejection if those alternative strategies should fail. This effort can disrupt marriage and family life, threaten the continuation or resumption of a satisfying work life, and otherwise take a heavy toll on people's quality of life. These kinds of outcomes have been little studied or measured in a systematic way, but they must be acknowledged. Fortunately, not all transplant recipients have to continue indefinitely in that mode because some are able to develop longer-term strategies to secure access to their medication. Figure 5-2 sketches some, but by no means all, of the consequences to the patient and to Medicare that may result after Medicare coverage for immunosuppressive drugs ceases.

Data about the effects of the Medicare coverage limit are sparse. Not surprisingly, no randomized studies compare the results for patients provided coverage and those not provided coverage for immunosuppressive drugs. One analysis based on a sample of 1990 Medicare records for 7,949 renal transplant patients showed that the rate of graft loss decreased steeply during the first six months after the operation (risk of rejection is highest just after the operation is performed), but then remained stable through the end of the year and beyond (Eggers, 1999; Eggers and Milan, 1998). Given that the time limit for Medicare coverage of immunosuppressants was one year in 1990, this analysis does not indicate any dramatic impact of coverage expiration. The data were not, however, stratified by beneficiary income or any income surrogate, and for technical reasons, the analysis may have been limited in its ability to detect all graft failures.

Another report, this time for a single kidney transplant center, describes a natural experiment on loss of Medicare coverage, again when the coverage limit was one year. For one group of patients who could manage some but not full payment, doses of cyclosporine were reduced. For a second group that had found no way to pay at all, cyclosporine was eliminated completely. The outcomes for these two groups were later compared to a third group of similar patients at the center who were able to finance their full dose of cyclosporine. Patients were followed, and otherwise cared for, through at least three years. Patients in the no-dose group exhibited more late-stage acute rejection than the reduced-dose or full-dose group. The reduced-dose and full-dose groups did not differ significantly. Although this was not a randomized, controlled trial, patients were matched, so the data suggest that it may be better to reduce the dose than discontinue it, if at all possible (Sanders et al., 1993). The results may also suggest that the optimum dose of immunosuppressive drugs has yet to be determined—and may be lower than now believed.

The same transplant center completed a further study on the relation of resources for purchasing cyclosporine to patient outcomes. This analysis was made possible by another natural experiment—initiatied by the National Organization for Rare Diseases (NORD) —of an indigent drug access program for cyclosporine. The study followed a group of NORD participants at the center who were socioeconomically matched with the no-dose group previously ob-

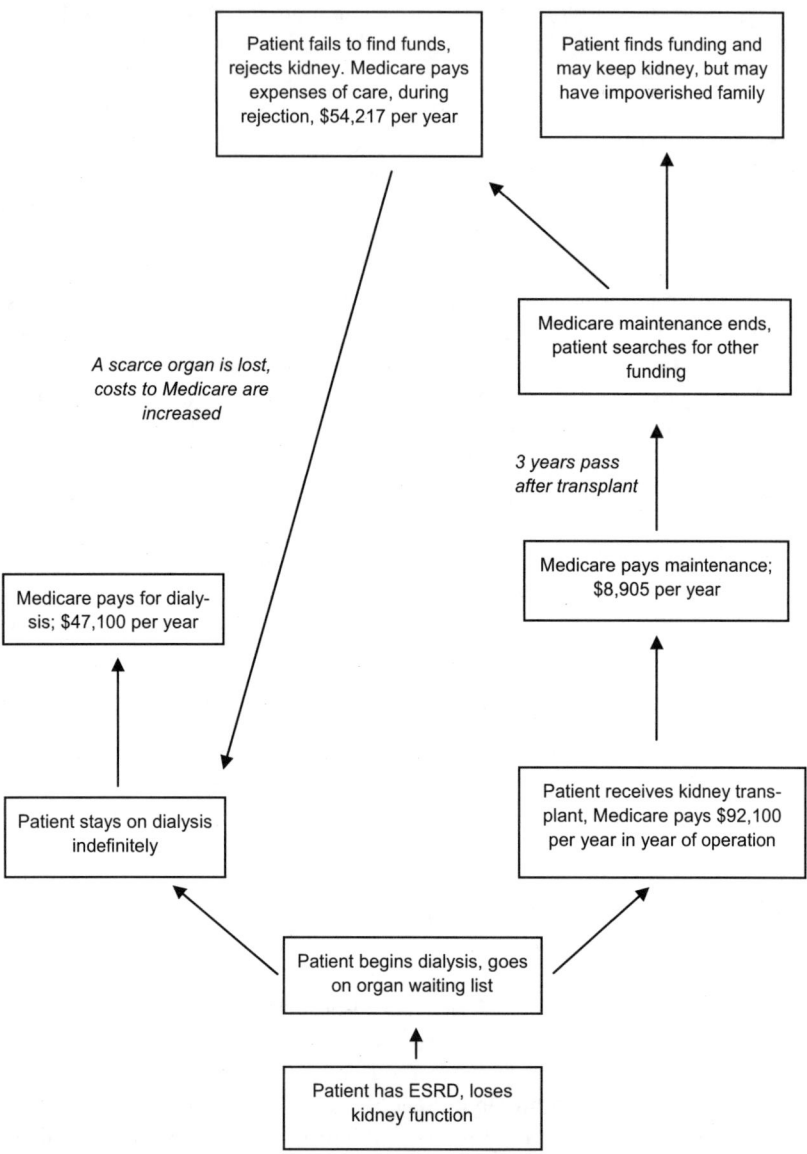

FIGURE 5-2 Possible consequences when a Medicare-eligible kidney transplant patient reaches the end of coverage and cannot locate other funds for immunosuppressive drugs. NOTE: Amounts represent costs to Medicare per patient in 1994.

served; both groups were then followed for an additional 2.5 to 5 years. The no-dose group and the NORD program participants had exhibited similar rates of acute rejection prior to the NORD intervention. After the intervention, members of the no-dose group experienced significantly more episodes of rejection, resulting in increased risk of graft loss; NORD program participants did not experience any increase in their episodes of rejection (Sanders et al., 1996). Further data suggesting that financially induced noncompliance is reversible were described at the committee workshop.[14] Researchers reported the results of an analysis of national data comparing renal graft survival at one and three years posttransplant for high- and low-income groups. When Medicare coverage was available for only one year, the high- and low-income transplant recipients had similar rates of graft survival at one year, but the high-income group had significantly better rates of graft survival at three years. When Medicare coverage was extended to three years, the high- and low-income groups had similar rates of survival at both one and three years posttransplant (Woodward et al., 1999). Like the study of the NORD intervention, this study showed a statistically significant association between better outcomes and better access to funding, whether through private means or public programs.

Another study relevant to some of these issues is underway, sponsored by the National Kidney Foundation in cooperation with George Mason University. Unfortunately, the results were not available before this report was completed.

To summarize, some level of noncompliance with prescribed medications may be an expected—if unfortunate—aspect of outpatient management of any illness. The evidence described above, although not based on strong controlled studies, suggests that for some groups of transplant patients the lack of Medicare coverage for medications is a factor contributing to noncompliance and worse patient outcomes, especially for low-income people without alternative insurance through a family member (or their own work). Some patients may badly need help in paying for their immunosuppressants, whereas others may be in less financial need (though perhaps still in need of help to locate and manage other coverage programs). [15]

The data reviewed did not address the less easily quantified burdens of coverage loss. These include its emotional toll and its diversion of the time and talent of so many individuals from other purposes to arranging access to medications. (The latter is described in Appendix D, Part 2 as the "survival paradox.")

---

[14]Mark Schnitzler, Ph.D., Washington University, St. Louis, presentation to the IOM Committee on Medicare Coverage Extensions at public workshop, Institute of Medicine, Washington, D.C., June 18, 1999.

[15]The Medicare program is not "means-tested," so the entitlement to coverage would be equally extended for any patient regardless of the other financial resources available to him or her.

Another factor to consider in estimating the effect of extending Medicare coverage is the effect such a decision might have on drug pricing. Although Medicare is today a major payer for immunosuppressive drug therapy for transplants, the time limit on coverage means that other parties including Medicaid, private insurers, patients and families, charitable organizations, and drug companies themselves participate in the overall financing of access. Depending on the specifics of the policy, eliminating the time limit on coverage would reduce the involvement of these parties to varying degrees.[16] This could affect manufacturers' pricing of the drugs and possibly the choice of drugs by physicians and patients. It might seem that if Medicare were the major if not the only buyer for this use, then it might be able to negotiate or otherwise secure better prices, at least when multiple sellers exist (which is not the case for drugs still under patent). This would, however, require potentially controversial legislative changes in the way Medicare pays for covered prescription drugs. The Balanced Budget Act of 1997 provided that the Health Care Financing Administration limit payments to the lower of the billed charge or 95 percent of the average wholesale price.

Congress could also establish a cap on Medicare payments per patient per year, with patients responsible for any amounts over the cap. Such a cap could, for example, be set initially at the level of the lowest-cost accepted or commonly prescribed multidrug immunosuppressive regimen. It could also be set arbitrarily based on budgetary considerations. Given some clinical flexibility in moving patients from higher-cost to lower-cost regimens, this could put pressure on manufacturers to reduce prices for the most expensive drugs. Undoubtedly, some patients who could not be managed with less expensive regimens would face substantial costs, although they would still benefit from the extension of coverage past the current 3-year limit. Whether existing private programs to help cover drug costs for those without coverage would be continued for those with partial coverage is unknown.

ESTIMATED COSTS TO MEDICARE OF EXTENDING COVERAGE

As discussed in Chapter 2, the cost estimation approach of the committee generally follows the generic practices (e.g., not discounting estimates to present value) employed by the Congressional Budget Office (CBO) in making estimates for Congress. A more detailed presentation of the committee's cost estimates and their associated assumptions and data sources appears in Appendix E, which was prepared by the Lewin Group in consultation with the committee and background paper author.

---

[16] The phenomenon is sometimes referred to as "crowd out."

The committee's estimates of Medicare costs are based on a series of assumptions, some of which have supporting evidence or data but others of which are best guesses based on committee judgment in the absence of such information. The estimates are intended to suggest the order of magnitude of the costs to Medicare of extending coverage, but they could be considerably higher or lower than what Medicare might actually spend were coverage policies changed. The tables in Appendix E allow readers to vary some of the assumptions and calculate alternative estimates.

Box 5-1 summarizes the assumptions and data used to develop the estimates. It includes one estimate that assumes coverage for immunosuppressive drugs is extended only for transplant recipients eligible for Medicare by reason of age or disability. A second estimate assumes that the drug coverage is also extended for currently covered "ESRD only" renal transplant recipients who lose other Medicare coverage after three years because they are not either disabled or at least age 65. For the five-year period 2000 to 2004, the total net estimated cost to Medicare of eliminating the three-year limit on coverage of immunosuppressive drugs for the first, smaller group would be $778.4 million, taking into account $553.9 million in savings from avoiding a return to dialysis for those with failed renal grafts. Adding the "ESRD only" group would raise the total net estimated cost to $1,060.1 million, taking into account $830.4 million in offsetting savings.

BOX 5-1 Summary of Estimated Costs to Medicare for Extending Coverage of Immunosuppressive Drugs After Transplant Operations

Coverage Model Assumptions

- Version 1: Coverage without time limits for immunosuppressants would be an entitlement of any solid organ transplant recipient who had had a transplant at least three years previously who was otherwise Medicare eligible by virtue of age or other disability.
- Version 2: Same, except that coverage for immunosuppressants would also be extended to renal transplant recipients who would not qualify by virtue of age or disability ("ESRD only").

Cost Estimate Assumptions for Years 2000–2004 (see also Appendix E)

- In 2000, Medicare pays $5,400 per patient per year for immunosuppressive drugs.
- Medicare payments increase at 4 percent per year for 2000–2004.
- Costs are not discounted to present value.
- The 20 percent Medicare Part B copayment is deducted as well as a 5% provider discount from the average wholesale price of the drugs.

Continued

BOX 5-1 *Continued*

Cost Estimate Assumptions for Years 2000–2004 (*continued*)

• Kidney transplants are assumed to be associated with offsets due primarily to avoidance of return to dialysis.
• Organs other than the kidney are assumed to include heart, liver, and lung transplants. No cost offsets due to treatment comparable to dialysis for these organ grafts.
• In 2000, approximately 75,000 kidney transplant patients have a graft that has survived three or more years, increasing at 10 percent per year for 2000–2004.
• In 2000, approximately 5,800 other organ transplant patients have a graft that has survived three or more years, increasing at different rates for different organs, all higher than 10 percent initially but assumed to decrease to a rate of 10 percent per year by 2004.
• Medicare secondary payer requirements would result in reductions based on 25% of beneficiary population assumed to be covered by employer health plan with primary payment responsibility.
• Potential savings to Medicaid are not included.

Data Sources

• Beneficiary population data are from Dr. Paul Eggers, HCFA Division of Beneficiaries Research.
• Average cost of immunosuppressive therapy from HCFA Office of the Actuary and paper authors.

Estimated Costs (in millions) to Medicare, Summed over 2000–2004

	Age and Disability Medicare Eligible	Age, Disability, and ESRD Medicare Eligible
Kidney transplants, gross	$1,120.2	$1,678.4
All other covered transplants, gross	212.1	212.1
Total gross costs	1,332.3	1,890.5
Kidney-related cost savings	−553.9	−830.4
5-year net cost to Medicare, all transplants	**778.4**	**1,060.1**

In order to estimate the cost to Medicare of eliminating the three-year limit on coverage of immunosuppressants for transplant recipients, the different clinical circumstances of renal and nonrenal transplant recipients must be taken into account. Most ESRD patients who receive renal transplants have an alternative treatment available, dialysis. Other transplant patients do not have an alternative long-term treatment; they either survive with a graft or die while waiting for a graft or later if the graft fails and retransplantation is not an option. Renal transplant is certainly preferred by most patients and physicians, but dialysis still exists as a life-extending option for someone whose graft fails.

The cost estimates assume that only a subset of renal transplant recipients who suffer graft failure after three years do so for reasons related to cost. As described earlier and in Appendix D, various factors contribute to graft rejection including lack of patient adherence to demanding drug regimens. After considering the very limited and inadequate information on the role of financial pressure, the committee estimated that one-third of renal graft failure might be attributed to lack of financial resources (2.5 percent of the 7 percent failure rate after three years).

Renal transplant recipients also differ from other patients because their ESRD diagnosis qualifies them for three years of posttransplant Medicare coverage without the need to meet the age or disability requirements that apply to others. This raises the question of how the three-year limit on immunosuppressive drugs would be eliminated for ESRD versus other Medicare-covered transplant recipients. For purposes of one estimate, the committee assumed that the time limit on coverage of immunosuppressive drugs would be eliminated only for those transplant recipients who stay eligible for Medicare coverage after three years by reason of age or disability. For purposes of the other estimate, the committee assumed that Congress would extend coverage to all Medicare-covered transplant recipients including those now qualified by virtue of ESRD diagnosis alone.

The committee assumed that costs would be offset by savings from extended primary-payer requirements for beneficiaries covered by employer health plans. As explained in Appendix E, the committee assumed for both the first and the second cost estimates that each of the relevant beneficiary populations would drop by 25 percent.

For the purpose of estimating costs for renal transplant recipients, the committee considered the likely cost of the immunosuppressive drugs required to maintain a renal graft compared to the cost of returning a patient with a failed graft to dialysis. The initial cost of a transplant is high relative to dialysis. Data presented at the committee workshop (Table 5-5) showed that Medicare's 1994 expenditures per ESRD patient (controlling for differences in patient survival) were highest for patients transplanted that year and lowest for patients who were maintaining grafts transplanted in previous years (Eggers, 1999). The yearly cost of dialysis was almost as high as the cost of treating someone for graft failure.

TABLE 5-5 Medicare Expenditure per
ESRD Patient, 1994

Situation	Medicare Expenditure
Kidney transplant	$92,100
Transplant maintenance	8,905
Maintained on dialysis	47,100
Graft failure	54,217

The "break-even" point for transplantation occurs when the total cost of a transplant and subsequent maintenance equals the cost of maintaining someone on dialysis for the same period of time. After the break-even point, maintaining someone with a kidney transplant costs the Medicare program less than maintaining someone on dialysis. According to Eggers (1999), the break-even point for Medicare occurred at 3.1 years in 1994, down from 4.6 years in 1989. That is, if the graft could be maintained for 3.1 years, then transplantation would become less expensive than dialysis would have been had the patient survived on dialysis for that period. The change between 1989 and 1994 probably reflects both changes in transplant care and the substantial increase in the cost of dialysis following the introduction of coverage for erythropoietin, a drug for dialysis-induced anemia. In sum, not only is maintaining a functioning transplant preferred by physicians and patients, it is clearly less costly over the long-term than maintaining a patient on dialysis.

In estimating the cost of extending coverage for immunosuppressive drugs, the gross cost of coverage for transplant recipient patients is not reduced by a premium offset as were the gross cost estimates in the preceding chapters. This is because the beneficiary premium (set by statute at 25 percent of total Part B expenditures) is based only on payments for the aged beneficiary population and most Medicare costs for transplant recipients are for people under age 65.

The committee was not asked to estimate savings to the federal–state Medicaid program that might result from elimination of Medicare's time limit on immunosuppressive drugs. In 1996, the CBO estimated that the federal share of Medicaid expenditures for Medicare–Medicaid-eligible beneficiaries would be reduced $6 million per year in 2000 and 2001 if the time limit on coverage of immunosuppressive drugs was eliminated for Medicare-eligible transplant patients (CBO, 1996). As explained in Appendix E, if the CBO estimates were adjusted to reflect inflation and this committee's coverage extension assumptions for the larger beneficiary population (including "ESRD only"), the estimated five-year savings (2000 to 2004) to the federal Medicaid program would total $49 million. Clearly, some patients and families would also benefit financially from the extension of Medicare coverage for immunosuppressive drugs, but the committee found no solid estimate of these benefits.

STATEMENTS OF OTHERS ON COVERAGE FOR IMMUNOSUPPRESSANTS

More policy attention has been devoted to renal transplantation than to the transplantation of other organs, reflecting the greater number of these operations and the longer experience with transplantation as a successful treatment modality in the case of ESRD. The disparity in the number of transplants of different types of organs may decrease as continuing developments in the technology of transplantation are reflected in the increased success rate of other types of transplants. At this time, policy statements by other groups tend to focus on renal transplantation.

The committee noted that a previous (IOM, 1991) report included coverage policy recommendations at the request of the Congress. In *Kidney Failure and the Federal Government*, the IOM committee then in place recommended that all ESRD patients who are citizens or resident aliens of the United States be eligible for Medicare coverage, that the time limit on coverage for immunosuppressive drugs be eliminated, and that other Medicare benefits also be extended to these patients without time limits. The earlier report did not address transplants of organs other than the kidney.

The Office of Technology Assessment (OTA) released a report, *Outpatient Immunosuppressive Drugs Under Medicare,* in 1991. OTA did not make recommendations to Congress, but, rather, analyzed a series of policy options. Regarding the time limit on coverage, OTA observed that if Congress decided to make a change in this aspect of Medicare law, it could either extend coverage for a limited time (which is what Congress eventually did) or eliminate the time limit altogether. OTA noted that extending coverage would reduce any inequity in access to transplants due to ability to pay and that eliminating the time limit completely would accomplish this best. OTA also noted that such a step would be likely to shift financing from other sources to Medicare.

In a 1997 position statement entitled *The Decade of Transplantation,* the American Society of Transplant Physicians (ASTP; since renamed American Society of Transplantation, AST) called for extending payment for immunosuppressive drugs for transplants from the current three years to the life of the graft. The AST argued that the ESRD program would experience dramatic savings by extending graft life through appropriate drug regimens. They did not give details on how these savings would be realized. Presumably, they would result from lower rates of graft rejection followed by return to dialysis or retransplantation.

The National Kidney Foundation (NKF) also advocates the elimination of the time limits on Medicare coverage. It too argues that this would save Medicare money.

COMMITTEE FINDINGS AND CONCLUSIONS

In developing its findings and conclusions, the committee benefited from the review of the literature presented in Appendix D and the discussion during a public workshop that included clinicians, researchers, and members of the public (see Appendix A). Unfortunately, little systematic research is available to assess the health and cost consequences of the current coverage limit on immunosuppressive drugs. The committee's findings, as discussed in this chapter, are summarized briefly below. Its conclusions about Medicare coverage follow:

Findings

Burden of Disease. The committee found strong evidence that organ transplants, the majority of which are kidney transplants, are increasingly common, with more than 20,000 performed per year and approximately 80,000 patients now living with functioning grafts. The committee found further strong evidence that virtually all transplant recipients require immunosuppressive drugs to avoid immunologic rejection of their grafts.

Effective Treatments Available. The committee found strong evidence that the immunosuppressive agents now available are effective in reducing organ rejection. Rates of long-term recipient survival with functioning grafts have increased, but patients who do not get adequate doses of immunosuppressive drugs have a higher rate of rejection than transplant recipients who can maintain the appropriate drug regimen.

Benefits of Drugs Outweigh Harms. The committee found strong evidence that although immunosuppressive agents can have serious side effects, their benefits to transplant patients outweigh the side effects. The committee noted that the chronic condition of immunosuppression is generally manageable under the supervision of experienced physicians. The alternative treatment for patients with ESRD, dialysis, does not provide the same quality of life as a functioning renal graft. The alternative for those with other kinds of organ failure is generally death.

Burden of Disease from Noncompliance. The committee found a body of literature that, although small and not including randomized controlled trials, was still persuasive that some otherwise functioning grafts are lost because of the patient's lack of compliance with the immunosuppressive drug regimen.

Coverage Effective in Reducing Noncompliance. The committee found a body of literature which, although small and not including randomized controlled trials, still suggested that lack of financial access to necessary drugs is one factor in lack of compliance with immunosuppressive drug regimens and such noncompliance contributes to graft failure and loss.

Benefits of Coverage Outweigh Harms. For the individual, the health and other benefits of drug coverage surely outweigh possible harms. The potential *harm* of extending Medicare coverage would involve not the transplant recipient but other Medicare beneficiaries who might benefit if the same resources were directed elsewhere within Medicare. A cost-effectiveness analysis could very well identify alternative uses of these resources that would result in more benefit (e.g., QALYs) for these resources, The committee recognized this trade-off as a critical issue, but also an issue beyond the scope of this report.

Possible Directions for Further Research

The committee was hampered by lack of evidence in several areas, including not only medical questions pertaining to transplantation but also factors affecting patient compliance with medical advice and the comparison of the costs of alternative treatments that receive substantial public funding. Given the cost and risks associated with long-term use of immunosuppressive drugs, the prospect of alternatives that are safer, less expensive, or both is obviously attractive.

For the present, a better understanding of the factors that support or obstruct compliance with therapeutic regimens would be helpful. Compliance is clearly a complex phenomenon that is difficult to study. However, because noncompliance puts pressure on an already scarce lifesaving resource, it is important to try to identify barriers to compliance that are amenable to mitigation through dose alteration, financial, educational, or other strategies. Research indicating that patients are more compliant just before contact with health care professionals suggests that research on practical, affordable ways of increasing such contacts might be productive.

For example, a considerable body of research involving telephone contact has accumulated in recent years, and attention is now being paid to the role of e-mail in changing communication between physicians and their patients. A 1996 IOM report discussed several applications of regular or even automated telephone patient monitoring programs while noting that the literature evaluating the effectiveness of telemedicine was sparse (IOM, 1996). Several other recent publications report encouraging results with telephone and/or other electronic contacts both to monitor clinical signs and to encourage compliance with drug regimens (Alemi et al., 1996, Finkelstein et al., 1996; Friedman et al., 1996, 1998; Hetzer et al., 1998); although other reports indicate that some applications have been less successful with some patient groups (Alemi et al., 1997).

The committee also encourages the National Kidney Foundation and George Mason University in their survey of kidney transplant patients. The survey may improve understanding of the impact of coverage on both patient compliance and other social and economic activities such as employment.

Conclusions

Good evidence supports patients' continued need for immunosuppressive therapy and the increased risk of graft loss if they cannot follow the prescribed drug regimen. **Given this evidence and the existing Medicare policy of supporting organ transplants, the rationale for eliminating the current time limits for coverage of immunosuppressive drugs for all solid organ transplant recipients is strong**. Although people who lose coverage often find ways to obtain sufficient drugs to maintain immunosuppression, experience and limited evidence suggest that some grafts—and some lives—are eventually lost for lack of coverage. The estimated five-year net cost to Medicare of eliminating the three-year limit on coverage would be approximately $778 million if extended coverage were limited to those eligible by virtue of age or disability, and $1.06 billion if the time limit was also removed for those who have been Medicare-eligible only by reason of an ESRD diagnosis.

In addition to the economic and possible clinical consequences of time-limited drug coverage for transplant recipients, the committee notes that current policy has societal implications. Organs are a scarce resource for which demand far outstrips supply. Every graft failure that results in retransplantation is a special burden on this limited supply. Beyond those immediately affected, the larger society of citizens has a strong interest in the successful maintenance of grafts to protect their potential access or that of their loved ones.

From a societal perspective, elimination of the time limit on coverage of immunosuppressive drugs for transplant patients presents some delicate ethical and policy considerations. On the one hand, recipients of organ transplants who are eligible for Medicare by reason of age, disability, or ESRD already have a drug benefit that few other classes of beneficiaries have, and ESRD-qualified Medicare beneficiaries are generally treated as a special group. On the other hand, termination of the drug benefit at the end of three years may result in more graft loss, more expenses for treatment of graft rejection and possible return to dialysis, and added demands for scarce organs for retransplantation. The committee returns to this issue in Chapter 6.

6

Future Directions

The preceding chapters of this report respond to the provisions of the Balanced Budget Act of 1997 that asked for an assessment of "the short- and long-term benefits, and costs to Medicare" of extending Medicare coverage for certain preventive and other services. This final chapter examines some broader concerns about the processes for making coverage decisions and the research and organizational infrastructure for this decisionmaking. It also briefly examines the limits of coverage as a means of improving health services and outcomes and the limits of evidence as a means of resolving policy and ethical questions. In addition, this chapter examines how current Medicare coverage of preventive services compares to the clinical practice recommendations of the U.S. Preventive Services Task Force.

LINKING EVIDENCE TO MEDICARE COVERAGE: THE CASE OF PREVENTIVE SERVICES

One criticism of Congress's service-by-service approach to coverage decisions about preventive services, prescription drugs, and other generally excluded categories of care is that it may favor services for high-profile conditions and technologies that have strong lobbying groups but not necessarily a strong evidence base. Another criticism is that the focus on covering specific services can distract policymakers, advocates, and clinicians from problems in the organization and delivery of services that limit the routine use of preventive services and other interventions known to be effective.

Congress first made an exception to the general coverage exclusion for preventive services in 1980 when it authorized Medicare coverage of pneumococcal pneumonia vaccine. Table 6-1 lists the preventive services that Congress has now authorized for coverage. For several of these services, Congress has waived application of the Part B deductible and 20 percent coinsurance. Frequency limits are also specified for several services, and coverage is sometimes conditional on the presence of certain risk factors.

All the covered services listed in the body of Table 6-1 involve either primary prevention (keeping people from developing disease) or secondary prevention (identifying risk factors or detecting disease early) as discussed in Chapter 3. The service noted in the footnote—outpatient self-management training and supplies for diabetics—falls in the category of tertiary preventive services, which is more typically described as patient management for those already diagnosed with a medical problem. The discussion below considers only primary and secondary preventive services.

Given Medicare's statutory goal of covering "medically necessary" services and the committee's experience with the work of the U.S. Preventive Services Task Force (USPSTF) in assessing evidence about the effectiveness of various

TABLE 6-1 Preventive Services Covered by Medicare

Service (effective date of coverage)	Special Provisions
Pneumococcol vaccine (1981)	No coinsurance; deductible not applied
Hepatitis B vaccine (1984)	High- or intermediate-risk beneficiaries
Cervical cancer screening by Pap smear (1990) and pelvic examination (1998)	Every 3 years for most beneficiaries; 20% coinsurance; deductible not applied
Influenza vaccine (1991)	No coinsurance, deductible not applied
Breast cancer screening by mammography (1991, 1998)	Every year for beneficiaries ≥ 40; 20% coinsurance, no deductible
Colorectal cancer screening (1998)	20% coinsurance, deductible applied; details differ for different tests and risk groups
Osteoporosis screening by bone densitometry (1998)	For high-risk beneficiaries; 20% coinsurance and deductible applied
Prostate cancer screening by prostate specific antigen (PSA) and digital rectal examination DRE (2000)	No cost sharing for PSA; 20% coinsurance; deductible for DRE

NOTE: In 1997, Congress also added coverage for outpatient self-management training and supplies for those diagnosed with diabetes.

SOURCE: HCFA, 1999b, *Carriers Manual,* Chapter 3 (which includes other details about coverage administration for these services).

services, it is reasonable to examine the match between the services recommended by the Task Force and those now covered by Medicare. As described earlier in this report, the Task Force is charged by the Department of Health and Human Services (DHHS) with making recommendations that rely extensively on rigorous assessment of scientific evidence about the benefits and harms of preventive services provided by physicians, nurse practitioners, and other clinicians. The Task Force is not charged with making recommendations about coverage of preventive services. Its published assessments to date have not included cost-effectiveness analyses, although such analyses are planned (David Atkins, personal communication, October 1999).

The list of preventive services now covered by Medicare excludes some services that the 1996 report of the U.S. Preventive Services Task Force recommended as part of a periodic health visit for asymptomatic people over age 64. The list also includes a few services that were not recommended by the Task Force. Table 6-2 lists the recommended services, which include 8 screening services and 15 counseling services.

The clinical screening services recommended by the Task Force for older persons but not covered by Medicare are blood pressure testing, height and weight checks, and screening for vision and hearing impairment and problem drinking. Some of these services, in particular, blood pressure tests, are routine parts of patient visits for many older people who see a physician or nurse practitioner for a variety of reasons, including screenings covered by Medicare and care for existing medical problems. About 90 percent of Medicare beneficiaries have at least one physician visit a year (HCFA, 1998a).

The other noncovered preventive services that the Task Force recommends for those over age 64 involve patient education and counseling about tobacco cessation, diet, alcohol, physical activity, seat belts, motorcycle and bicycle helmets, firearms, fall prevention, hormone replacement therapy, sexually transmitted diseases, CPR training, dental visits and dental hygiene, smoke detectors, and settings for hot water heaters. It should be noted that some education and counseling recommendations were "based on good evidence of the effectiveness of counseling per se" whereas others were made "primarily on the basis of a strong link between behavior and disease" (USPSTF, 1996, p. xxvi). Recommendations based only on the latter rationale, which were described as such, included counseling or education about physical activity, seat belt and helmet use, dental hygiene, sexually transmitted diseases, firearms, smoke detectors, and water heaters. Because Medicare beneficiaries often have one or more chronic health problems such as high blood pressure or arthritis, many Medicare-covered physician visits are likely to involve some attention to tobacco, diet, physical activity, and other risk factors covered in the Task Force list.

TABLE 6-2 Interventions Considered and Recommended by USPSTF for Periodic Health Examinations for Persons Age 65 and Older

SCREENING	**Injury Prevention**
Blood pressure	Lap/shoulder belts
Height and weight	Motorcycle and bicycle helmets
Fecal occult blood test and/or sigmoid-	Fall prevention
oscopy	Safe storage/removal of firearms
Mammogram ± clinical breast exam	Smoke detector
(women ≤ 69 years old)	Set hot water heater to <120°F–130°F
Papanicolaou (Pap) test (women)	CPR training for household members
Vision screening	
Assess for hearing impairment	**Dental Health**
Assess for problem drinking	Regular visits to dental care provider
	Floss, brush with fluoride toothpaste
COUNSELING	daily
Substance Use	
Tobacco cessation	**Sexual Behavior**
Avoid alcohol/drug use while driving,	STD prevention: avoid high-risk sexual
swimming, boating, etc.	behavior, use condoms
Diet and Exercise	**IMMUNIZATIONS**
Limit fat and cholesterol; maintain caloric	Pneumococcal vaccine
balance; emphasize grains, fruits, vege-	Influenza
tables	Tetanus-diphtheria (Td) boosters
Adequate calcium intake (women)	
Regular physical activity	**CHEMOPROPHYLAXIS**
	Discuss hormone prophylaxis (women)

NOTE: CPR = cardiopulmonary resuscitation; STD = sexually transmitted disease.

SOURCE: Table 4, p. xviii, USPSTF, 1996.

When Congress approved a number of additional preventive services for coverage in 1997, it included two services that were not among those recommended by the USPSTF. Specifically, the Task Force judged the evidence insufficient to recommend for or against osteoporosis screening by bone densitometry. Further, it judged the evidence sufficient to recommend that men *not* be screened for prostate cancer. Concern about such issues led the committee to consider coverage decisionmaking for preventive and other services more generally.

To the extent that Medicare covers such services, it gives them a special prominence that could divert patients, clinicians, and others (1) from undertaking more beneficial actions and (2) from adequately considering the potential of some preventive services to harm people who undergo unnecessary testing or treatment based on false positive screening results. Some argue that preventive services should ordinarily face stricter scrutiny than treatment services because rather than responding to sick people who need treatment, they invite healthy people to receive care. Any untoward effect of a preventive service (e.g., vaccine reaction, false positive screening result leading to unnecessary testing and treatment) puts healthy people at risk.

Some have proposed that Congress delegate decisions about preventive services coverage to the USPSTF. Such delegation could be a bigger step than Congress wishes to take at this time. Moreover, such a step could damage still evolving efforts to develop credible, evidence-based recommendations for clinical care. For example, if recommendations of the Task Force were sufficient to "qualify" a service for Medicare coverage, this could put a great deal more lobbying pressure on the citizen experts who serve on that group. Also, the Task Force is not intended or constituted to consider the cost and other implications of its recommendations for the Medicare program.

An alternative would be for Congress to direct DHHS to continue to support the Task Force and the Agency for Health Care Policy and Research (AHCPR) in rigorously assessing the evidence base for clinical preventive services and in evaluating the cost-effectiveness of these services. For services recommended for inclusion in a periodic health examination, Congress could then direct the Health Care Financing Administration (HCFA) through the new Medicare Coverage Advisory Committee to consider costs, cost-effectiveness, and feasibility in the context of the Medicare program. HCFA could also be directed to publish its recommendations in the *Federal Register* for public comment just as it now publishes its proposed coverage decisions. In addition, HCFA could, as it does now, ask AHCPR and private technology assessment organizations to review evidence for any preventive services not already evaluated by USPSTF or to reevaluate services for which new evidence or cost concerns had emerged. One objective of this general approach would be to retain the Task Force's focus on clinical care recommendations and let HCFA focus on coverage. Regardless of where responsibility for coverage decisions is located, the information, methods, and processes used should provide decisionmakers with the best available data and analyses on the effectiveness, costs, and cost-effectiveness of health services.

STRENGTHENING THE INFRASTRUCTURE FOR COVERAGE DECISIONS

The committee's application of the analytic framework outlined in Chapter 2 reinforced its view that this evidence-based approach can be a powerful tool for guiding clinical and policy decisions. For both new technologies and current practices, it helps make clear the extent to which there is good evidence about the benefits and harms of a particular intervention and points those who conduct and fund research toward important health problems and interventions for which good evidence does not exist. It puts pressure on clinicians to abandon practices that are clearly not beneficial and to apply and recommend practices that have been identified as worthwhile. It likewise supports governments and others who pay for care in revising coverage, reimbursement, quality assessment, and related policies to discourage nonbeneficial services and encourage effective care.

The work reported here also makes clear the value of public and private efforts to build a stronger infrastructure for clinical, public health, and other health care decisions. The term "infrastructure" here means

1. clinical, epidemiological, health services, and other research that helps clinicians and policymakers judge the extent to which different health care strategies are effective in improving health outcomes and have benefits that exceed harms;

2. methods for conducting valid research, measuring outcomes accurately and meaningfully, summarizing data usefully, assessing resource implications of decisions, and otherwise helping ensure the credibility and utility of research to clinicians, policymakers, and others; and

3. organizational structures and procedures for initiating and managing knowledge-building efforts, effectively applying knowledge to clinical and policy decisions, and then monitoring results to guide future activities.

Commitment to Technology Assessment

The fluctuating policy support for technology assessment and evidence-based recommendations for clinical practice and coverage policy is a continuing concern. Even within the past decade, political controversies over assessments of scientific evidence have threatened the survival of AHCPR (e.g., see Butler, 1996; de Jong, 1995; Kahn, 1998) and put advisory groups within the National Institutes of Health at odds with each other (e.g., see Taubes, 1997a,b). The Health Care Financing Administration has had a variety of problems relating to budget constraints and workloads, disagreements about the role of cost-effectiveness analyses, challenges to its coverage advisory process, and other matters. Congress eliminated its own technology advisory agency (the OTA) in 1995 (Leary, 1995). Nonetheless, the last decade has still seen both the creation of more formal, continuing links between government and nongovernmental expertise and the expansion of tools for communicating with health professionals and the public about the evidence base for health services (Gaus, 1997; Graham, 1998).

To tackle the weaknesses in the infrastructure for coverage decisionmaking and improve the value of Medicare spending will require resources. For example, adding new tasks for HCFA or other agencies without adding new resources could do more harm than good if agencies simply reroute resources from quality monitoring or other important administrative responsibilities. Although additional resources for infrastructure improvements would be minuscule compared to the total budget for Medicare or the National Institutes of Health, they nonetheless could be difficult to commit under budget neutrality rules.

Examples of Specific Infrastructure Weaknesses

In addition to broader concerns about the depth of commitment to the conduct and use of technology assessments and effectiveness research, the committee was also struck by certain specific weaknesses in the foundation for both clinical and coverage decisionmaking. One such weakness is the still-limited use in clinical research of *outcomes measures that are meaningful to patients and consumers*. Meaningfulness relates to the kinds of benefits and harms identified, the magnitude of the effect of an intervention on an outcome, and individual preferences about different outcomes. Much is assumed but relatively little is known about how individuals perceive the possible benefits and harms of different health services. Physiological measures are important and convenient but not sufficient for assessing whether interventions improve health as people actually experience it (e.g., see Fleming and DeMets, 1996; Psaty, 1999).

A related concern is the even sparser *work to assess individual and societal preferences for the outcomes of different health interventions*. Clinicians, policymakers, and health services researchers may impute their own values to patients and the public, but there is reason to question this approach. A number of investigators have documented disagreement in values or preferences, for example, when patient, family, and physician responses are compared on preferences about care at the end of life (Lynn et al., 1995, 1997; SUPPORT Principal Investigators, 1995).

Without sound preference or utility information, the usefulness of cost-effectiveness analyses and other kinds of comparisons may be compromised. The calculation of quality-adjusted life years or similar summary measures of health status depends not only on evidence about the benefits and harms of interventions but also on information about how people value these outcomes.

Just as knowledge of people's preferences is limited so is *knowledge of people's understanding of the possible harms* as well as the possible benefits of screening or other interventions. Even when special efforts have been made to present risk information clearly, a number of studies have found that people vary greatly in their ability to accurately interpret quantitative information about health risks and benefits and that misinterpretations are common (e.g., see Hux and Naylor, 1995; Ransohoff and Harris, 1997; Schwartz et al., 1997; Woloshin et al., 1999a). If people do not understand such information, then informed decisionmaking may be an illusion.

Effective methods for communicating information to patients and consumers and helping them make informed decisions can also be considered part of the infrastructure for health care decisionmaking. These methods are crucial to the still evolving *concept of shared decisionmaking*, which is intended to strengthen patient involvement in care decisions, especially in "close call" situations when the evidence about benefits and harms of different interventions is weak and patient perceptions are variable or poorly understood (Flood et al., 1996; Morgan et al., 1997; Pauker and Kassirer, 1997; Woolf, 1997). At its most formal, shared decisionmaking is a process in which the clinician (1) describes the available options and their associated benefits and harms (including their likelihood and magnitude and the quality of the evidence on which the estimates are based); (2) checks patient understanding of the information; (3) presents a recommendation if asked; and (4) helps the patient to assess the information and the importance of possible outcomes in his or her own life and, then, make a decision. Further research is needed to evaluate the effectiveness and feasibility of specific methods and techniques for accomplishing the shared decisionmaking tasks just described.

Role of Cost and Cost-Effectiveness Analyses

In addition to strengthening the information and technical foundations for cost and cost-effectiveness analyses, the role of these analyses in coverage decisionmaking needs further attention. Currently, the extent to which cost, cost-effectiveness, or both are explicitly considered in coverage decisions varies depending on who makes the decision and whether the decision involves a new technology or a previously excluded service. For example:

- When legislators consider preventive care, dental services, and other interventions that are now statutorily excluded from Medicare coverage, costs, if not cost-effectiveness, are routinely weighed in decisions to extend coverage.
- When HCFA makes coverage determinations about new technologies that fit under existing categories of covered services, its decisions are not directly governed by the "budget neutrality" rules that Congress has adopted for itself.
- When HCFA considers new technologies, it applies criteria of effectiveness that are not systematically applied to established technologies.

During the first three decades following the establishment of Medicare, Congress appeared to be sensitive to issues of clinical effectiveness and cost-effectiveness. For example, at the behest of Congress, the now defunct Office of Technology Assessment (OTA) undertook analyses of the cost-effectiveness of several preventive services. Congress also authorized DHHS to undertake preventive services demonstration projects that included assessments of cost-effectiveness. A study of coverage exceptions from 1965 to 1990 identified evidence of favorable cost-effectiveness ratios as one factor differentiating services for which Congress had approved coverage from those not approved (Schauffler, 1993).

Attempts by HCFA to include cost-effectiveness among the explicit criteria for coverage decisionmaking have so far been unsuccessful.[1] The point is not that resources should be allocated for cost-effectiveness analyses for all currently covered services (a massive task) or that cost-effectiveness should be the only criterion for coverage decisions. It is, rather, that the current process makes it difficult to compare the expected benefits, harms, and costs—that is, to judge the probable value—of different health care decisions. Similarly, the procedure relied on by Congress for estimating the costs to Medicare of covering a new service—although necessary for understanding budgetary implications—provides a very incomplete picture of the value for money of such an action.

Although the weakness of our knowledge base is one obstacle to systematic comparisons of health care services and technologies, other factors probably play a greater role in decisionmaking. Policies that would make high costs (or cost-effectiveness) an explicit factor in coverage decisions tend to be controversial, especially if the insurance is provided without regard to income and if the decision involves an already-covered category of services. Certainly, much of the controversy about managed care plans focuses on the ways these organizations factor costs into decisions about the care available to their enrollees. In contrast, it seems easier politically to accept high costs (without respect to cost-effectiveness) as a reason for not making public or private health insurance itself available to those who lack such coverage altogether.

Within these political constraints, it is still possible to take some steps that make more apparent the trade-offs involved in coverage decisions. A small step in this direction would be for Congress to encourage and support AHCPR, HCFA, and other relevant agencies in preparing cost-effectiveness analyses for informational purposes, if not for coverage decisionmaking. For example, as suggested in Chapter 4, Congress could direct the Health Care Financing Administration to develop evidence-based recommendations for covering dental care in conjunction with certain serious medical conditions and treatments. Similarly, as suggested above, for the preventive services recommended by the USPSTF, Congress could direct the Health Care Financing Administration to assess these services in the context of the Medicare program and then make coverage recommendations. This would provide Congress systematic analyses of the potential benefits, harms, and costs of covering additional preventive services.

---

[1] For durable medical equipment, HCFA regulations provide that if a contractor determines that there is a medically appropriate and realistically feasible alternative pattern of care for which payment could be made, payment should be based on the reasonable charge for this alternative rather than a higher cost alternative for which a claim has been submitted (HCFA, 1999b, *Carriers Manual,* section 2100.2). This "least costly alternative" criterion may also be applied at a contractor's discretion to other services (HCFA, 1999b, *Program Integrity Manual,* chapter 3, section 3.1.1).

In addition, the committee's work has suggested some directions for research related to the specific clinical services and conditions reviewed here. For example, the discussion of skin cancer screening has suggested the importance of more research on the methods of identifying and targeting high-risk individuals for education and, possibly, screening. It also points to the opportunities for learning from the screening research of other nations and, by implication, the importance of the growing worldwide network of evidence-based medicine initiatives and communication. The discussion of "medically necessary dental services" has illustrated important gaps in evidence about how dental problems and dental care affect outcomes for people with a number of life-threatening medical problems. The discussion of immunosuppressive drugs for transplant recipients points to our still limited understanding of patient nonadherence to treatment recommendations.

Linking Evidence to Recommendations

Despite steps taken by public and private organizations to improve information and processes for coverage decisionmaking, no common standards of evidence govern the multiple decisionmakers now involved. This is particularly true for the early stages when innovative technologies first come to the attention of health plans.

Moreover, the criteria for making coverage recommendations or decisions may not be explicit or public, despite calls for health plans to be more rigorous and open about these criteria (e.g., see IOM, 1989). For each of the conditions examined, the committee's review of statements by other organizations revealed both substantive disagreement and differences in the extent to which recommendations were accompanied by descriptions of the supporting evidence.

Such variability is not surprising given variations in the processes used by different organizations to develop their recommendations. All use some degree of expert judgment and consensus, but the role of evidence in informing judgment is not at all clear in many cases. This makes it difficult to identify the basis for inconsistent recommendations and judge their credibility. One additional reason for explicitly linking practice or coverage recommendations to evidence reviews is that such reviews—along with judgments about the population burden of disease, costs, and productive avenues for research—can help decisionmakers set priorities for future biomedical, clinical and health services research.

THE LIMITS OF COVERAGE

Even those fortunate enough to have coverage from Medicare or other sources often do not receive recommended preventive (or other) services (e.g., see Jaen et al., 1994; Morrissey et al., 1995; Roos et al., 1999). In some cases, beneficiaries fail to seek these services or their physicians fail to provide, recommend, or discuss these services. For services that involve referrals to other clinicians or specialized facilities, people may fail to follow up for a variety of reasons including forgetfulness, time demands, and cost.

The fact that coverage fails to guarantee use of effective services is not, of course, an argument for not covering them. It is, however, an argument for paying attention to noncoverage obstacles to care and to strategies for overcoming such obstacles. Such strategies aim to strengthen the organizational infrastructure for disease prevention and health promotion.

In particular, many have recognized the obstacles to implementing recommended clinical preventive measures in primary care settings and have supported practical programs and research to address these obstacles (Wolfe et al., 1996). For example, the DHHS initiative "Put Prevention into Practice" has developed a set of materials for the physician office or clinic including patient education brochures, a handbook for clinicians, posters for waiting and examination rooms, "alert" stickers for medical records, and reminder postcards (AHCPR, 1998). It cannot, of course, be assumed that such materials, even if ordered, will be used or, if used, will be effective (McVea et al., 1996).

Moreover, community-based preventive programs may be more successful (and less expensive) in getting services to high-risk groups than coverage or other approaches that rely on people visiting a physician (Roos et al., 1999). This is, for example, suggested by data from Canadian provinces that have developed community-based screening programs, in part to reach people who do not use covered preventive services under the government health insurance program (de Grasse et al., 1999; Olivotto et al., 1999).

One claim in favor of beneficiary enrollment in health maintenance organizations (HMOs) is that some of the obstacles to preventive care may be more effectively tackled in HMOs and similar health plans than in fee-for-service health care (e.g., see Heiser and St. Peter, 1997; Mandelson and Thompson, 1998). For example, these organizations can, in principle, mobilize their information systems to identify enrolled members who have not received preventive services from the plan and then use reminder systems to prompt these members to seek or accept recommended services. Likewise, they can use their information systems to track clinician performance in providing recommended services and then, as appropriate, employ educational efforts (e.g., evidence-based practice guidelines), performance feedback, peer comparison data, and other strategies to encourage clinicians to provide or advise recommended services.[2] For

---

[2]In addition, because the provision of certain preventive services is fairly easy to track, their provision is frequently monitored by groups assessing and comparing the performance of health plans, for example, the National Committee for Quality Assurance (NCQA, 1999). If services not demonstrated to be effective are covered and monitored, some plans could divert resources from other more effective services that were not

interventions with relatively short-term outcomes, health plans may also be able to assess health as well as utilization outcomes, although enrollment turnover can complicate such assessments.

Studies generally show higher use of preventive services in HMOs compared to fee-for-service medicine (Gordon et al., 1998). The degree to which higher-risk individuals are more effectively reached in managed care programs is, however, less clear and, thus, an important question for further research (Amonkar et al., 1999; Schauffler and Rodriguez, 1993).

In the process of examining the obstacles to the implementation of preventive services recommendations, decisionmakers may decide that one strategic step is to set priorities for the delivery of preventive services and focus resources on higher-priority services. For example, a health plan might work to increase the use of clearly effective services, especially in higher-risk groups with lower levels of utilization, while providing marginally beneficial or disputed services only to those who request and still want such services after a discussion of potential benefits and harms (Thompson, 1996).

As is true for health care services themselves, the effectiveness of organizational efforts to improve the delivery of services cannot be assumed. Although evaluation is expensive and often difficult, especially when controlled studies are attempted, organizational initiatives also need to be evaluated.

THE LIMITS OF EVIDENCE

Lack of evidence was one difficulty this committee faced in reaching conclusions. In addition, the committee encountered a number of policy and ethical questions that could not be ignored, although their thorough examination was beyond the group's charge.

For example, the committee is hardly the first to note the many complexities created by Medicare coverage distinctions for people with and without end-stage renal disease (ESRD); for ESRD patients on dialysis versus those who receive kidney transplants; for kidney versus other transplant candidates or recipients; and for Medicare-covered transplant recipients versus other beneficiaries needing expensive outpatient drugs (IOM, 1991). Because Medicare now covers immunosuppressive drugs for up to three years after transplantation and because government policy more generally promotes guardianship of organs before and after transplantation, it seems straightforward to argue for elimination of the three-year limit. Fairly quickly, however, the question arises about whether this is fair, given that the lives and well-being of many Medicare beneficiaries with other medical problems depend on expensive prescription drugs that would continue to be excluded from coverage.

---

included in performance monitoring systems in order to invest in providing services that would count toward their performance score.

The case of immunosuppressive drugs highlights the frustrations that policymakers and clinicians can encounter in trying to develop rational and consistent coverage policies on an incremental basis as innovative technologies emerge and new evidence about established technologies accumulates. Despite such problems with incremental policy development, recent experiences with more global efforts to define a total package of covered services for Americans covered by public and private health insurance have had their own problems. These problems reflect, in part, the larger failure of comprehensive national health care reform in the early 1990s (e.g., see Budetti, 1997; Feder and Levitt, 1995; Iglehart, 1995; Yankelovich, 1995). The most comprehensive state initiative—which was undertaken by policymakers and citizens in Oregon—has been cut back in scope and has not prompted much imitation in other states (Bodenheimer, 1997a,b; Ham, 1998; Jacobs et al., 1999; Leichter, 1999). Efforts to define a comprehensive package of basic benefits present formidable technical, intellectual, and cultural challenges. Certainly, when all services are, in principle, "on the table," divisive debates among advocates of different services become more likely.

For clinical preventive services, the incremental adoption of exceptions to Medicare's general exclusion of coverage has probably had some positive aspects. The exclusion may have been originally motivated on grounds that preventive services were relatively inexpensive and could be budgeted. Subsequent attempts to breach the exclusion have encouraged efforts to systematically assess—rather than assume—the effectiveness and cost-effectiveness of specific clinical preventive services. Such analyses appear to have helped persuade decisionmakers to authorize coverage for effective services and even to favor some of these services over treatment services by waiving beneficiary cost sharing. At the same time, however, Congress has authorized coverage for certain services for which evidence is inconclusive or disputed.

More generally, whether to consider cost-effectiveness in coverage decisions about preventive and other services raises political and ethical questions that have important implications for the ways in which limited resources are distributed among different worthy purposes. Evidence cannot usually answer such fundamental political and ethical questions. It can, however, often clarify the rationales and potential consequences of different answers and help policymakers and their constituents assess the actual consequences—for good and ill—of their decisions.

References

AAD (American Academy of Dermatology). What Is Skin Cancer? 1994a. http://www. aad.org/SkinCancerNews/WhatIsSkinCancer. Accessed July 6, 1999.

AAD. ABCDs of Melanoma Detection. 1994b. http://www.aad.org/SkinCancerNews/ WhatIsSkinCancer. Accessed July 6, 1999.

AAFP (American Academy of Family Practice). Information from Your Family Doctor: How to Prevent Skin Cancer. 1998. http://www.aafp.org/patientinfo/980915a.html. Accessed July 6, 1999.

Abbasoglu, O., M.F. Levy, B.B. Brkic, G. Testa, D.R. Jeyarajah, R.M. Goldstein, et al. Ten Years of Liver Transplantation: An Evolving Understanding of Late Graft Loss. *Transplantation* 64(12):1801–1807, 1997.

ACPM (American College of Preventive Medicine). Policy Statement: Screening for Skin Cancer. *American Journal of Preventive Medicine* 14(1):80–82, 1998. http:// www.acpm.org. Accessed July 6, 1999.

ACS (American Cancer Society). *Cancer Facts and Figures—1999*. Atlanta: ACS, 1999a.

ACS. *Skin Cancer—Melanoma: Detection and Symptoms.* 1999b. Last updated 4/26/1999. http://www3.cancer.org/cancerinfo/main_cont.asp?st=ds&ct=50. Accessed July 7, 1999.

ACS. *Skin Cancer—Nonmelanoma: Detection and Symptoms.* 1999c. Last updated 1/11/99 http://www3.cancer.org/cancerinfo/main_cont.asp?st=ds&ct=51. Accessed July 7, 1999.

AHA (American Heart Association). 1999 Heart and Stroke Statistical Update: Major Cardiovascular Diseases. 1999. http://www.americanheart.org/statistics. Accessed August 24, 1999.

AHCPR (Agency for Health Care Policy and Research, U.S. Department of Health and Human Services). *Put Prevention into Practice: Overview.* 1998. http://www.ahcpr. gov/ppip. Accessed August 1, 1999.

Albandar, J.M., and A. Kingman. Gingival Recession, Gingival Bleeding, and Dental Calculus in Adults 30 Years of Age and Older in the United States. *Journal of Periodontology* 70(1):30–43, 1999.

142 EXTENDING MEDICARE COVERAGE

Albert, V.A., H.K. Koh, A.C. Geller, D.R. Miller, M.N. Prout, and R.A. Lew. Years of
Potential Life Lost: Another Indicator of the Impact of Cutaneous Malignant Melanoma on Society. *Journal of the American Academy of Dermatology* 23:308–310,
1990.

Alemi, F., S.A. Alemagno, J. Goldhagen, L. Ash, B. Finkelstein, A. Lavin, et al. Com-
puter Reminders Improve On Time Immunization Rates. *Medical Care* 34(10
Suppl.):OS45–51, 1996.

Alemi, F., M. Jackson, T. Parren, L. Williams B. Cavor, S. Llorens, and M. Mosavel.
Participation in Teleconference Support Groups: Application to Drug-Using Preg-
nant Patients. *Journal of Medical Systems* 21(2):119–125, 1997.

Amonkar, M.M., S. Madhavan, S.A. Rosenbluth, and K.J. Simon. Barriers and Facilita-
tors to Providing Common Preventive Screening Services in a Managed Care Setting. *Journal of Community Health* 24(3):229–247, 1999.

Anderson, G., M.A. Hall, and T.R. Smith. When Courts Review Medical Appropriations.
Medical Care 36(8):295–302, 1998.

Arndt, K.A., P. Leboit, J. Robinson, and B.Wintroub. *Cutaneous Medicine and Surgery:
An Integrated Program in Dermatology.* Philadelphia: W.B. Saunders, 1995.

ASDS (American Society for Dermatological Surgery). *Skin Cancer Fact Sheet.* http://
www.asds-net.org/scfactsheet.html. Accessed July 7, 1999.

Bagley, G.P., and K. McVearry. Medicare Coverage for Oncology Services. *Cancer*
82(10 Suppl.):1991–1994, 1998.

Bailar, J.C., III. The Promise and Problems of Meta-Analysis. *New England Journal of
Medicine* 337(8):559–561, 1997.

Balch, C.M., S.J. Soong, A.A. Bartolucci, M.M. Urist, C.P. Karakousis, T.J. Smith, et al.
Efficacy of an Elective Regional Lymph Node Dissection of 1 to 4 mm Thick Melanomas for Patients 60 Years of Age and Younger. *Annals of Surgery* 224(3):255–
263, 1996.

Ball, R.M. What Medicare's Architects Had in Mind. *Health Affairs* 14(4):62–72. 1995.

Bame, S.I. Treatment Regime Complexity and Patient Compliance. Abstract presented at
the 1995 Association for Health Services Research Annual Meeting on Medical Effectiveness and Patient Outcomes Research: What Works in Health Care, Chicago,
June 5–6, 1995.

Barratt, A., L. Irwig, P. Glasziou, R.G. Cumming, A. Raffle, N. Hicks, et al. Users'
Guides to the Medical Literature: XVII. How to Use Guidelines and Recommenda-
tions About Screening. Evidence-Based Medicine Working Group. *Journal of the
American Medical Association* 281(21):2029–2034, 1999.

Beck, J. R. Garcia, G. Heiss, P.S. Vokonas, and S. Offenbacher. Periodontal Disease and
Cardiovascular Disease. *Journal of Periodontology* 67:1123–1137, 1996.

Bedwinek, J.M., L.J. Shukovsky, G.H. Fletcher, and T.E. Daley. Osteoradionecrosis in
Patients Treated with Definitive Radiotherapy for Squamous Cell Carcinomas of the
Oral Cavity and Naso- and Oropharynx. *Radiology* 119:665–667, 1976.

Bekker, H., J. Thornton, C. Airey, J. Connelly, J. Hewison, M. Robinson, et al. Informed
Decision Making: An Annotated Bibliography and Systematic Review. *Health
Technology Assessment* 3(1):1–156, 1999.

Bergmann, O.J. Oral Infections and Septicemia in Immunocompromised Patients with
Hematologic Malignancies. *Journal of Clinical Microbiology* 26(10):2105–2109,
1988.

Bergmann, O.J. Oral Infections and Fever in Immunocompromised Patients with Hae-matologic Malignancies. *European Journal of Clinical Microbiology and Infectious Diseases* 8(3):207–213, 1989.

Bergthold, L.A. Medical Necessity: Do We Need It? *Health Affairs* 14(4):180–190, 1995.

Berlin, J.A., E. Abrutyn, B.L. Strom, J.L. Kinman, M.E. Levison, O.M. Korzeniowski, et al. Incidence of Infective Endocarditis in the Delaware Valley. *American Journal of Cardiology* 76(12):933–936, 1995.

Berry, N.J., D. Burns, G. Wannamethee, J.E. Grundy, S.F. Lui, H.G. Prentice, and P.D. Griffiths. Seroepidemiological Studies on the Acquisition of Antibodies to Cyto-megalovirus, Herpes Simplex Virus and Human Immunodeficiency Virus Among General Hospital Patients and Those Attending a Clinic for Sexually Transmitted Diseases. *Journal of Medical Virology* 24:385–393, 1988.

Berwick, M., C.B. Begg, J.A. Fine, G.C. Roush, and R.L. Barnhill. Screening for Cuta-neous Melanoma by Skin Self-Examination. *Journal of the National Cancer Insti-tute* 88(1):17–23, 1996.

Beumer, J., R. Harrison, B. Sanders, and M. Kurrasch. Osteoradionecrosis: Predisposing Factors and Outcomes of Therapy. *Head and Neck Surgery* 6(4):819–827, 1984.

Blettner, M., W. Sauerbrei, B. Schlehofer, T. Scheuchenpflug, and C. Friedenreich. Tra-ditional Reviews, Meta-Analyses and Pooled Analyses in Epidemiology. *Interna-tional Journal of Epidemiology* 28(1):1–9, 1999.

Bloom, B., H.C. Gift, and S.S. Jack. *Dental Services and Oral Health: United States 1989.* National Center for Health Statistics. Vital Health Statistics 10(183), 1992.

Bodenheimer, T. The Oregon Health Plan—Lessons for the Nation. First of Two Parts. *New England Journal of Medicine* 337(9):651–655, 1997a.

Bodenheimer, T. The Oregon Health Plan—Lessons for the Nation. Second of Two Parts. *New England Journal of Medicine* 337(10):720–723, 1997b.

Bodey, G.P., V. Rodriquez, H.Y. Chang, and G. Narboni. Fever and Infection in Leuke-mic Patients: A Study of 494 Consecutive Patients. *Cancer* 41:1610–1622, 1978.

Bonow, R.O., B.Carabello, A.C. de Leon, Jr., L.H. Edmunds, Jr., B.J. Fedderly, M.D. Freed, et al. ACC/AHA Guidelines for the Management of Patients with Valvular Heart Disease: A Report of the American College of Cardiology/American Heart Association Task Force on Practice Guidelines (Committee on Management of Pa-tients with Valvular Heart Disease). *Journal of the American College of Cardiology* 32:1486–1588, 1998.

Borowski, B., E. Benhamou, J.L. Pico, A. Laplanche, J.P. Margainaud, and M. Hayat. Prevention of Oral Mucositis in Patients Treated with High-Dose Chemotherapy and Bone Marrow Transplantation: A Randomised Controlled Trial Comparing Two Protocols of Dental Care. *European Journal of Cancer: Oral Oncology* 30B:93–97, 1994.

Breslow, L., and A.R. Somers. The Lifetime Health Monitoring Program: A Practical Approach to Preventive Medicine. *New England Journal of Medicine* 296:601–608, 1977.

Budetti, P.P. Health Reform for the 21st Century? It May Have to Wait Until the 21st Century. *Journal of the American Medical Association* 277(3):193–198, 1997.

Burton, R., and B. Armstrong. Recent Incidence Trends Imply a Nonmetastasizing Form of Invasive Melanoma. *Melanoma Research* 4:107–113, 1995.

Burton, R.C., C. Howe, L. Adamson, A.L. Reid, P. Hersey, A. Watson, et al. General Practitioner Screening for Melanoma: Sensitivity, Specificity, and Effect of Training. *Journal of Medical Screening* 5:156–561, 1998.

Butler, R.N. A Spineless Attack on the AHCPR. Agency That Is the Backbone of Science and Medical Cost Containment Is in Jeopardy. *Geriatrics* 51(4):9–10, 1996.

Buto, K.A. Decisionmaking in the Health Care Financing Administration. Pp. 87–95 in *Adopting New Medical Technology.* Institute of Medicine. Washington, D.C.: National Academy Press, 1994.

Byles, J.E., D. Hennrikus, R. Sanson-Fisher, and P. Hersey. Reliability of Naevus Counts in Identifying Individuals at High Risk of Malignant Melanoma. *British Journal of Dermatology* 130(1):51–56, 1994.

Cameron, C.A., C. S. Litch, M. Liggett, and S. Heimberg. National Alliance for Oral Health Consensus Conference on Medically Necessary Oral Health Care: Legal Issues. *SCD Special Care in Dentistry* 15(5):192–200, 1995.

Capilouto, E.I., J. Piette, B.A. White, and J. Fleishman. Perceived Need for Dental Care Among Persons Living with Acquired Immunodeficiency Syndrome. *Medical Care* 29:745–754, 1991.

Carroll, R.W., G.E. Peters, and D.J. Halvorson. Head and Neck Cancer: An Update. Available online at http://cancernet.nci.nih.gov/ord/news-reports/workshops/head-neck960927.html. Accessed July 16, 1999. *Federal Practitioner Supplement* June 1998.

Cassileth, B.R., W.H. Clark, Jr., E.J. Lusk, B.E. Frederick, C.J. Thompson, and W.P. Walsh. How Well Do Physicians Recognize Melanoma and Other Problem Lesions? *Journal of the American Academy of Dermatology* 14(4):555–560, 1986.

CBO (Congressional Budget Office). Letter to Representative Charles Canaday from June E. O'Neill with attached cost estimate for proposal to eliminate time limitation on benefits for immunosuppressive drugs under the Medicare program. July 3, 1996.

CDC (Centers for Disease Control and Prevention). *CDC Guidelines: Improving the Quality.* Atlanta: Centers for Disease Control and Prevention, 1996.

CDC. Dental Service Use and Dental Insurance Coverage—United States, Behavioral Risk Factor Surveillance System. *Mortality and Morbidity Weekly Report* 46(50):1199–1203, 1997. http://www.cdc.gov/mmwr/preview/mmwrhtm1/00050448.htm. Accessed September 21, 1999.

Cecka, J.M. The UNOS Scientific Renal Transplant Registry—Ten Years of Kidney Transplants. *Clinical Transplantation* 1–14, 1997.

Chan, L., J.N. Doctor, R.F. MacLehose, H. Lawson R.A. Rosenblatt, L.M. Baldwin, and A. Jha. Do Medicare Patients with Disabilities Receive Preventive Services? A Population-Based Study. *Archives of Physical Medicine and Rehabilitation* 80(6): 642–646, 1999.

Chan, M., and S.A. Hunt. Heart Retransplantation. *Cardiology Review* 6(6):350–355, 1998.

Cohen, R.A., B. Bloom, G. Simpson, and P.E. Parsons. Access to Health Care. Part 3: Older Adults. *Vital and Health Statistics* 10(198):1–32, 1997.

Conway, T.E. What Is Currently Available in Terms of Medically Necessary Oral Health Care. *SCD Special Care in Dentistry* 15(5):187–191, 1995.

Cook, M.G., T.J. Clarke, S. Humphreys, A. Fletcher, K.M. McLaren, et al. The Evaluation of Diagnostic and Prognostic Criteria and the Terminology of Thin Cutaneous

Malignant Melanoma by the CRC Melanoma Pathology Panel. *Histopathology* 28(6):497–512, 1996.

Cool, N., J.E. Faunal, and P. Kronholm. The Role of Medication Noncompliance and Adverse Drug Reactions in Hospitalizations of the Elderly. *Archives of Internal Medicine* 150(4):841–845, 1990.

Coons, S.J., S.L. Sheahan, S.S. Martin, J. Hendricks, C.A. Robbins, and J.A. Johnson. Predictors of Medication Noncompliance in a Sample of Older Adults. *Clinical Therapy* 16(1):110–117, 1994.

Corona, R., A. Mele, M. Amini, G. DeRosa, G. Coppola, P. Piccardi, et al. Interobserver Variability on the Histopathologic Diagnosis of Cutaneous Melanoma and Other Pigmented Skin Lesions. *Journal of Clinical Oncology* 14:1218–1123, 1996.

Cramer, J.A. Relationship Between Medication Compliance and Medical Outcomes. *American Journal of Health-System Pharmacy* 52(14 Suppl. 3):S27–S29, 1995.

CRC (Cancer Research Campaign) Melanoma Pathology Panel. A Nationwide Survey of Observer Variation in the Diagnosis of Thin Cutaneous Malignant Melanoma Including the MIN Terminology. *Journal of Clinical Pathology* 50(3):202–205, 1997.

CTFPHE (Canadian Task Force on the Periodic Health Examination). The Periodic Health Examination. *Canadian Medical Association Journal* 121(9):1193–1254, 1979.

Cunningham, R. Policymakers Grapple with Foundations of Process for Coverage Decisions, Appeals. *Medicine and Health Perspectives* 53(18 Suppl.): 1–4, 1999.

Curi, M.M., and L.L. Dib. Osteoradionecrosis of the Jaws: A Retrospective Study of the Background Factors and Treatment in 104 cases. *Journal of Oral and Maxillofacial Surgery* 55(6):540–544; discussion: 545–546.

Dajani, A.S., K.A. Taubert, W. Wilson, A.F. Bolger, A. Bayer, P. Ferrieri, et al. Prevention of Bacterial Endocarditis. Recommendations by The American Heart Association. *Journal of the American Medical Association* 277(22):1794–1801, 1977.

Dans, A.L., L.F. Dans, G.H. Guyatt, and S. Richardson. Users' Guides to the Medical Literature: XIV. How to Decide on the Applicability of Clinical Trial Results to Your Patient. Evidence-Based Medicine Working Group. *Journal of the American Medical Association* 279(7):545–549, 1998.

Davidson, B.L. A Controlled Comparison of Directly Observed Therapy vs Self-Administered Therapy for Active Tuberculosis in the Urban United States. *CHEST* 114(5):1239–1243, 1998.

DeGrasse, C.E., A.M. O'Connor, J. Boulet, N. Edwards, H. Bryant, and K. Briethaupt. Changes in Canadian Women's Mammography Rates Since the Implementation of Mass Screening Programs. *American Journal of Public Health* 89(6):927–929, 1999.

De Jong, R.H. Backfire: AHCPR Practice Guideline for Acute Low Back Pain. *Journal of the South Carolina Medical Association* 91(11):465–468, 1995.

Dennis, L. K. Analysis of the Melanoma Epidemic, Both Apparent and Real: Data from the 1973 Through 1994 Surveillance, Epidemiology, and End Results Program Registry. *Archives of Dermatology* 135(3):275–280, 1999.

De Rooij, M.J., F.H. Rampen, L.J. Schouten, and H.A. Neumann. Skin Cancer Screening Focusing on Melanoma Yields More Selective Attendance. *Archives of Dermatology* 131:422–425, 1995.

De Rooij, M.J., F.H. Rampen, L.J. Schouten, and H.A. Neumann. Factors Influencing Participation Among Melanoma Screening Attenders. *Acta Dermato-Venereologica* 77:467–470, 1997.

Detsky, A.S., G. Naglie, M.D. Krahn, D. Naimark, and D.A. Redelmeier. Primer on Medical Decision Analysis: Part 1—Getting Started. *Medical Decision Making* 17(2):123–125, 1997.

Dew, M.A., R.L. Kormos, L.H. Roth, S. Murali, A. DiMartini, and B.P. Griffith. Early Post-Transplant Medical Compliance and Mental Health Predict Physical Morbidity and Mortality One to Three Years After Heart Transplantation. *Journal of Heart Lung Transplant* 18(6):549–562, 1999.

DHHS (U.S. Department of Health and Human Services). Review of EPOGEN Reimbursement (A-01-97-00509), November 24, 1997.

Donabedian, A. *Benefits in Medical Care Programs.* Cambridge, Mass.: Harvard University Press, 1976.

Drangsholt, M.T. A New Causal Model of Dental Diseases Associated with Endocarditis. *Annals of Periodontology* 3(1):184–196, 1998.

Dreizen, S., L.R. Brown, T.E. Daly, and J.B. Drane. Prevention of Xerostomia-Induced Dental Caries in Irradiated Cancer Patients. *Journal of Dental Research* 56:99–104, 1977.

Dreizen, S., G.P. Bodey, and M. Valdivieso. Chemotherapy-Associated Oral Infections in Adults with Solid Tumors. *Oral Surgery, Oral Medicine and Oral Pathology* 55(2): 113–120, 1983.

Dreizen, S., K.B. McCredie, G.P. Bodey, and M.J. Keating. Quantitative Analysis of the Oral Complications of Antileukemia Chemotherapy. *Oral Surgery, Oral Medicine and Oral Pathology* 62(6):650–653, 1986.

Drummond, M.F., W.S. Richardson, B.J. O'Brien, M. Levine, and D. Heyland. Users' Guides to the Medical Literature: XIII. How to Use an Article on Economic Analysis of Clinical Practice. A. Are the Results of the Study Valid? Evidence-Based Medicine Working Group. *Journal of the American Medical Association* 277(19): 1552–1557, 1997.

Durack, D.T. Antibiotics for Prevention of Endocarditis During Dentistry: Time to Scale Back. *Annals of Internal Medicine* 129(10):829–831, 1998.

Eckman, M.H., H.J. Levine, D.N. Salem and S.G. Pauker. Making Decisions About Antithrombotic Therapy in Heart Disease: Decision Analytic and Cost-Effectiveness Issues. *CHEST* 108(4 Suppl.):457S–470S, 1998.

Eddy, D.M. *Common Screening Tests.* Philadelphia: American College of Physicians, 1991.

Eddy, D.M. Breast Cancer Screening in Women Younger than 50 Years of Age: What's Next? *Annals of Internal Medicine* 127(11):1035–1036, 1997.

Eddy, D.M., and the Council of Medical Specialty Societies Task Force on Practice Policies. *A Manual for Assessing Health Practices and Designing Practice Policies.* Philadelphia: American College of Physicians, 1992.

Eggers, P. Presentation to the IOM Committee on Medicare Coverage Extensions at Public Workshop, Institute of Medicine, Washington, D.C., June 18, 1999.

Eggers, P., and R. Milan. Cost Comparison of Dialysis and Transplantation. Abstract presented at the Immunosuppression Conference in Organ Transplantation: Patient

Access to Long-Term Care. *American Society of Transplant Physicians,* December 4, 1998.

Elwood, J.M. Screening for Melanoma and Options for Its Evaluation. *Journal of Medical Screening* 1:22–38, 1994.

Elwood J.M. Screening for Melanoma. Pp. 129–146 in *Advances in Cancer Screening,* A.B. Miller, ed. Boston: Kluwer Academic Publishers, 1996.

Emanuel, E.J., and L.L. Emanuel. Four Models of the Physician–Patient Relationship. *Journal of the American Medical Association* 267:2221–2226, 1992.

Epstein, D.S., J.R. Lange, S.B. Gruber, M. Mofid, and S.E. Koch. Is Physician Detection Associated with Thinner Melanomas? *Journal of the American Medical Association* 281:640–643, 1999.

Epstein, J.B., and M.M. Schubert. Oral Mucositis in Myelosuppressive Cancer Therapy. *Oral Surgery, Oral Medicine and Oral Pathology* 88(3):273–276, 1999.

Epstein, J.B., F.L. Wong, and P. Stevenson-Moore. Osteoradionecrosis: Clinical Experience and a Proposal for Classification. *Journal of Oral and Maxillofacial Surgery* 45:104–110, 1987.

Epstein, J.B., L. Vickars, J. Spinelli. and D. Reece. Efficacy of Chlorhexidine and Nystatin Rinses in Prevention of Oral Complications in Leukemia and Bone Marrow Transplantation. *Oral Surgery, Oral Medicine and Oral Pathology* 73(6):682–689, 1992.

Epstein, J.B., E.H. van der Meij, S.M. Emerson, N.D. Le, and P. Stevenson-Moore. Compliance with Fluoride Gel Use in Irradiated Patients. *Special Care in Dentistry* 15:218–222, 1995.

Epstein, J.B., E.H. van der Meij, R. Lunn, and P. Stevenson-Moore. Effects of Compliance with Fluoride Gel Application on Caries and Caries Risk in Patients After Radiation Therapy for Head and Neck Cancer. *Oral Surgery, Oral Medicine and Oral Pathology* 82(3):268–275, 1996.

Faulkner, E. *Accident and Health Insurance.* New York: McGraw-Hill Book Company, 1940.

Faulkner, L.A., and H.H. Schauffler. The Effect of Health Insurance Coverage on the Appropriate Use of Recommended Clinical Preventive Services. *American Journal of Preventive Medicine* 13(6):453–458, 1997.

Feder, J., and L. Levitt. Steps Toward Univeral Coverage. *Health Affairs (Millwood)* 14(1):140–149, 1995.

Federman, D.G., J. Concato, P.V. Caralis, G.E. Hunkele and R.S. Kirsner. Screening for Skin Cancer in Primary Settings. *Archives of Dermatology* 133(11):1423–1425, 1997.

Feingold, E. *Medicare: Policy and Politics.* San Francisco: Chandler Publishing Company, 1966.

Feldman, S.R., P.M. Williford, and A.B. Fleischer, Jr. Lower Utilization of Dermatologists in Managed Care: Despite Growth in Managed Care, Visits to Dermatologists Did not Decrease: An Analysis of National Ambulatory Medical Care Survey Data, 1990–1992. *Journal of Investigational Dermatology* 107(6):860–864, 1996.

Ferretti, G.A., R.C. Ash, A.T. Brown, M.D. Parr, E.H. Romond, and T.T. Lillich. Control of Oral Mucositis and Candidiasis in Marrow Transplantation: A Prospective, Double-Blind Trial of Chlorhexide Digluconate Oral Rinse. *Bone Marrow Transplant* 3(5):483–493, 1988.

Fink, A., J. Kosecoff, M. Chassin, and R.H. Brook. Consensus Methods: Characteristics and Guidelines for Use. *American Journal of Public Health* 74(9):979–983, 1984.

Finkelstein, S.M., M. Snyder, C. Edin-Stibbe, L. Chlan, B. Prasad, P. Dutta, et al. Monitoring Progress After Lung Transplantation from Home-Patient Adherence. *Journal of Medical Engineering and Technology* 20(6):203–210, 1996.

Fleming, T.R., and D.L. DeMets. Surrogate End Points in Clinical Trials: Are We Being Misled? *Annals of Internal Medicine* 125:605–613, 1996.

Flood, A.B., J.E. Wennberg, R.F. Nease, Jr., F.J. Fowler, Jr., J. Ding, and L.M. Hynes. The Importance of Patient Preference in the Decision to Screen for Prostate Cancer. *Journal of General Internal Medicine* 11(6):377–378, 1996.

Fontana, S.A., L.C. Baumann, C. Helberg, and R.R. Love. The Delivery of Preventive Services in Primary Care Practices According to Chronic Disease Status. *American Journal of Public Health* 87(7):1190–1196, 1997.

Foxman, B., R.B. Valdez, K.N. Lohr, G.A. Goldberg, J.P. Newhouse, and R.H. Brook. The Effect of Cost Sharing on the Use of Antibiotics in Ambulatory Care: Results from a Population-Based Randomized Controlled Trial. *Journal of Chronic Diseases* 40(5):429–437, 1987.

Freedberg, K. Screening for Melanoma: A Cost-Effectiveness Analysis. *Journal of American Academy of Dermatology,* 41(5 Pt 1):738–745, 1999.

Friedman, R.H., L.E. Kazis, A. Jette, M.B. Smith, J. Stollerman, et al. A Telecommunications System for Monitoring and Counseling Patients with Hypertension. Impact on Medication Adherence and Blood Pressure Control. *American Journal of Hypertension* 9(4 Pt 1):285–292, 1996.

Friedman, R.H., J. Stollerman, L. Rozenblyum, D. Belfer, A. Selim, D. Mahoney, and S. Steinbach. A Telecommunications System to Manage Patients with Chronic Disease. *Medinfo* 9(Pt. 2):1330–1334, 1998.

Friedman, R.J., D.S. Rigel, and A.W. Kopf. Early Detection of Malignant Melanoma: The Role of Physician Examination and Self-Examination of the Skin. *CA: A Cancer Journal for Clinicians* 35(3):130–151, 1985.

Gaston, R.S. Role of Medication Non-Adherence in Late Allograft Failure. Abstract presented at the Immunosuppression Conference in Organ Transplantation: Patient Access to Long-Term Care. American Society of Transplant Physicians, Philadelphia, December 4, 1998.

Gaus, C. From Theory to Practice: AHCPR's New Mission. *Health Systems Review* 30(1):35–37, 1997.

Geisse, J.K. Biopsy Techniques for Pigmented Lesions of the Skin. *Pathology* 2(2):181–193, 1994.

Gerbert, B., A. Bronstone, M. Wolff, T. Maurer, T. Berger, S. Pantilat, and S.J. McPhee. Improving Primary Care Residents' Proficiency in the Diagnosis of Skin Cancer. *Journal of General Internal Medicine* 13(2):91–97, 1998.

German, P.S., L.C. Burton, S. Shapiro, D.M. Steinwachs, I. Tsuji, et al. Extended Coverage for Preventive Services for the Elderly: Response and Results in a Demonstration Population. *American Journal of Public Health* 85(3):379–386, 1995.

Gershenwald, J.E., M.I. Colome, J.E. Lee, P.F. Mansfield, C. Tseng, et al. Patterns of Recurrence Following a Negative Sentinel Lymph Node Biopsy in 243 Patients with Stage I or II Melanoma. *Journal of Clinical Oncology* 16(6):2253–2260, 1998.

Glass, F.L., J.A. Cottam, D.S. Reintgen, and N.A. Fenske. Lymphatic Mapping and Sentinel Node Biopsy in the Management of High-Risk Melanoma. *Journal of American Academy of Dermatology* 39(4 Pt 1):603–610, 1998.

Gold, M.R., J.E. Siegel, L.B. Russell, and M.C. Weinstein, eds. *Cost-Effectiveness in Health and Medicine.* New York: Oxford University Press, 1996.

Gordon, N.P., T.G. Rundall, and L. Parker. Type of Health Care Coverage and the Likelihood of Being Screened for Cancer. *Medical Care* 36(5):636–645, 1998.

Graham, J. Perspectives. AHCPR's Evidence-Based Centers: Will Their Findings Guide Clinical Practice? *Medicine and Health* 52(32: Suppl.):1–4, 1998.

Green, A., G. Williams, R. Neale, V. Hart, D. Leslie, P. Parsons, et al. Daily Sunscreen Application and Betacarotene Supplementation in Prevention of Basal-Cell and Squamous-Cell Carcinomas of the Skin: A Randomised Controlled Trial. *Lancet* 354(9180):723–729, 1999.

Greenberg, M. Prechemotherapy Dental Treatment to Prevent Bacteremia. *NCI Monographs* 9:49–50, 1990.

Greenberg, M., S.G. Cohen, J.C. McKitrick, and P.A. Cassileth. The Oral Flora as a Source of Septicemia in Patients with Acute Leukemia. *Oral Surgery* 53:32–36, 1982.

Greenstein, S., and B. Siegal. Odds Probabilities of Compliance and Noncompliance in Patients with a Functioning Renal Transplant: A Multicenter Study. *Transplantation Proceedings* 31:280–281, 1999.

Greer, J.W., P.W. Eggers, R. Milam, and N.R. Powe. Medicare Payment for Recombinant Erythropoietin (EPO): Costs, Access, and Outcomes in a Single Payer Market. Abstract presented at the 1992 Annual Meeting on Implications for Policy, Management and Clinical Practice. *Association for Health Services Research,* June 7–9, 1992.

Grossi, S.G., and R.J. Genco. Periodontal Disease and Diabetes Mellitus: A Two-Way Relationship. *Annals of Periodontology* 3(1):51–61, 1998.

Grossi, S.G., F.B. Skrepcinski, T. DeCaro, D.C. Robertson, A.W. Ho, and R.J. Genco. Treatment of Periodontal Disease in Diabetics Reduces Glycated Hemoglobin. *Journal of Periodontology* 68:713–719, 1997.

Guyatt, G.H., D.L. Sackett, J.C. Sinclair, R. Hayward, D.J. Cook, and R.J. Coork. Users' Guides to the Medical Literature. IX: A Method for Grading Health Care Recommendations. Evidence-Based Medicine Working Group. *Journal of the American Medical Association* 274(22):1800–1804, 1995.

Guyatt, G.H., D.J. Cook, D.L. Sackett, M. Eckman, and S. Pauker. Grades of Recommendations for Antithrombotic Agents. *Chest* 114:441S–444S, 1998.

Guyatt, G.H., J. Sinclair, D.J. Cook, and P. Glasziou. Users' Guides to the Medical Literature: XVI. How to Use a Treatment Recommendation. Evidence-Based Medicine Working Group and the Cochran Applicability Working Group. *Journal of the American Medical Association* 281(19):1836–1843, 1999.

Hadorn, D.C., D. Baker, J.S. Hodges, and N. Hicks. Rating the Quality of Evidence for Clinical Practice Guidelines. *Journal of Clinical Epidemiology* 49(7):749–754, 1996.

Halpern, A.C., and L.M. Schuchter. Prognostic Models in Melanoma. *Seminars in Oncology* 24(1 Suppl. 4):S2–S7, 1997.

Ham, C. Retracing the Oregon Trail: The Experience of Rationing and the Oregon Health Plan. *British Medical Journal* 316(7149):1965–1969, 1998.

Harris, J.M., Jr., S.J. Salasche, and R.B. Harris. Using the Internet to Teach Melanoma Management Guidelines to Primary Care Physicians. *Journal of Evaluation in Clinical Practice* 5(2):199–211, 1999.

Harris, R. *A Sacred Trust*. Baltimore: Penguin Books, 1969. (Reprint: Originally published by The New American Library, Inc. New York, 1966.)

HCFA (Health Care Financing Administration, U.S. Department of Health and Human Services). Criteria and Procedures for Making Medical Services Coverage Decisions That Relate to Health Care Technology. *Federal Register* 54:4302–4318, 1989.

HCFA. *A Profile of Medicare: Medicare Chartbook*. Baltimore, Md.: U.S. Department of Health and Human Services, 1998a.

HCFA. Description of FY 1999 Legislative Proposals. 1998b. Available at http://www. hcfa.gov/reg/budget99.htm. Accessed July 7, 1999.

HCFA. Information Clearinghouse: Medicare National Enrollment Trends, 1966–1998. 1999a. http://www.hcfa.gov/stats/stats.htm. Accessed August 17, 1999.

HCFA. Medicare and Medicaid Program Manuals, 1999b. http://www.hcfa.gov/pubforms/ htmltoc.htm. Accessed various dates from June 1, 1999, to November 1, 1999.

Heenan, P.J., L.R. Matz, J.B. Blackwell, G.R. Kelsall, A. Singh, et al. Inter-Observer Variation Between Pathologists in the Classification of Cutaneous Malignant Melanoma in Western Australia. Histopathology 8(5):717–729, 1984.

Heiser, N.A., and R.F. St. Peter. Improving the Delivery of Clinical Preventive Services to Women in Managed Care Organizations: A Case Study Analysis. *Joint Commission Journal of Quality Improvement* 23(10):529–547, 1997.

Helfand, M., and S.G. Pauker. Influence Diagrams: A New Dimension for Decisionmaking. *Medical Decision Making* 17(3):351–352, 1997.

Hetzer, R., E.V. Potapov, J. Muller, M. Loebe, M. Hummel, Y. Weng, et al. Daily Noninvasive Rejection Monitoring Improves Long-Term Survival in Pediatric Heart Transplantation. *Annals of Thoracic Surgery* 66(4):1343–1349, 1998.

Hill, D. Efficacy of Sunscreens in Protection Against Skin Cancer. *Lancet* 354(9180): 699–700, 1999.

HIMA (Health Industry Manufacturers Association). Overview of Change in the National Medicare Coverage Process. Washington, D.C., April 30, 1999.

Hochwald, S.N., and D.G. Coit. Role of Elective Lymph Node Dissection in Melanoma. *Seminars in Surgical Oncology* 14(4):276–282, 1998.

Hollister, M.C., and J.A. Weintraub. The Association of Oral Status with Systemic Health, Quality of Life, and Economic Productivity. *Journal of Dental Education* 57(12):901–912, 1993.

Holmstrom, H. Surgical Management of Primary Melanoma. *Seminars in Surgical Oncology* 8(6):366–369, 1992.

HSR (*Health Systems Review* [journal]). A Technology Anthology: Recent Writings and Remarks on the State-of-the-Art. 30(2):58–62, 1997.

Hux, J.E., and C.D. Naylor. Communicating the Benefits of Chronic Preventive Therapy: Does the Format of Efficacy Data Determine Patients' Preferences for Therapeutic Outcomes? *Medical Decision Making* 15(2):152–157, 1995.

Iglehart, J.K. A New Era: Modest Reform and Managed Care. *Health Affairs (Millwood)* 14(2):5–6, 1995.

IOM (Institute of Medicine). *Assessing Medical Technologies*. Washington, D.C.: National Academy Press, 1985.

IOM. *Controlling Costs, Changing Patient Care: The Role of Utilization Management*. Washington, D.C.: National Academy Press, 1989.

IOM. *Clinical Practice Guidelines: Directions for a New Program*. Washington, D.C.: National Academy Press, 1990a.

IOM. *Consensus Development at the NIH: Improving the Program*. Washington, D.C.: National Academy Press, 1990b.

IOM. *Improving Consensus Development for Health Technology Assessment: An International Perspective*. Washington, D.C.: National Academy Press, 1990c.

IOM. *Kidney Failure and the Federal Government*. Washington, D.C.: National Academy Press, 1991.

IOM. *Guidelines for Clinical Practice: From Development to Use*. Washington, D.C.: National Academy Press, 1992.

IOM. *Employment and Health Benefits: A Connection at Risk*. Washington D.C.: National Academy Press, 1993.

IOM. *Dental Education at the Crossroads*. Washington, D.C.: National Academy Press, 1995a.

IOM. *Setting Priorities for Clinical Practice Guidelines*. Washington, D.C.: National Academy Press, 1995b.

IOM. *Telemedicine: A Guide to Assessing Telecommunications in Health Care*. Washington, D.C.: National Academy Press, 1996.

IOM. *Summarizing Population Health: Directions for the Development and Application of Population Metrics*. Washington, D.C.: National Academy Press, 1998.

IOM/NRC (Institute of Medicine/National Research Council*). Exposure of the American People to Iodine-131 from Nevada Nuclear-Bomb Tests*. Washington, D.C.: National Academy Press, 1999.

Jackson, A., C. Wilkinson, M. Ranger, R. Pill, and P. August. Can Primary Prevention or Selective Screening for Melanoma Be More Precisely Targeted Through General Practice? A Prospective Study to Validate a Self Administered Risk Score. *British Medical Journal* 316(7124):34–38; discussion 38–39, 1998.

Jacobs, C. Current National Coverage of Immuosuppression Medication. Abstract presented at the Immunosuppression Conference in Organ Transplantation: Patient Access to Long-Term Care. American Society of Transplant Physicians, Philadelphia, December 4, 1998.

Jacobs, L., T. Marmor, and J. Oberlander. The Oregon Health Plan and the Political Paradox of Rationing: What Advocates and Critics Have Claimed and What Oregon Did. *Journal of Health Politics, Policy, and Law* 24(1):161–180, 1999.

Jaen, C.R., K.C. Stange, and P.A. Nutting. Competing Demands of Primary Care: A Model for the Delivery of Clinical Preventive Services. *Journal of Family Practice* 38(2):166–171, 1994.

Jonna, B.P., R.J. Delfino, W.G. Newman, and W.D. Tope. Positive Predictive Value for Presumptive Diagnoses of Skin Cancer and Compliance with Follow-Up Among Patients Attending a Community Screening Program. *Preventive Medicine* 27:611–616, 1998.

Kahn, C.N., III. The AHCPR After the Battles. *Health Affairs* 17(1):109–110, 1998.

Kahn, C.N., and H. Kuttner. Budget Bills and Medicare Policy. *Health Affairs* 18(1):37–47, 1999.

Kahn, H.S., L.M. Tatham, A.V. Patel, M.J. Thun, and C.W. Heath, Jr. Increased Cancer Mortality Following a History of Nonmelanoma Skin Cancer. *Journal of the American Medical Association* 280(10):910–912, 1998.

Kahn, K.L., E.B. Keeler, M.J. Sherwood, W.H. Rogers, D. Draper, S.S. Bentow, et al. Comparing Outcomes of Care Before and After Implementation of the DRG-Based Prospective Payment System. *Journal of the American Medical Association* 264(15):1984–1988, 1990.

Kaiser Family Foundation. *Medicare Managed Care.* 1998. Washington, D.C. http://www.kff.org/content/archive/2052/mngcare.html. Accessed July 9, 1999.

Karagas, M.R. Occurrence of Cutaneous Basal Cell and Squamous Cell Malignancies Among Those with a Prior History of Skin Cancer. The Skin Cancer Prevention Study Group. *Journal of Investigational Dermatology* 102(6):10S–13S, 1994.

Karagas, M.R., T.A. Stukel, E.R.Greenberg, J.A. Baron, L.A. Mott, and R.S. Stern. Risk of Subsequent Basal Cell Carcinoma and Squamous Cell Carcinoma of the Skin Among Patients with Prior Skin Cancer. *Journal of the American Medical Association* 267(24): 3305–3310, 1992.

Karagas, M.R., E.R.Greenberg, L.A. Mott, J.A. Baron, and V.L. Ernster. Occurrence of Other Cancers Among Patients with Prior Basal Cell and Squamous Cell Skin Cancer. *Cancer Epidemiology Biomarkers and Prevention* 7(2):157–161, 1998.

Karakousis, C.P. Therapeutic Node Dissections in Malignant Melanoma. *Seminars in Surgical Oncology* 14(4):291–301, 1998.

Karakousis, C.P., C.M. Balch, M.M. Urist, M.M. Ross, T.J. Smith, and A.A. Bartolucci. Local Recurrence in Malignant Melanoma: Long-Term Results of the Multiinstitutional Randomized Surgical Trial. *Annals of Surgical Oncology* 3(5):446–452, 1996.

Kasiske, B.L., E.L. Ramos, R.S. Gaston, M.J. Bia, G.M. Danovitch, P.A. Bowen, et al. The Evaluation of Renal Transplant Candidates: Clinical Practice Guidelines. Patient Care and Education Committee of the American Society of Transplant Physicians. *Journal of American Society of Nephrology* 6(1):1–34, 1995.

Kassirer, J.P., and S.G. Pauker. The Toss-Up. *New England Journal of Medicine* 305: 1467–1469, 1981.

Kassirer, J.P., A.J. Moskowitz, J. Lau, and S.G. Pauker. Decision Analysis: A Progress Report. *Annals of Internal Medicine* 106(2):275–291, 1987.

Kastrissios, H., N.T. Flowers, and T.F. Blaschke. Introducing Medical Students to Medication Noncompliance. *Clinical Pharmacology and Therapeutics* 59(5):577–582, 1996.

Keeler, E.B., R.H. Brook, G.A. Goldberg, C.J. Kamberg, and J.P. Newhouse. How Free Care Reduced Hypertension in the Health Insurance Experiment. *Journal of the American Medical Association* 254(14):1926–1931, 1985.

Kelly, J.W., R.W. Sagebiel, W. Calderon, L. Murillo, R.L. Dakin, and M.S. Blois. The Frequency of Local Recurrence and Microsatellites as a Guide to Reexcision Margins for Cutaneous Malignant Melanoma. *Annals of Surgery* 200(6):759–763, 1984.

Keys, H.M., and J.P. McCasland. Techniques and Results of a Comprehensive Dental Care Program in Head and Neck Cancer Patients. *International Journal of Radiation Oncology, Biology and Physics* 1(9–10):859–965, 1976.

Kirsner, R.S., S. Muhkerjee, and D.G. Federman. Skin Cancer Screen in Primary Care: Prevalence and Barriers. *Journal of the American Academy of Dermatology* 41:564–566, 1999.

Kittler, H., M. Seltenheim, M. Vawid, H. Pehamberger, K. Wolff, and M. Binder. Morphologic Changes of Pigmented Skin Lesions: A Useful Extension of the ABCD Rule for Dermatoscopy. *Journal of American Academy of Dermatology* 40(4):558–562, 1999.

Koh, H.K., D.R. Miller, A.C. Geller, R.W. Clapp, M.B. Mercer, et al. Who Discovers Melanoma? *Journal of the American Academy of Dermatology* 26:914–919, 1992.

Koh, H.K., L.A. Norton, A.C. Geller, Ting Sun, D.S. Rigel, et al. Evaluation of the American Academy of Dermatology's National Skin Cancer Early Detection and Screening Program. *Journal of the American Academy of Dermatology* 34:971–978, 1996.

Lagnado, L. Transplant Patients Ply Illicit Market for Drugs. *Wall Street Journal,* June 21, 1999, p.1.

Landis, S.H., T. Murray, S. Bolden, and P.A. Wingo. Cancer Statistics. *CA—A Cancer Journal for Clinicians* 49:8–31, 1999.

Lau, J., J.P. Ioannidis, and C.H. Schmid. Quantitative Synthesis in Systematic Reviews. *Annals of Internal Medicine* 127(9):820–826, 1997.

Laupacis, A., D. Feeny, A.S. Detsky, and P.X. Tugwell. How Attractive Does a New Technology Have to Be to Warrant Adoption and Utilization? Tentative Guidelines for Using Clinical and Economic Evaluations. *Canadian Medical Association Journal* 146(4):473–481, 1992.

Laupacis, A., P. Keown, N. Pus, H. Krueger, B. Ferguson, C. Wong, and N. Muirhead. A Study of the Quality of Life and Cost-Utility of Renal Transplantation. *Kidney International* 50(1):235–242, 1996.

Lave, J.R., D.G. Ives, N.D. Traven, and L.H. Kuller. Evaluation of a Health Promotion Demonstration Program for the Rural Elderly. *Health Services Research* 31(3):261–281, 1996.

Leary, W.E. Congress's Science Agency Prepares to Close Its Doors. *New York Times,* Sept. 24, 1995, p. 26.

Leichter, H.M. Oregon's Bold Experiment: Whatever Happened to Rationing? *Journal of Health Politics, Policy and Law* 24(1):147–160, 1999.

Levy-Polack, M.P., P. Sebelli, and N.L. Polack. Incidence of Oral Complications and Application of a Preventive Protocol in Children with Acute Leukemia. *Special Care in Dentistry* 18(5):189–193, 1998.

Lieu, T.A., M.D. Smith, P.W. Newacheck, D. Langthorn, P. Venkatesh, and R. Herradora. Health Insurance and Preventive Care Sources of Children at Public Immunization Clinics. *Pediatrics* 93(3):373–378, 1994.

Limeback, H. Implications of Oral Infections on Systemic Diseases in the Institutionalized Elderly with a Special Focus on Pneumonia. *Annals of Periodontology* 3(1): 262–275, 1998.

Limpert, G.H. Skin-Cancer Screening: A Three Year Experience That Paid for Itself. *Journal of Family Practice* 40:471–475, 1995.

Lockhart, P.B., and J. Clark, Pretherapy Dental Status of Patients with Malignant Conditions of the Head and Neck. *Oral Surgery, Oral Medicine and Oral Pathology* 77:235–241, 1994.

Lohr, K.N., and S. Carey. Assessing "Best Evidence": Issues in Grading the Quality of Studies for Systematic Reviews. *Joint Commission Journal of Quality Improvement* 25(9):470–479, 1999.

Lohr, K.N., R.H. Brook, R.H., C.J. Kamberg, G.A. Goldberg, A. Leibowitz, et al. Use of Medical Care in the Rand Health Insurance Experiment. Diagnosis- and Service-Specific Analyses in a Randomized Controlled Trial. *Medical Care* 24(Suppl.):S1–S87, 1986.

Lynn, J., J.M. Teno, and F.E. Harrell, Jr. Accurate Prognostications of Death: Opportunities and Challenges for Clinicians. *Western Journal of Medicine* 163(3):250–257, 1995.

Lynn, J., J.M. Teno, R.S. Phillips, R.S. Phillips, A.W. Wu, N. Desbiens, J. Harrold, et al. Perceptions by Family Members of the Dying Experience of Older and Seriously Ill Patients. *Annals of Internal Medicine* 126(2):97–106, 1997.

MacIntyre, D. *Voluntary Health Insurance and Rate Making.* Ithaca, N.Y.: Cornell University Press, 1962.

Malm, H.M. Medical Screening and the Value of Early Detection: When Unwarranted Faith Leads to Unethical Recommendations. *Hastings Center Report* 29(1):26–37, 1999.

Mandelson, M.T., and R.S. Thompson. Cancer Screening in HMOs: Program Development and Evaluation. *American Journal of Preventive Medicine* 14(3 Suppl.):26–32, 1998.

Marcus, P.A., A. Joshi, J.A. Jones, and S.M. Morgano. Complete Edentulism and Denture Use for Elders in New England. *Journal of Prosthetic Dentistry* 76(3):260–266, 1996.

Markmann, J.F., J.S. Markowitz, H. Yersiz, M. Morrisey, D.G. Farmer, D.A. Farmer, et al. Long-Term Survival After Retransplantation of the Liver. *Annals of Surgery* 226(4):408–418; discussion 418–420, 1997.

Marmor, T. *The Politics of Medicare.* Chicago: Aldine Publishing Company, 1973. (Reprint: Originally published by Routledge & Kegan Paul Ltd., 1970.)

Marquis, M.S., and S.H. Long. Reconsidering the Effect of Medicaid on Health Care Services Use. *Health Services Research* 30(6):791–808, 1996.

Marx, R.E., R.P. Johnson, and S.N. Kleine. Prevention of Osteoradionecrosis: A Randomized Prospective Clinical Trial of Hyperbaric Oxygen Versus Penicillin. *Journal of the American Dental Association* 111:49–54, 1985.

McGee, R., M. Elwood, M.J. Sneyd, S. William, and M. Tilyard. Recognition of Skin Cancers [letter; comment]. *New Zealand Medical Journal* 107(988):439–440, 1994a.

McGee, R., M. Elwood, S. Williams, and F. Lowry. Who Comes to Skin Checks? *New Zealand Medical Journal* 107:58–60, 1994b.

McPhee, S.J., and S.A. Schroeder. Promoting Preventive Care: Changing Reimbursement Is not Enough. *American Journal of Public Health* 77(7):780–781, 1987.

McVea, K., B.F. Crabtree, J.D. Medder, J.L. Susman, L. Lukas, H.E. McIlvain, et al. An Ounce of Prevention? Evaluation of the "Put Prevention into Practice" Program. *Journal of Family Practice* 43(4):361–369, 1996.

Merenstein, D., H. Rabinowitz, and D.Z. Louis. Health Care Plan Decisions Regarding Preventive Services. *Archives of Family Medicine* 8(4):354–356, 1999.

Migliorati, C.A., and M.M. Koller. HIV Disease: Medical and Dental Aspects and Trends for the Future. A Literature Review. *Schweizer Monatsschrift Zahnmedizin* 104(5): 565–577, 1994.

Mittelbronn, M.A., D.L. Mullins, F.A. Ramos-Caro, and F.P. Flowers. Frequency of Pre-Existing Actinic Keratosis in Cutaneous Squamous Cell Carcinoma. *International Journal of Dermatology* 37(9):677–681, 1998.

MMWR (*Morbidity and Mortality Weekly Report*). Use of Clinical Preventive Services by Medicare Beneficiaries Aged > r = 65 Years—United States, 1995. *Morbidity and Mortality Weekly Report* 46(48):1138–1143, 1997. (Published erratum appears in *MMWR* 47(14):287–289, 1998.)

MMWR. Total Tooth Loss Among Persons Aged Greater Than or Equal to 65 Years—Selected States, 1995–1997. *Morbidity and Mortality Weekly Report* 48(10):206–210, 1999. http://www.cdc.gov/epo/mmwr/preview/mmwrhtml/00056723.htm. Accessed July 16, 1999.

Moher, D., and B. Pham. Meta-Analysis: An Adolescent in Need of Evidence and a Watchful Eye. *Annals of Medicine* 31(3):153–155, 1999.

Morgan, M.W., R.B. Deber, H.A. Llewellyn-Thomas, P. Gladstone, R.J. Cusimano, and K. O'Rourke. A Randomized Trial of the Ischemic Heart Disease Shared Decision Making Program: An Evaluation of a Decision Aid [abstract]. *Journal of General Internal Medicine* 12:62, 1997.

Morrissey, J.P., R.P. Harris, J. Kincade-Norburn, C. McLaughlin, J.M.Garrett, A.M. Jackman, et al. Medicare Reimbursement for Preventive Care. Changes in Performance of Services, Quality of Life, and Health Care Costs. *Medical Care* 33(4):315–331, 1995.

Mulrow, C., and D. Cook. *Synthesis of Best Evidence for Health Care Decisions*. Philadelphia: American College of Physicians, 1998.

Mulrow, C., and A. Oxman, eds. *Cochrane Collaboration Handbook* (version 3.0.2 updated 1997). Oxford, England: The Cochrane Collaboration, 1997. http://hiru.mcmaster.ca/cochrane/cochrane/revhb302.htm. Accessed July 9, 1999.

Murray, C.G., J. Herson, T.E. Daly, and S. Zimmerman. Radiation Necrosis of the Mandible: A 10-Year Study. Part I. Factors Influencing the Onset of Necrosis. *International Journal of Radiation Oncology, Biology and Physics* 6:543–548, 1980a.

Murray, C.G., J. Herson, T.E. Daly, and S. Zimmerman. Radiation Necrosis of the Mandible: A 10-Year Study. Part II. Dental Factors: Onset, Duration and Management of Necrosis. *International Journal of Radiation Oncology, Biology and Physics* 6:549–553, 1980b.

Myers, R.A.M., and R.E. Marx. Use of Hyperbaric Oxygen in Postradiation Head and Neck Surgery. *NCI Monographs* 9:151–157, 1990.

NCHS (National Center for Health Statistics). Vital and Health Statistics. Series II, No. 27. *Loss of Teeth in Adults, United States—1960–1962*. DHEW Pub. No. (HRA) 74-1280, 1973.

NCI (National Cancer Institute). Adult Hodgkin's Disease. *PDQ Cancer Information Summaries:Treatment—Health Professionals*. 1999a. Last updated September 1999. http://cancernet.nci.nih.gov/pdq/pdq_treatment.shtml. Accessed October 20, 1999.

NCI. Melanoma. *PDQ Cancer Information Summaries: Treatment—Health Professionals.* 1999b. Last updated June 1999. http://cancernet.nci.nih.gov/pdq/pdq_treatment.shtml. Accessed July 3, 1999.

NCI. Melanoma. *PDQ Cancer Information Summaries: Treatment—Patients.* 1999c. Last updated June 1999. http://cancernet.nci.nih.gov/pdq/pdq_treatment.shtml. Accessed July 3, 1999.

NCI. Nonmelanoma Skin Cancers. *PDQ Cancer Information Summaries: Treatment—Professionals.* 1999d. Last updated July 1999. http://cancernet.nci.nih.gov/pdq/pdq_treatment.shtml. Accessed July 31, 1999.

NCI. Nonmelanoma Skin Cancers, Actinic Keratoses. *PDQ Cancer Information Summaries: Treatment—Health Professionals.* 1999e. http://cancernet.nci.nih.gov/pdq/pdq_treatment.shtml. Last updated June 1999. Accessed September 21, 1999.

NCI. Screening for Skin Cancer. *PDQ Cancer Information Summaries: Screening and Prevention—Health Professionals.* 1999f. http://cancernet.nci.nih.gov/pdq/pdq_screening.shtml. Last updated June 1999. Accessed July 3, 1999.

NCQA (National Committee for Quality Assurance). *State of Managed Care Quality.* Washington, D.C.: NCQA, 1999.

NHPF. (National Health Policy Forum). *Medicare Coverage and Technology Diffusion: Past, Present and Future.* Issue Brief 722. Washington, D.C.: George Washington University, July 9, 1998.

NHPF. *Medical Necessity and Evolving Standards of Care.* Issue Brief 739. Washington, D.C.: George Washington University, May 11, 1999.

NIDCR (National Institute of Dental and Craniofacial Research). Oral Complications of Cancer Treatment: What the Oral Health Team Can Do. http://www.aerie.com/nohicweb/campaign/den_fact.htm. Accessed July 26, 1999.

NIDR (National Institute for Dental Research). *The National Survey of Oral Health in U.S. Employed Adults and Seniors: 1985–86.* NIH Pub. No. 87-2868. Bethesda, Md., August 1987.

Niewald, M. O. Barbie, K. Schnabel, M. Engel, M. Schedler, C. Nieder, and W. Berberichl. Risk Factors and Dose–Effect Relationship for Osteoradionecrosis After Hyperfractionated and Conventionally Fractionated Radiotherapy for Oral Cancer. *British Journal of Radiology* 69:847–851, 1996.

NIH (National Institutes of Health). Consensus Development Conference Statement: Oral Complications of Cancer Therapies: Diagnosis, Prevention, and Treatment. *Journal of the American Dental Association* 119:179–183, 1989.

NIH. Diagnosis and Treatment of Early Melanoma. NIH Consensus Statement Online. 10(1):1–26, 1992. http://odp.od.nih.gov/consensus/cons/088/088_intro.htm. Accessed July 7, 1999.

NIHCM (National Institute for Health Care Management). Making Coverage Decisions About Emerging Technologies. Proceedings of a Symposium, Washington, D.C., February 11, 1999. Fairfax, Va.: NIHCM Foundation, 1999.

O'Brien, B.J., D. Heyland, W.S. Richardson, M. Levine, and M.F. Drummond. Users' Guides to the Medical Literature. XIII. How to Use an Article on Economic Analysis of Clinical Practice. B. What Are the Results and Will They Help Me in Caring for My Patients? Evidence-Based Medicine Working Group. *Journal of the American Medical Association* 277(22):1802–1806, 1997.

Olivotto, I.A., L. Kan, D. Mates, and S. King. Screening Mammography Program of British Columbia: Pattern of Use and Health Care System Costs. *Canadian Medical Association Journal* 160(3):337–341, 1999.

Ostchega, Y. Preventing and Treating Cancer Chemotherapy's Oral Complications. *Nursing* 10(8):47–52, 1980.

OTA (Office of Technology Assessment). *Cost-Effectiveness of Influenza Vaccination.* Washington, D.C.: U.S. Government Printing Office, 1981.

OTA. *Screening for Open-Angle Glaucoma in the Elderly.* Washington, D.C.: U.S. Government Printing Office, 1988.

OTA. *Costs and Effectiveness of Cholesterol Screening in the Elderly.* Washington, D.C.: U.S. Government Printing Office, 1989.

OTA. *Costs and Effectiveness of Cervical Cancer Screening in Elderly Women.* Washington, D.C.: U.S. Government Printing Office, 1990a.

OTA. *Preventive Health Services for Medicare Beneficiaries: Policy and Research Issues.* Washington, D.C.: U.S. Government Printing Office, 1990b.

OTA. *Outpatient Immunosuppressive Drugs Under Medicare.* Washington, D.C.: U.S. Government Printing Office, September 1991.

OTA. *Benefit Design in Health Care Reform: Clinical Preventive Services.* Washington, D.C.: U.S. Government Printing Office, 1993.

OTA. *Identifying Health Technologies That Work: Searching for Evidence.* Washington, D.C.: U.S. Government Printing Office, 1994.

Overholser C.D., D.E. Peterson, S.A. Bergman, and L.T. Williams. Dental Extractions in Patients with Acute Nonlymphocytic Leukemia. *Journal of Oral Maxillofacial Surgery* 40(5):296–298, 1982.

Owens, D.K., R.D., Shachter, and R.F. Nease. Representation and Analysis of Medical Decision Problems with Influence Diagrams. *Medical Decision Making* 17(3):241–262, 1997.

Pallasch, T.J., and J. Slots. Antiobiotic Prophylaxis and the Medically Compromised Patient. *Periodontology 2000* 10:107–138, 1996.

Paris, W., S. Dunham, B. Nour, and A. Sebastian. Medication Non-Adherence and Its Relation to Financial Barriers. INTEGRIS Oklahoma Transplantation Institute. Abstract presented at the Immunosuppression Conference in Organ Transplantation: Patient Access to Long-Term Care. American Society of Transplant Physicians, December 4, 1998.

Pauker, S.G., and N.F. Col. Clinical Decision Making. Pp. 2517–2526 in *Merck Manual of Diagnosis and Therapy*, 17th Ed., M.H. Beers and R. Berkow, eds. Whitehouse Station, N.J.: Merck Research Laboratories, 1999.

Pauker, S.G., and J.P. Kassirer. Contentious Screening Decisions: Does the Choice Matter? *New England Journal of Medicine* 336(17):1243–1244, 1997.

Pauker S.G., and R.I. Kopelman. Clinical Problem-Solving: Some Familiar Trade-Offs. *New England Journal of Medicine* 331(22)1511–1514, 1994.

Peterson, D.E. Pretreatment Strategies for Infection Prevention in Chemotherapy Patients. *NCI Monographs* 9:61–71, 1990.

Peterson, D.E., and S.T. Sonis. Oral Complications of Cancer Chemotherapy: Present Status and Future Studies. *Cancer Treatment Reports* 66(6):1251–1256, 1982.

Powe, N.R., R.I. Griffiths, G.F. Anderson, G. deLissovoy, A.J. Watson, et al. Medicare Payment Policy and Recombinant Erythropoietin Prescribing for Dialysis Patients. *American Journal of Kidney Diseases* 22(4):557–567, 1993.

Powell-Griner, E., J. Bolen, and S. Bland. Health Care Coverage and Use of Preventive Services Among the Near Elderly in the United States. *American Journal of Public Health* 89(6):882–886, 1999.

PPRC (Physician Payment Review Commission). *Annual Report to Congress.* Washington, D.C., 1989.

PPRC (Physician Payment Review Commission). *Annual Report to Congress.* Washington, D.C., 1995.

Preston, D.S., and R.S. Stern. Nonmelanoma Cancers of the Skin. *New England Journal of Medicine* 327(23):1649–1662, 1992.

Psaty, B.M., N.S. Weiss, C.D. Furberg, T.D. Koepsell, D.S. Siscovick, F.R. Rosendaal, et al. Surrogate End Points, Health Outcomes, and the Drug-Approval Process for the Treatment of Risk Factors for Cardiovascular Disease. *Journal of the American Medical Association* 282(8):786–790, 1999.

Raiz, L.R., K.M. Kitty, M.L. Henry, and R.M. Ferguson. Medication Compliance Following Renal Transplantation. *Transplantation* 68(1):51–55, 1999.

Rampen, F.H., J.I. Casparie-van Velsen, B.E. van Huystee, L.A. Kiemeney, and L.J. Schouten. False-Negative Findings in Skin Cancer and Melanoma Screening. *Journal of the American Academy of Dermatology* 33:59–63, 1995.

Ransohoff, D.F., and R.P. Harris. Lessons from the Mammography Screening Controversy: Can We Improve the Debate? *Annals of Internal Medicine* 127(11):1029–1034, 1997.

Rebelsky, M.S., C.H. Sox, A.J. Dietrich, B.R. Schwab, C.E. Labaree, and N. Brown-McKinney. Physician Preventive Care Philosophy and the Five-Year Durability of a Preventive Services Office System. *Social Science and Medicine* 43(7):1073–1081, 1996.

Richard, M.A., J.J. Grob, M.F. Avril, M. Delaunay, X. Thirion, et al. Melanoma and Tumor Thickness: Challenges of Early Diagnosis. *Archives of Dermatology* 135(3): 269–274, 1999.

Richard, P., G. Amador Del Valle, P. Moreau, N. Milpied, M.P. Felice, T. Daeschler, et al. Viridans Streptococcal Bacteraemia in Patients with Neutropenia. *Lancet* 345(8965):1607–1609, 1995.

Rigel, D.S., R.J. Friedman, A.W. Kopf, R. Weltman, P.G. Prioleau, B. Safai, et al. Importance of Complete Cutaneous Examination for the Detection of Malignant Melanoma. *Journal of the American Academy of Dermatology* 14(5 Pt 1):857–860, 1986.

Rintala, E. Incidence and Clinical Significance of Positive Blood Cultures in Febrile Episodes of Patients with Hematological Malignancies. *Scandinavian Journal of Infectious Diseases* 26:77–84, 1994.

Roberts, G.J. Dentists Are Innocent! "Everyday" Bacteremia Is the Real Culprit: A Review and Assessment of the Evidence That Dental Surgical Procedures are a Principal Cause of Bacterial Endocarditis in Children. *Pediatric Cardiology* 20:317–325, 1999.

Roos, D.E., S. Dische, and M.I. Saunders. The Dental Problems of Patients with Head and Neck Cancer Treated with CHART. *Oral Oncology, European Journal of Cancer* 32B:176–181, 1996.

Roos, L.L., D. Traverse, and D. Turner. Delivering Prevention: The Role of Public Programs in Delivering Care to High-Risk Populations. *Medical Care* 37(6 Suppl.): JS264–JS278, 1999.

Rubin, R.H., and N.E. Tolkoff-Rubin. Opportunistic Infections in Renal Allograft Recipients. *Transplant Proceedings* 20(6 Suppl. 8):12–18, 1988.

Russell, L.B. Proposed: A Comprehensive Health Care System for the Poor. *Brookings Review* 7:13–20, 1989.

Russell, L.B. *Educated Guesses: Making Policy About Medical Screening Tests.* Berkeley, Calif.: University of California Press, 1994.

Rutkauskas, J.S. Medically Necessary Oral Care, Medicare, Medicaid, Managed Care, and Mayhem [editorial]. *SCD Special Care in Dentistry* 15(5):176–177, 1995.

Sabin, S., B. Rao, A.W. Kopf, D.S. Rigel, R. Nossa, I.J. Rahman, et al. Predicting Ten-Year Survival of Patients with Primary Cutaneous Melanoma: Corroboration of a Prognostic Model. *Cancer* 80(8):426–431, 1997.

Sackett, D.L., W.S. Richardson, W.M. Rosenberg, and R.B. Hynes. *Evidence-Based Medicine: How to Practice and Teach EBM.* New York: Churchill Livingstone, 1997.

Sanders, C.E., J.J. Curtis, B.A. Julian, R.S. Gaston, P.A. Jones, et al. Tapering or Discontinuing Cyclosporine for Financial Reasons—A Single-Center Experience. *American Journal of Kidney Diseases* 21(1):9–15, 1993.

Sanders, C.E., B.A. Julian, R.S. Gaston, M.H. Dejerhoi, A.G. Diethelm, and J.J. Curtis. Benefits of Continued Cyclosporine Through an Indigent Drug Program. *American Journal of Kidney Diseases* 28(4):572–577, 1996.

Sbarbaro, J.A. Of Pride and Program Planning—A Lesson in Reality. *CHEST* 114(15): 1229–1238, 1998.

Sbarbaro, J.A., and S. Johnson. Tuberculous Chemotherapy for Recalcitrant Outpatients Administered Directly Twice Weekly. *American Review of Respiratory Disease* 97:895–903, 1968.

Scannapieco, F.A., and J.M. Mylotte. Relationships Between Periodontal Disease and Bacterial Pneumonia. *Journal of Periodontology* 67(10 Suppl.):1114–1122, 1996.

Schauffler, H.H. Disease Prevention Policy Under Medicare: A Historical and Political Analysis. *American Journal of Medicine* 9(2):1226–1230, 1993.

Schauffler, H.H., and T. Rodriguez. Managed Care for Preventive Services: A Review of Policy Options. *Medical Care Review* 50(2):153–198, 1993.

Scheinkopf, L.J. *Thinking for a Change: Putting the TOC Thinking Processes to Use.* Boca Raton, Fla.: St. Lucie Press, 1999.

Schimpff, S.C. Oral Complications of Cancer Therapies. Surveillance Cultures. *NCI Monographs* (9):37–42, 1990.

Schwartz, L.M., S. Woloshin, W.C. Black, and H.G. Welch. The Role of Numeracy in Understanding the Benefit of Screening Mammography. *Annals of Internal Medicine* 127(11):966–972, 1997.

Schwartz, R.A. The Actinic Keratosis. A Perspective and Update. *Dermatologic Surgery* 23(11):1009–1019, 1997.

SEER (Surveillance, Epidemiology and End Results), National Cancer Institute. Cancer Statistics Review 1973–1996 Initial Content. 1999. Last updated November 5, 1999. http://www.seer.ims.nci.nih.gov/Publications/CSR1973_1996. Accessed June 2, 1999.

Shaughnessy, P.W., R.E. Schlenker, and D.F. Hittle. Home Health Care Outcomes Under Capitated and Fee-for-Service Payment. *Health Care Financing Review* 16:197–222, 1994.

160 EXTENDING MEDICARE COVERAGE

Siegal, B.R., and S.M. Greenstein. Postrenal Transplant Compliance from the Perspective of African-Americans, Hispanic-Americans, and Anglo-Americans. *Advances in Renal Replacement Therapy* 4(1):46–54, 1997.

Siegel, J.E., M.C. Weinstein, and G.W. Torrance. Reporting Cost-Effectiveness Studies and Results, Pp. 276–303 in *Cost-Effectiveness in Health and Medicine,* M.R. Gold, J.E. Siegel, L.B. Russell, and M.C. Weinstein, eds. New York: Oxford University Press, 1996.

Sisson, S., J. Tripp, W. Paris, D.K.C. Cooper, and N. Zuhdi. Medication Noncompliance and Its Relationship to Financial Factors After Heart Transplantation [letter]. *Journal of Heart and Lung Transplantation* 13(5):930, 1994.

Siu, A.L., F.A. Sonnenberg, W.G. Manning, G.A. Goldberg, E.S. Bloomfield, J.P. Newhouse, and R.H. Brook. Inappropriate Use of Hospitals in a Randomized Trial of Health Insurance Plans. *New England Journal of Medicine* 315(20):1259–1266, 1986.

Slade, G.D., A.J. Spencer, D. Locker, R.J. Hunt, R.P. Strauss, and J.D. Beck. Variations in the Social Impact of Oral Conditions Among Older Adults in South Australia, Ontario, and North Carolina. *Journal of Dental Research* 75(7):1439–1450, 1996.

Solberg, L.E., M.L. Brekke, and T.E. Kottke. Are Physicians Less Likely to Recommend Preventive Services to Low-SES Patients? *Preventive Medicine* 26(3):350–357, 1997.

Somacarrera, M.L. M. Lucas, V. Cuervas-Mons, and G. Hernandez. Oral Care Planning and Handling of Immunosuppressed Heart, Liver, and Kidney Transplant Patients. *Special Care in Dentistry* 16(6):242–246, 1996.

Somers, A.R., and H.M. Somers. National Health Insurance: Story with a Past, Present, and Future. Pp. 179–197 in *Health and Health Care: Policies in Perspective,* A.R. Somers and H.M. Somers, eds. Germantown, Md.: Aspen Systems Corporation, 1977a.

Somers, A.R., and H.M. Somers. National Health Insurance: Criteria for an Effective Program and a Proposal. Pp. 192–203 in *Health and Health Care: Policies in Perspective,* A.R. Somers and H.M. Somers, eds. Germantown, Md.: Aspen Systems Corporation, 1977b.

Somers, H.M., and A.R. Somers. *Doctors, Patients, and Health Insurance.* Washington, D.C.: The Brookings Institution, 1961.

Somers, H.M., and A.R. Somers. *Medicare and the Hospitals: Issues and Prospects.* Washington, D.C.: The Brookings Institution, 1967.

Sonis, S., and J. Clark. Prevention and Management of Oral Mucositis Induced by Antineoplastic Therapy. Oncology 5(12):11–88, 1991.

Sox, H.C., Jr. *Common Diagnostic Tests: Use and Interpretation.* Philadelphia: American College of Physicians, 1987.

Spitzer, T.R., F. Delmonico, N. Tolkoff-Rubin, S. McAfee, R. Sackstein, S. Saidman, et al. Combined Histocompatibility Leukocyte Antigen-Matched Donor Bone Marrow and Renal Transplantation for Multiple Myeloma with End Stage Renal Disease: The Induction of Allograft Tolerance Through Mixed Lymphohematopoietic Chimerism. *Transplantation* 68(4):480–484, 1999.

Starr, P. *The Social Transformation of American Medicine.* New York: Basic Books, 1982.

Steckelberg, J.M., L.J. Melton III, D.M. Ilstrup, M.S. Rouse, and W.R. Wilson. Influence of Referral Bias on the Apparent Clinical Spectrum of Infective Endocarditis. *American Journal of Medicine* 88(6):582–588, 1990.

Stevens, R. *In Sickness and in Wealth: American Hospitals in the Twentieth Century.* New York: Basic Books, 1989.

Straume, O., and L.A. Akslen. Independent Prognostic Importance of Vascular Invasion in Nodular Melanomas. *Cancer* 78(6):1211–1219, 1996.

Strauss, R.P., and R.J. Hunt. Understanding the Value of Teeth to Older Adults: Influence on the Quality of Life. *Journal of American Dental Association* 124(1):105–110, 1993.

Strickland, D. Perspectives. House Subcommittee Vote Signals AHCPR Reprieve. *Faulkner & Gray's Medicine and Health* 49(29Suppl.):1–4.

Strom, B.L., E. Abrutyn, J.A. Berlin, J.L. Kinman, R.S. Feldman, P.D. Stolley, et al. Dental and Cardiac Risk Factors for Infective Endocarditis. A Population-Based, Case-Control Study. *Annals of Internal Medicine* 129(10):761–769, 1998.

SUPPORT Principal Investigators. A Controlled Trial to Improve Care for Seriously Ill Hospitalized Patients: The Study to Understand Prognoses and Preferences for Outcomes and Risks of Treatments (SUPPORT). *Journal of the American Medical Association* 274:1591–1598, 1995.

Suresh, J.A., C.W. Stratton, and J.S. Drummer. Lactobacillus Bacteremia: Description of the Clinical Course in Adult Patients Without Endocarditis. *Clinical Infectious Diseases* 23:773–778, 1996.

Sutton, A.J., K.R. Abrams, D.R. Jones, T.A. Sheldon, and F. Song. Systematic Reviews of Trials and Other Studies. *Health Technology Assessment* 2(19):1–276, 1998.

Swerlick, R.A., and S. Chen. The Melanoma Epidemic: Is Increased Surveillance the Solution or the Problem? *Archives of Dermatology* 132:881–884, 1996.

Swerlick, R.A., and S. Chen. The Melanoma Epidemic: More Apparent than Real? *Mayo Clinic Proceedings* 72:559–564, 1997.

TAC (Technology Advisory Committee), Health Care Financing Administration. Minutes of November 5 and 6 meeting. 1996. http://www.hcfa.gov/events/1196min.htm. Accessed July 26, 1999.

Taira, D.A., D.G. Safran, T.B. Seto, W.H. Rogers, and A.R. Tarlov. The Relationship Between Patient Income and Physician Discussion of Health Risk Behaviors. *Journal of the American Medical Association* 278(17):1412–1417, 1997.

Taubes, G. NCI Reverses One Expert Panel, Sides with Another. *Science* 276:27–28, 1997a.

Taubes, G. The Breast-Screening Brawl. *Science* 275(5303):1056–1059, 1997b.

Terezhalmy, G.T., T.J. Safadi, D.L. Longworth, and D.D. Muehrcke. Oral Disease Burden in Patients Undergoing Prosthetic Heart Valve Implantation. *Annals of Thoracic Surgery* 63(2):402–404, 1997.

Thomas, L., P. Tranchand, F. Bgerard, T. Secchi, C. Colin, and G. Moulin. Semiological Value of ABCDE Criteria in the Diagnosis of Cutaneous Pigmented Tumors. *Dermatology* 197(1):11–17, 1998.

Thomas R.M., and R.A. Amonette. Mohs Micrographic Surgery. *American Family Physician/GP* 37(3):135–142, 1988.

Thompson, R.S. What Have HMOs Learned About Clinical Prevention Services? An Examination of the Experience at Group Health Cooperative of Puget Sound. *Milbank Quarterly* 74(4):469–509, 1996.

Toljanic, J.A., J.F. Bedard, R.A. Larson, and J.P. Fox. A Prospective Pilot Study to Evaluate a New Dental Assessment and Treatment Paradigm for Patients Scheduled to Undergo Intensive Chemotherapy for Cancer. *Cancer* 85(8):1843–1848, 1999.

UNOS (United Network for Organ Sharing). 1998 Annual Report of the U.S. Scientific Registry for Transplant Recipients and the Organ Procurement and Transplanting Network: Transplant Data: 1988–1997. DHHS/HRSA, Richmond, Va.,: UNOS 1999a. Available at http://www.unos.org/fram_default.asp?category=newsdata.

UNOS. UNOS Critical Data: Waiting List. Richmond, Va.: UNOS, 1999b. http://www.unos.org/newsroom/critdata_wait.htm. Accessed October 5, 1999.

Urquhart, J. Patient Non-Compliance with Drug Regimens: Measurement, Clinical Correlates, and Economic Impact. *European Health Journal* 17(Suppl. A):8–15, 1996.

U.S. House of Representatives, Committee on Ways and Means. *1997 Medicare and Health Care Chartbook.* Washington, D.C.: U.S. Government Printing Office, 1997.

U.S. House of Representatives, Committee on Ways and Means. *1998 Green Book: Overview of Entitlement Programs.* Washington, D.C.: U.S. Government Printing Office, 1998.

USPSTF (U.S. Preventive Services Task Force). *Guide to Clinical Preventive Services.* Baltimore, Md.: Williams & Wilkins, 1990.

USPSTF. *Guide to Clinical Preventive Services,* 2nd Ed. Washington, D.C.: U.S. Department of Health and Human Services, 1996.

USRDS (U.S. Renal Data System): Excerpts from USROS 1998 Annual Data Report. *American Journal of Kidney Diseases* 32(Suppl. 1):S1–S162, 1998.

Van Der Meer, J.T.M., J. Thompson, H.A. Valkenburg, and M.F. Michel. Epidemiology of Bacterial Endocarditis in the Netherlands. I. Patient Characteristics. *Archives of Internal Medicine* 151:1863–1868, 1992a.

Van Der Meer, J.T.M., J. Thompson, H.A. Valkenburg, and M.F. Michel. Epidemiology of Bacterial Endocarditis in the Netherlands. II. Antecedent Procedures and Use of Prophylaxis. *Archives of Internal Medicine* 151:1869–1873, 1992b.

Wahlin, Y.B. Effects of Chlorhexide Mouth Rinse on Oral Health in Patients with Acute Leukemia. *Oral Surgery, Oral Medicine and Oral Pathology, Oral Radiology and Endodontics* 68(3):279–287, 1989.

Waid, M.O. Overview of the Medicare and Medicaid Programs. *Health Care Financing Review: Medicare and Medicaid Statistical Supplement* 1–19, 1998.

Weese, C.B., and M.R. Krauss. A "Barrier-Free" Health Care System Does not Ensure Adequate Vaccination of 2-Year-Old Children. *Archives of Pediatric Adolescent Medicine* 149(10):1130–1135, 1995.

Weinstock, M.A., M.G. Goldstein, C.E. Dube, A.R. Rhodes, and A.J. Sober. Basic Skin Cancer Triage for Teaching Melanoma Detection. *Journal of American Academy of Dermatology* 34(6):1063–1066, 1996.

Weisdorf, D.J., B. Bostrom, D. Raether, M. Mattingly, P. Walker, B. Pihlstrom, et al. Oropharyngeal Mucositis Complicating Bone Marrow Transplantation: Prognostic Factors and the Effect of Chlorhexidine Mouth Rinse. *Bone Marrow Transplantation* 4(1):89–95, 1989.

Westerdahl, J., H. Anderson, H. Olsson, and C. Ingvar. Reproducibility of a Self-Administered Questionnaire for Assessment of Melanoma Risk. *International Journal of Epidemiology* 25(2):245–251, 1996.

Westfelt, E., H. Rylander, G. Blohme, P. Jonasson, and J. Linhe. The Effect of Periodontal Therapy in Diabetics. Results After 5 Years. *Journal of Clinical Periodontology* 23:92–100, 1996.

White, A. The Costs and Consequences of Neglected Medically Necessary Oral Care. *SCD Special Care in Dentistry* 15(5):180–186, 1995.

White, J. Uses and Abuses of Long-Term Medicare Cost Estimates. *Health Affairs* 18(1): 63–79, 1999.

Whited, J.D., and J.M. Grichnik. Does This Patient Have a Mole or a Melanoma? *Journal of the American Medical Association* 279:696–701, 1998.

Wolfe, R.A., V.B. Ashby, E.L. Milford, A.O. Ojo, R.E. Ettenger, L.Y. Agodoa, P.J. Held, and F.K. Port. Comparison of Mortality in All Patients on Dialysis, Patients on Dialysis Awaiting Transplantation, and Recipients of a First Cadaveric Transplant. *New England Journal of Medicine* 341(23):1725–1730, 1999.

Woloshin, S., and L.M. Schwartz. The U.S. Postal Service and Cancer Screen—Stamps of Approval? *New England Journal of Medicine* 340(11):884–887, 1999b.

Woodward, R.S., M.A. Schnitzler, J.A. Lowell, G.G. Singer, D.S. Cohen, E.L. Spitnagel, et al. Medicare's Extended Immunosuppression Coverage Improved Graft Survival. Abstract submitted for the 32nd Annual Meeting of the American Society of Nephrology, Miami Beach, Fla., November 2–8, 1999.

Woloshin, S., L.M. Schwartz, W.C. Black, and H.G. Welch. Women's Perceptions of Breast Cancer Risk: How You Ask Matters. *Medical Decision Making* 19(3):221–229, 1999a.

Woolf, S.H. Should We Screen for Prostate Cancer? Men over 50 Have a Right to Decide for Themselves. *British Medical Journal* 314:989–990, 1997.

Woolf, S.H., J. Steven, and R.S. Lawrence. *Health Promotion and Disease Prevention in Clinical Practice.* Baltimore, Md.: Lippincott, Williams and Wilkins, 1996.

WPSIC (Wisconsin Physician Services Insurance Corporation). Dental Services, Policy No. DENT-002, June 14, 1996. *Wisconsin Medicare Part B Policy Manual.* 1996. http://www.wpsic.com:80/medicare/policy/dent-002.html. Accessed July 26, 1999.

Yankelovich, D. The Debate That Wasn't. The Public and the Clinton Plan. *Health Affairs (Millwood)* 14(1):7–23, 1995.

Yonayama, T., M. Yoshida, R. Matsui, H. Sasaki, and the Oral Care Working Group. Oral Care and Pneumonia. *Lancet* 354:615, 1999.

Zeldin, G., J. Magyars, A. Klein, and P.J. Thuluvath. Immunization, Screening for Malignancy, and Health Maintenance in the Liver Transplant Recipient [abstract]. *American Society of Transplant Surgeons*, 1998. http://www.a-s-t.org/abstracts98/196.htm. Accessed July 6, 1999.

APPENDIX A

Study Activities

Consistent with the provisions in the Balanced Budget Act of 1997, the Institute of Medicine (IOM) created a seven-person committee that was charged with studying the effects of expanded Medicare coverage in the areas of skin cancer screening, medically necessary dental care, and elimination of the time limitation for coverage of immunosuppressive drugs for transplant patients. The committee included specialists in public health, dermatology, transplantation, hospital dentistry, health policy, and cost-effectiveness analysis. From February 1999 to August 1999 the committee met five times. A workshop in April focused on medically necessary dental services, and workshops in June focused on skin cancer screening and immunosuppressive drugs. These workshops, which were open to the public, included presentations on the evidence base for these interventions, the estimated costs to Medicare of extending coverage, and other relevant topics. Public statements and comments were invited. Agendas follow in this appendix. In addition, four background papers were commissioned by the committee, and these are included as Appendixes B–E of this report.

The other two topics specified in the Balanced Budget Act were certain nutrition services and routine patient care costs in clinical trials. Two separate committees were created to examine these topics. Their reports, *Extending Medicare Reimbursement in Clinical Trials* and *The Role of Nutrition Therapy in Maintaining the Health of the Nation's Elderly: Evaluating Coverage of Nutrition Services for Medicare Beneficiaries,* are also available from the National Academy Press, including on-line at www.nap.edu.

INSTITUTE OF MEDICINE
COMMITTEE ON MEDICARE COVERAGE EXTENSIONS
WORKSHOP ON MEDICALLY NECESSARY DENTAL CARE

May 19–20, 1999, Washington, D.C.

Agenda

Wednesday, May 19

9:00   **Welcome, Introductions, Workshop Overview**
        Robert S. Lawrence, M.D., Committee Chair,
          Johns Hopkins University School of Hygiene and Public Health
        Marilyn J. Field, Ph.D., Study Director, Institute of Medicine

        Background and Logistics
        Following each presentation there will be a discussion and comments
        by invited discussants, registered members of the audience, and the
        audience at large.

9:30   **Remarks on Current Dental Care Issues**
        Current Coverage for Oral Health Care by Medicare
        Health Care Financing Administration

9:45   Dushanka V. Kleinman, D.D.S., M.Sc.D.
        Deputy Director, National Institute of Dental and Craniofacial Research

        Caswell Evans, D.D.S., M.P.H.
        Executive Editor and Project Director, Surgeon General's Report on
          Oral Health, National Institute of Dental and Craniofacial Research

        Charles (Bud) Conklin, D.D.S.
        Director, Carilion Dental Care, Roanoke, Virginia
        Speaking for the Federation of Special Care Organizations in Dentistry

11:00   **Review Issues of Defining "Medically Necessary Dental Care"**
        Alexander White, D.D.S., Dr.P.H., M.P.H., M.S., Lead Author,
          Commissioned Paper, Kaiser Permanente Center for Health Research

1:00   **Care for Lymphoma or Leukemia**
        James A. Lipton, D.D.S., Ph.D.
          National Institute of Dental and Craniofacial Research
        Lead Discussant: Dr. Kathryn Atchison

1:50   **Head and Neck Cancers**
Lauren Patton, D.D.S.
University of North Carolina, Chapel Hill
Lead Discussant: Dr. Carter Van Waes

2:50   **Organ Transplants**
William G. Kohn, D.D.S.
Centers for Disease Control and Prevention
Lead Discussant: Dr. Michele Saunders

3:40   **Valve Repair**
Alexander White, D.D.S., Dr.P.H., M.P.H., M.S.
Kaiser Permanente Center for Health Research
Lead Discussant: Dr. David Pearle

4:30   General discussion led by Dr. Lawrence, assisted by Dr. White

5:00   **ADJOURN**

Thursday, May 20, 1999

8:30   **Public Statements and Discussion**
Attendees wishing to make public statements are requested to notify a
staff member.

9:00   **Methods of Cost Analysis**
Allen Dobson, Ph.D., and Joan DaVanzo, Ph.D., M.S.W.
The Lewin Group, Inc.

10:15   **Further Discussion**

12:00   **ADJOURN**

Other Participants and Observers: Akintoye Adelakun, M.D., Health Care
Financing Administration Fellow; Robert E. Barsley, D.D.S.; Randy Burk-
holder, HBK Publishing; Jodi Chappell, Academy of Osseointegration; Robert
Collins, D.M.D., International and American Association for Dental Research;
Jesse Kerns, M.P.P., The Lewin Group, Inc., Gina Luke, American Association
of Dental Schools; Chris Maynard, HBK Publishing; Craig Palmer, ADA News;
Ira R. Parker, D.D.S., University of California at San Diego.

INSTITUTE OF MEDICINE
COMMITTEE ON MEDICARE COVERAGE EXTENSIONS
WORKSHOP ON SKIN CANCER SCREENING

June 17, 1999, Washington, D.C.

Agenda

8:30   **Welcome, Introductions, Workshop Overview, Charge to the Committee**
Robert S. Lawrence, M.D., Committee Chair,
   Johns Hopkins University School of Hygiene and Public Health
Marilyn J. Field, Ph.D., Study Director, Institute of Medicine

Public Statements and Discussion
Attendees wishing to make formal public statements are requested to
notify a staff member.

9:00   **Epidemiology of Skin Cancer**
Marianne Berwick, Ph.D.
Associate Attending Epidemiologist, Memorial Sloan Kettering
   Cancer Center

9:30   **Current Approaches to Screening for Skin Cancer**
Alan Geller, R.N., M.P.H.
Associate Director, Cancer Prevention and Control Center, Boston
   University, School of Medicine

10:00   **General Discussion and Questions**

10:30   **Presentation of Draft Commissioned Paper**
Mark Helfand, M.D., Lead Author, Commissioned Paper
Assistant Professor, Oregon Health Sciences University

11:00   **Discussion/Questions**
Discussants
Lowell A. Goldsmith, M.D.
Dean, School of Medicine and Dentistry, University of Rochester

Alan Moshell, M.D.
Chief, Skin Diseases Branch, National Institute of Arthritis and
Musculoskeletal and Skin Diseases

12:30   **Cost-Effectiveness of Screening for Melanoma**
        Kenneth A. Freedberg, M.D., M.Sc.
        Associate Professor of Medicine and Public Health, Boston Medical
            Center

1:00   **Cost Estimations of Screening Medicare Beneficiaries for
        Skin Cancer**
        Allen Dobson, Ph.D.
        Senior Vice President, The Lewin Group, Inc.

1:30   **Public Comment**
        American Academy of Dermatology
        June Robinson, M.D., Secretary Treasurer

1:45   **General Discussion and Questions**

2:30   **ADJOURN**

Other Participants and Observers: Clifford Amend, M.D., Blue Cross/Blue
Shield of Maryland; Joseph Chin, M.D., Health Care Financing Administration;
Joan DaVanzo, Ph.D., The Lewin Group, Inc.; Karen Eden, Ph.D., Oregon
Health Sciences University; Cheryl Hayden, American Academy of Dermatol-
ogy; Jesse Kerns, M.P.P., Study Consultant, The Lewin Group, Inc.; William
Larsen, Health Care Financing Administration; Donald R. Miller, Sc.D., Boston
University; Katharine Pirotte, Health Care Financing Administration.

Appendix A continues

INSTITUTE OF MEDICINE
COMMITTEE ON MEDICARE COVERAGE EXTENSIONS
WORKSHOP ON IMMUNOSUPPRESSIVE DRUG THERAPY

June 18, 1999, Washington, D.C.

Agenda

8:30   Welcome, Introductions, Workshop Overview, Charge to the Committee
Robert S. Lawrence, M.D., Committee Chair, Johns Hopkins
  University School of Hygiene and Public Health
Marilyn J. Field, Ph.D., Study Director, Institute of Medicine

Public Statements and Discussion
Attendees wishing to make public statements are requested to notify a staff member.

8:45   Presentation of Draft Commissioned Paper and Remarks on Compliance
Dr. Robert S. Gaston, M.D., Author, Commissioned Paper
Associate Professor, Division of Nephrology, University of Alabama at
  Birmingham

9:30   Parallel Considerations for Liver Transplants
Michael R. Lucey, M.D.
Associate Professor of Medicine, Medical Director, Liver
  Transplantation Program, Hospital of the University of Pennsylvania

9:45   Coverage Options/Strategies Beyond Medicare Coverage
Cheryl Jacobs, MSW, LICSW
Clinical Transplant Social Worker, Fairview University Transplant
  Services, Minneapolis

10:00   General Discussion and Questions

11:00   Cost Considerations
Paul W. Eggers, Ph.D., Director, Division of Beneficiaries Research,
  Health Care Financing Administration

11:30   General Discussion and Questions

1:00   **Cost Estimations**
       Allen Dobson, Ph.D.
       Senior Vice President, The Lewin Group, Inc.

1:30   **Public Comment**
       Mark Schnizler, Ph.D., Graduate Program in Health Administration,
       Washington University, St. Louis

       National Kidney Foundation: transAction Council
       Dr. Andrew Silverman, Pharm.D.
       Pharmacotherapy Specialist, Transplantation Services, Tampa
          General Hospital

2:00   **General Discussion and Questions**

2:30   **ADJOURN**

Other Participants and Observers: Clifford Amend, M.D., Blue Cross and
Blue Shield of Maryland; Dolph Chianchiano, National Kidney Foundation;
Joseph Chin, M.D., Health Care Financing Administration; Julia Christensen,
Congressional Budget Office; Lauren Geyer, Health Care Financing Administration; Melody Hughson, Hoffman-La Roche; Kim Jackson, Transplant Recipients International Organization; Jesse Kerns, M.P.P., The Lewin Group, Inc.;
Lizzy O'Hara, Congressman Boggs's Office; Linda Ohler, National Association
of Transplant Coordinators; Jackie Sheidan, Health Care Financing Administration; Alex Shipman, Covance; Andy Swire, Pharmaceutical Research and Manufacturers of America; Patricia Weitzkittel, American Nephrology Nurses Association; Stacey Windham, Congressman Canady's Office; Troy Zimmerman,
National Kidney Foundation.

APPENDIX B

Screening for Skin Cancer

Mark Helfand, M.D., M.P.H.,[*] Susan Mahon, M.P.H., and
Karen Eden, Ph.D.

INTRODUCTION

In the United States in 1999, approximately one million new cases of basal cell and squamous cell carcinoma, and about 44,000 new cases of malignant melanoma, are expected to be diagnosed.[1] Malignant melanoma is often lethal, and its incidence in the United States has increased rapidly over the past two decades. Nonmelanoma skin cancer is seldom lethal but, if advanced, can cause severe disfigurement and morbidity.

Advanced melanoma and invasive squamous cell carcinoma of the skin occur most often in the elderly, especially elderly men. Early detection and treatment of melanoma might reduce mortality, while early detection and treatment of squamous cell carcinoma and basal cell carcinoma might prevent major disfigurement, reduce the need for expensive reconstructive surgery, and to a lesser extent, prevent mortality.

In this paper, we examine published data on the effectiveness of screening for skin cancer by a physician. Specifically, we examine the accuracy of the tests used for screening, the diagnostic yield of screening in the general population, and evidence that treatment of cancers found by screening improves outcomes.

We use the term "screening" to denote a systematic effort to detect unsuspected disease by performing a total-body skin examination or by assessing the risk for skin cancer in all patients seen in the primary care setting. We did not

This evidence review was developed for the Institute of Medicine and the U.S. Preventive Services Task Force and was reviewed and approved by both groups. This paper may differ slightly in format from the version that will be released by the Task Force (expected early in 2000).

[*]Assistant Professors (Helfand and Eden) and Research Assistant (Mahon), Oregon Health Sciences University, Division of Medical Informatics/Outcomes.

examine the effect of skin surveillance on children or on patients with familial syndromes that confer a high risk of melanoma.

We also did not examine the value of routine diagnosis and treatment of skin cancer in clinical practice. In everyday primary care, the clinician sees the skin of every patient's face and, in many, the extremities, chest, and back. Clinicians almost universally agree that incidental discovery of a suspicious skin lesion should prompt an evaluation, including a skin biopsy and a thorough inspection of the skin. The data we reviewed about screening do not address the value of attention to the skin as part of conscientious clinical care.

Other strategies to prevent skin cancer, such as *promotion and counseling* to reduce risky health behaviors and *skin self-examination*, are not addressed in this review. However, many studies combine screening with health promotion programs, and screening may itself contribute to primary prevention, since it provides the physician with an opportunity to increase awareness of skin cancer and to demonstrate examination techniques that patients can apply themselves.

EPIDEMIOLOGY AND BURDEN OF SUFFERING

Melanoma

In the United States, the lifetime risk of being diagnosed with melanoma is 1.74 percent in white men and 1.28 percent in white women. The lifetime risk of dying of melanoma is 0.36 percent in men and 0.21 percent in women. Between 1973 and 1995, the incidence of melanoma in the United States increased about 4 percent per year, from 5.7 per 100,000 in 1973 to 13.3 per 100,000 in 1995, according to data from the Surveillance, Epidemiology, and End Results program (SEER) of the National Cancer Institute.[2] By comparison, the overall rate in Queensland, Australia is 55 per 100,000.

The elderly and, in particular, elderly men bear a disproportionate burden of morbidity and mortality from melanoma. As shown in Figure B-1, older men have the highest incidence of invasive melanoma. In 1995, the age-adjusted incidence rate was 68.7 per 100,000 in white men over age 65 and 30.6 per 100,000 in white women over 65. Men over 65 years of age, who constitute 5.2 percent of the U.S. population, have 22 percent of newly diagnosed malignant melanomas each year; women over 65 who constitute 7.4 percent of the population, have 14 percent.

Melanoma in the elderly is not only more common, but also more lethal than in younger populations. In Australia, where for many years public education about melanoma has been intense, 75 percent of "thick" (>3 mm) melanoma lesions and 75 percent of deaths occur in people over 50 years of age; 50 percent of deaths occur in men over 50.[3] Similarly, in the United States, about 50 percent of deaths from melanoma are in men over 50 years of age.[2] Figure B-2

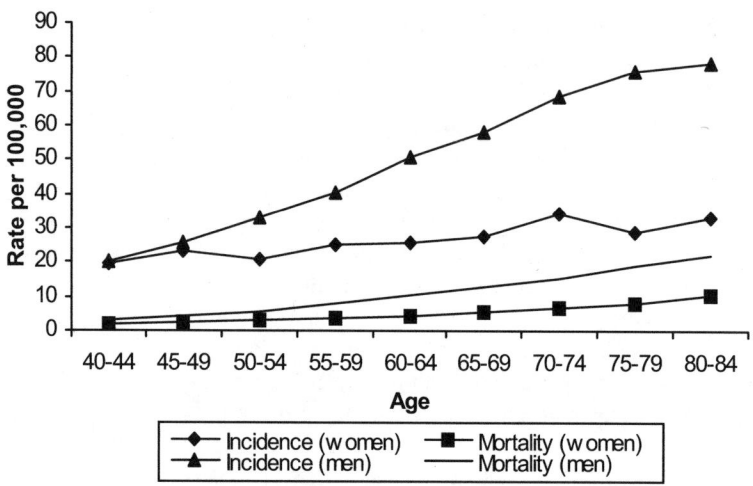

FIGURE B-1 Melanoma age-specific incidence and mortality.

shows that melanoma in the elderly, particularly elderly men, is more likely to be detected in advanced stages. For men in their 40s, for example, there are six times as many cancers diagnosed as deaths; for men in their 70s, there are about four cancers diagnosed per death. Some experts argue that the elderly, particularly elderly men, may have lower "skin awareness" and lower rates of skin self-examination, resulting in higher rates of advanced melanoma.[4]

Overall mortality from melanoma has increased. Between 1973 and 1995, overall mortality rates for melanoma increased by 1.3 percent per year, from 1.6 per 100,000 in 1973 to 2.2 per 100,000 in 1995. Nearly all of the increase was in white men (2.2 to 3.6 percent), especially older white men. Five-year survival for melanoma has improved to 88 percent currently from 80 percent 20 years ago. During this time, the rate of diagnosis of "early" or thin melanoma increased sharply, but so did the incidence of thicker (>3 mm) melanomas.[5]

Changes over time in ascertainment, diagnostic criteria, self-examination, and registry procedures make it difficult to draw reliable inferences about the effectiveness of early detection from epidemiologic data.[5-7] In an analysis of trends in Australia and New Zealand, Burton and colleagues noted that although there has been a huge increase in the incidence of very thin melanomas, the incidence of thick melanomas has increased as well.[8] Some experts interpret this to mean that increased surveillance in the population may detect a relatively unaggressive, unimportant type of thin melanoma.[7-10] Increased detection of these very thin, nonmetastasizing melanomas would increase the incidence and five-year survival rates for melanoma but would have little impact on mortality. However, in contrast to prostate and thyroid cancers, in which a large

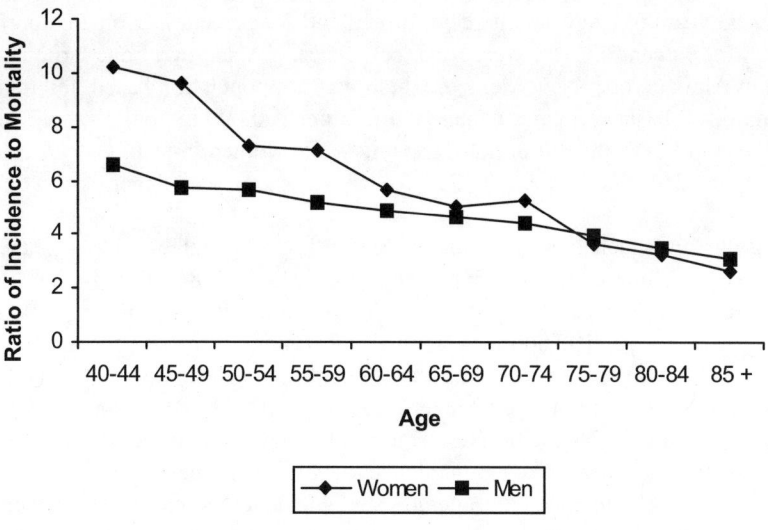

FIGURE B-2 Ratio of incidence to mortality by age.

reservoir of unaggressive cancers are known to exist, longitudinal studies of melanoma have not established the frequency or existence of histologically malignant, but behaviorally benign, melanoma in the general population.

Nonmelanoma Skin Cancer

Rates of nonmelanoma skin cancer in the United States are difficult to determine, since these cancers are not typically tracked by cancer registries. Cancer registries in Denmark and Canada do include nonmelanoma skin cancers. In British Columbia, Canada, the age-standardized incidence rate for basal cell cancer in men was 70.7 per 100,000 in 1973, increasing to 120.4 per 100,000 in 1987.[11] In women, basal cell cancer incidence increased from 61.5 to 92.2 per 100,000 over the same period. Squamous cell cancer incidence rose from 16.6 to 31.2 per 100,000 in men and from 9.4 to 16.9 per 100,000 in women.

Population-based surveys show substantial variation among geographic areas. In Queensland, Australia in the early 1990s, the age-adjusted incidence rates of basal cell carcinoma among men and women were 2,074 and 1,579 per 100,000 per year, respectively.[12] Squamous cell carcinoma occurred at half the rate of basal cell carcinoma among men and at about one-third the rate among women. In Geraldton, Western Australia, the estimated incidence of basal cell carcinoma was 1,335 per 100,000 in men and 817 per 100,000 in women.[13] In that community, the prevalence of nonmelanoma skin cancer in men and women under 65 years of age was 7 percent in men and 4.7 percent in women; approximately 90 percent of these were basal cell cancers. A survey of one large health plan in Albuquerque, New Mexico, which was not population based, found age-standardized basal cell cancer rates of 1,073 per 100,000 in non-Hispanic white men and 415 per 100,000 in non-Hispanic white women. Squamous cell cancer rates were 214 and 50 per 100,000 for non-Hispanic white men and women, respectively.

Rates are much lower in other U.S. studies. A population-based study in Rochester, Minnesota, covering the years 1976–1984 found that age-standardized incidence rates per year of basal cell cancer were 175 per 100,000 in men and 124 per 100,000 in women.[14,15] Rates of squamous cell cancer were 63.1 per 100,000 in men and 22.5 per 100,000 in women. Rates of both basal cell cancer and squamous cell cancer increased with advancing age. A population-based study of NMSC in New Hampshire suggests that incidence rates are increasing. This study looked at incidence rates for two time periods, 1979–1980 and 1993-1994.[16] In men, the age-adjusted incidence of basal cell cancer increased from 170 per 100,000 in 1979–1980 to 310 per 100,000 in 1993–1994; and in women basal cell cancer incidence rose from 91 to 166 per 100,000 over the same period. For squamous cell cancer, incidence rates in men rose from 29 to 97 per 100,000 over these periods, and in women, squamous cell cancer incidence rose from 7 to 32 per 100,000.

NATURAL HISTORY, DIAGNOSIS, AND STAGING OF SKIN CANCER

Melanoma

There are four major subtypes of melanoma: superficial spreading, nodular, lentigo maligna melanoma, and acral lentiginous melanoma.[17] Superficial spreading melanoma, the most common subtype in whites, is usually diagnosed at an early (thin) stage before there is a high risk of metastasis. Nodular melanoma is the second most common subtype in whites. Nodular melanomas are difficult for patients to find and are usually diagnosed in a more advanced stage.[18] The natural history of nodular melanoma is controversial.[19] The prevailing view is that nodular melanoma is characterized by rapid, early vertical growth and lack of an identifiable radial growth phase.

To determine which skin lesions are suspicious for melanoma, some clinicians in the United States use the ABCD checklist for detecting melanoma.[20] With this system, pigmented lesions are classified as suspicious for melanoma if they have an asymmetric shape; an irregular border that is scalloped, uneven, or ragged; varied color; or a diameter larger than 6 mm. Some add a fifth criterion (ABCDE) for elevation or enlargement. Some clinicians in the United Kingdom use a seven-point checklist that includes change in mole size, shape, and color; crusting or bleeding; sensory change; and a mole greater than 7 mm in diameter.[20]

Once a lesion suspected to be cancer is identified, one of several biopsy techniques is employed to obtain tissue for analysis. The pathological diagnosis of suspicious pigmented lesions can be difficult, especially for borderline and in situ neoplasms. In one recent study, four histopathologists evaluated 140 slides and classified each lesion as "melanoma" or "other pigmented lesion"; they were in agreement on diagnoses for 74 percent (kappa = .61) of the slides.[21] Similarly, when eight expert pathologists (recruited based on publications and reputations) classified 37 slides as "benign," "malignant," or "indeterminate," they had complete agreement, or only one discordant, on 62 percent (kappa = .50) of the cases.[22]

Stage is the most important prognostic factor in melanoma. The American Joint Commission on Cancer Classification, which is based on the TNM (tumor, node, metastasis) system, describes the stages from I to IV. Stage I is a primary tumor less than 1.5 mm in thickness with no regional lymph node metastases; Stage II is a primary tumor 1.5–4.0 mm in thickness with no regional lymph node metastases; Stage III is any primary tumor with regional lymph node metastases or in-transit metastases; and Stage IV is any primary tumor with distant metastases.[23] According to SEER data through 1995, five-year relative survival rates for localized, regional, and distant disease were 96 percent, 59 percent, and 12 percent, respectively.[2]

The thickness of the primary tumor is the strongest predictor of prognosis. To measure thickness of a melanoma, the pathologist uses a device called a "micrometer," similar to a small ruler under the microscope. This technique is called the Breslow measurement.[24] In general, melanomas less than 1 mm in depth have a very small chance of metastasizing. Five-year survival for those with melanomas between 1.5 mm and 4 mm is approximately 70 percent, and for those with melanomas thicker than 4 mm, it is about 45 percent. Thickness of the melanoma also guides the choice of therapy.

Nonmelanoma Skin Cancers

Basal cell carcinoma and squamous cell carcinoma are the most common forms of skin cancer. Despite their very high incidence they account for less than 0.1 percent of cancer deaths. There are several morphological types of basal cell cancer, such as nodular, ulcerative, and plaque-like but regardless of type, metastasis is very rare. Basal cell carcinoma can be locally destructive and frequently recurs.

Squamous cell cancers usually occur on chronically sun-exposed areas of the skin, especially the face, ears, or backs of the hands. Squamous cell cancer has the potential to metastasize and may account for up to 20 percent of deaths from skin cancer. A large primary tumor (>2 cm) is associated with an increased risk of metastasis.

Most studies of the natural history of nonmelanoma skin cancer have been done in selected patients who have an elevated risk due to environmental exposures, such as Psorolen plus ultraviolet-A (UV–A) radiation for psoriasis.[25,26] Patients with these exposures may constitute a substantial proportion of all patients who die of metastatic squamous cell cancer.[27] Very elderly men are also overrepresented among patients who die of squamous cell cancer. While there is strong suspicion on clinical grounds that advanced locally invasive or metastatic nonmelanoma skin cancers result from medical neglect, careful studies of the rate of progress of nonmelanoma skin cancers in the elderly are lacking.

RECOMMENDATIONS OF SECOND TASK FORCE AND OTHERS

Current recommendations of professional societies regarding screening for skin cancer vary. The American Cancer Society recommends skin examination every three years for people between 20 and 40 years of age and yearly for anyone over 40. The American College of Preventive Medicine and the U.S. Preventive Services Task Force[28] recommend total body skin examination in high-risk individuals who see a physician for other reasons, but they do not recommend routine screening. All of these organizations advise some form of public or patient education to change behaviors that may increase the risk of skin cancer and increase the likelihood of early self-detection.

ANALYTIC FRAMEWORK AND KEY QUESTIONS

Before the consequences of screening can be estimated, a necessary first step is to formulate the screening problem by specifying the population that screening is intended to reach; the screening tests, follow-up tests, and treatments that will be used; and the types of outcomes that will be affected by screening.

The analytic framework in Figure B-3 shows the interventions, intermediate outcome measures, and health outcome measures we examined. The accompanying key questions (Figure B-4) correspond to the numbered arrows in the analytic framework and articulate the main questions that guided our literature review and that are addressed in the results section of this appendix.

We studied screening in the general adult population and in the elderly, the group with the highest prevalence of and mortality from skin cancer. We have included studies of both *mass-screening* and *case-finding* programs to detect and treat melanoma and nonmelanoma skin cancer in the general population. In *mass-screening* programs, self-selected individuals respond to an invitation to undergo a total-body skin examination. Those with suspicious skin lesions are

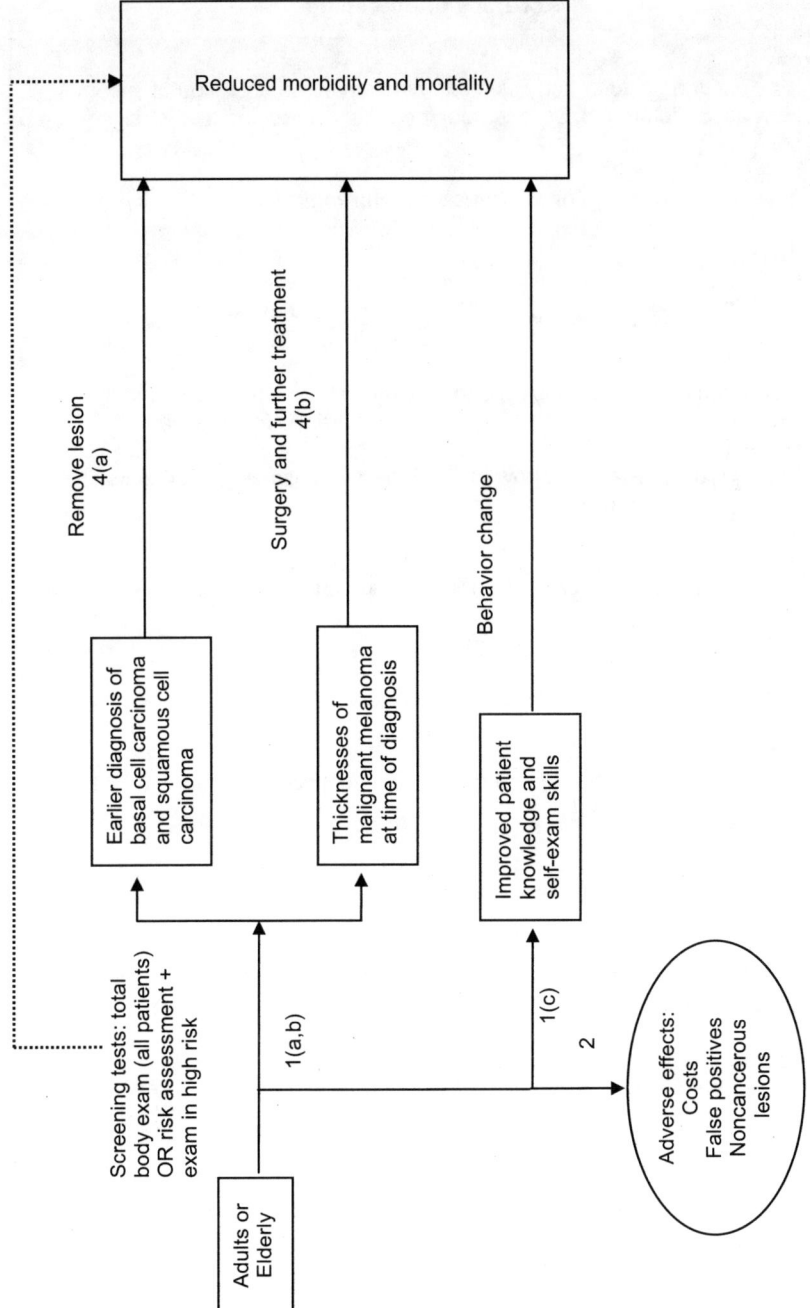

FIGURE B-3 Screening for skin cancer: Analytic framework.

Accuracy of Screening

Arrow 1a
1. How accurate is total-body skin examination in the detection of cancer?
2. How accurate are risk-assessment tools as a screening test for skin cancer?

Consequences of Screening

Arrow 1b
1. How often does screening detect suspicious lesions?
2. How often does screening result in a diagnosis of melanoma?
3. How often does screening result in a diagnosis of nonmelanoma skin cancer?
4. How often does screening lead to referral for follow-up and biopsy?
5. How do characteristics of the screening program affect the yield of screening?
6. Compared to usual care, how much earlier does screening detect skin cancers and precancerous lesions?

Arrow 1c
What is the effect of screening on patients' skin knowledge and self-care behavior?

Arrow 2
What are the adverse effects of screening?

Arrow 3
Is there direct evidence that screening for skin cancers leads to reduced morbidity and mortality?

Effectiveness of Early Treatment

Arrow 4a
Does treatment of non-melanoma skin cancer found by screening reduce morbidity and mortality?

Arrow 4b
Does treatment of malignant melanoma found by screening reduce morbidity and mortality?

FIGURE B-4 Key questions.

referred to their primary care physician or to a specialist for further evaluation. In *case-finding* programs, a total-body skin examination is offered to individuals who see a primary care physician for other reasons. A total-body skin examination may be offered to every individual or to selected individuals considered at high risk of skin cancer. Because the great majority of Medicare beneficiaries do see a physician each year, case-finding in physicians' offices might reach high-risk patients, especially elderly men, who are less likely than other groups to respond to an invitation to be screened in a mass screening program.

We sought studies of the accuracy of two methods of screening for skin cancer (*Arrow 1a*): (1) performing a total-body skin examination in all patients seen in the primary care setting, and (2) assessing the risk for skin cancer in all patients, followed by a total-body skin examination in those found to be at high risk. The primary aim of these strategies is earlier detection of melanoma, for which an examination confined to areas not covered by clothing is likely to miss a high proportion of potentially lethal cancers.[29] To assess the accuracy of these methods, both for melanoma and for nonmelanoma skin cancer, we sought studies that used these initial tests to screen in the general population or in the elderly and then confirmed positive screening test results with skin biopsy results.

We examined the consequences of screening on detection of squamous cell carcinoma, basal cell carcinoma, and malignant melanoma (*Arrow 1b*). Specifically, we examined how often patients are found to have skin cancer, how often suspected skin cancer is confirmed by biopsy, and at what stage cancer is found.

In addition to early detection, screening itself might confer a potential benefit by improving patients' knowledge and self-examination skills. We therefore sought evidence about the effect of screening on patients' health beliefs and practices regarding skin cancer prevention (*Arrow 1c*). We also considered the adverse effects of screening, including the frequency and consequences of false positive examinations or biopsies and the diagnosis of noncancerous lesions that may not require treatment (*Arrow 2*).

In considering outcomes, we sought, but did not find, direct evidence from controlled studies of the effect of screening on health outcomes (*Arrow 3, dotted line*) such as mortality and quality of life. In the absence of randomized trials of screening, these links may be made by studies of the association between delay of diagnosis and the outcome of cancer or of the outcomes of screened versus nonscreened populations.

Note that we did not examine the effectiveness or adverse consequences of various treatments for skin cancer, but rather investigated the evidence that detection of earlier cancers by screening in the general population is associated with reduced mortality and morbidity.

METHODS

Literature Review

To find relevant articles on screening for skin cancer, we searched the MEDLINE database for papers published in 1994 or later, using the search string in Addendum B-1 (see page 214). We conducted monthly updates during the course of the project. We included studies if they contained data on yield of screening, screening tests, risk factors, risk assessment, effectiveness of early detection, or cost-effectiveness.

Two reviewers evaluated abstracts for inclusion. The reviewers also searched the reference lists of relevant reviews. Of 54 included studies, 5 contained data on accuracy of screening tests, 24 contained data on yield of screening, 8 contained data on stage or thickness of lesions found through screening, 11 addressed risk assessment, and 7 addressed the effectiveness of early detection (some studies addressed more than one topic) (see Addendum B-2, page 215). We retrieved the full text of these articles and abstracted the data as described below. In addition, we retrieved the full text of 47 studies of various risk factors for skin cancer. We read these articles but did not systematically abstract them.

We identified the most important studies from before 1994 from the *Guide to Clinical Preventive Services, Second Edition;*[28] from high-quality reviews published in 1994 and 1996;[30,31] from reference lists of recent studies; and from experts. We found that many relevant publications from before 1994 were preliminary results of programs discussed in greater detail in more recent publications.

Data Extraction and Synthesis

We abstracted the following descriptive information from full-text, published studies of screening and recorded it in an electronic database: study type (mass screening, population based, case finding, other); setting (hospital, community, specialty clinic, primary care, other); population (percent white, age), recruitment (volunteers, invitation, random sampling), screening test (total-body skin examination, partial skin examination, lesion-specific examination, other); examiner (dermatologist, primary care physician, other); advertising targeted at high-risk groups or not targeted; reported risk factors of participants; and procedure for referring patients found to have a positive screen.

We also abstracted the number and probability of the following events from each study: referrals for skin examination; compliance with referral; suspected basal cell cancers, squamous cell cancers, actinic keratoses, and melanoma; confirmed melanoma and melanoma in situ; negative screening examinations; biopsies performed; the number with confirmed melanoma and number with suspicious melanoma; and the number with confirmed melanoma and number of all suspicious lesions. When available, the type, stage, and thickness of lesions found through screening were also recorded.

For studies that reported test performance, we also recorded the definition of a suspicious lesion, the "gold standard" determination of disease, the number of true positive, false positive, true negative, and false negative test results. To analyze data from these studies, we defined sensitivity as the proportion of people with a histologic diagnosis of skin cancer who had a positive test result— that is, a suspicious lesion on examination. Specificity was defined as the proportion of people who did not have skin cancer who had no suspicious lesions detected during the skin exam.

The positive predictive value (PV+) was computed in two ways to account for noncompliance in studies. The lower bound (Low PV+) of the predictive value was computed by dividing the number of patients with confirmed skin cancer by the number of patients who were diagnosed with a suspicious lesion. The upper bound (High PV+) was computed by dividing the number of patients with confirmed skin cancer by the number of patients who had biopsies. If the study provided sufficient detail, we calculated the PV+ of examination for each type of skin cancer. Most studies, however, did not report results in sufficient detail; for these, we combined the results for different types of skin cancer.

We calculated likelihood ratios (LRs) for each study. The LR for a positive test was calculated using the formula

$$LR = [High\ PV/(1 - High\ PV)]/[p(cancer)/(1 - p(cancer)],$$

where p(cancer) is the observed prevalence of disease, estimated as p(cancer) = (number of true positives + number of false negatives)/(number of patients screened).[32]

This formula was derived from the odds ratio form of Bayes' theorem.[33] The advantage of using the odds ratio form is that LR can be computed in studies that reported findings only for patients with positive tests. The computation is based on the following,

$$Posttest\ odds = pretest\ odds \times likelihood\ ratio.$$

In computing the LRs, we used the High PV+, which included only those patients who went on for biopsy. We assumed that the High PV+ was more representative of screening in a primary care setting. These patients would be more likely to follow through with a biopsy than those attending a mass screening.

In studies that did not measure the false negative rate, we assumed that there were no false negative results. The observed prevalence was computed by dividing the number of patients with true positive results by the number of screened patients. If there were, in fact, patients in these studies with false negative results, the observed prevalence was underreported. Since computation of the LR depends on an accurate measure of prevalence, LRs computed with an underreported prevalence are inflated. We performed a sensitivity analysis to record the effect on the estimate of LR when the number of false negatives and the prevalence were varied over a reasonable range of values.

RESULTS

Accuracy of Screening Tests

Before considering the consequences of screening, we raised and attempted to answer the following questions about the accuracy of the screening tests most commonly used in detecting skin cancers. The numbers and letters in parentheses relate to the arrows in the analytic framework (Figure B-3) and the related key questions (Figure B-4).

How accurate is total-body skin examination in the detection of skin cancer? (Arrow 1a, Q1)

Screening Studies

Table B-1 summarizes five recent prospective studies of the accuracy of skin examination in screening programs. In all of the studies the participants were self-selected individuals who responded to an advertisement that may have emphasized skin cancer risk factors. In some studies, total-body skin examinations were performed on all participants; in others, the examination focused on specific lesions identified by the patient. In all but one study,[34] the skin exams were conducted by dermatologists.

In these studies, a positive screening test result was defined as the clinical diagnosis of a suspicious skin lesion. Histologic diagnosis on skin biopsy was the gold standard for determination of disease. In four of the studies, skin examination was considered positive if the lesion was suspicious of any skin cancer.[34–38] In these studies, from 4.2 to 28.4 percent of subjects had suspicious lesions, and from 1 percent to 6 percent proved to have skin cancer. Basal cell cancer accounted for 74–93 percent of the confirmed skin cancer cases; melanoma, 7–27 percent; and squamous cell cancer, 0–4 percent of the skin cancer cases. This suggests that basal cell cancers contributed heavily to the summary estimates of the accuracy of skin examination reported in these studies.

Work-up bias was present in all of these studies—that is, only suspicious lesions were biopsied. This design permits measurement of the positive predictive value of screening, but not of the false negative rate. In Table B-1, High PV+ estimates (as defined in the methods section, above) for all types of skin cancer values ranged from 0.30 to 0.58, indicating that between 30 and 58 percent of patients found to have a suspicious lesion were eventually diagnosed to have skin cancer on biopsy.[34–38] The variation in High PV+ may be related to variation in the prevalence of disease, which in turn could be related to the type of patients recruited (high risk or not targeted).

The Low PV+ (also defined in the methods section) takes into account the effect of noncompliance with the recommendation to have a biopsy done. The two smallest studies[34,37] had great differences between the lower and upper estimates of predictive value. In both of these small studies the percentage of patients with suspicious lesions was high (21 percent[34] and 28 percent[37]), but the percentage of those patients who went on for biopsy was low (36 percent[37] and 65 percent[34]). The clinicians in these studies appeared to have less rigid criteria for diagnosing skin cancer from skin exams than did clinicians in the other, larger studies, since they were four times as likely to find a suspicious lesion. Low PV+ results may better represent the actual impact of mass screening, in which the patient must comply with referral to a physician for biopsy in order for screening to affect follow-up and treatment.

The last study shown in Table B-1 focuses on detection of melanoma in self-selected individuals.[39] The study demonstrated that dermatologists found lesions suspicious for melanoma in a very small proportion of individuals. In this study, 282,555 members of the general public were recruited for free examinations without regard to risk factors for skin cancer. Clinical suspicion was classified as "suspected melanoma" or "rule-out melanoma." Only 0.3 percent (n = 763) of the participants had a clinical diagnosis of suspected melanoma at the skin examination. Of the 679 patients who went on for biopsies, 130 patients had melanoma (PV+ = 0.191). Although the use of a lower cutoff, rule-out melanoma, identified an additional 234 patients with melanoma, an additional 2,316 patients without melanoma were biopsied and the predictive value was 0.09. Interestingly, compliance with biopsy was significantly lower for participants given a diagnosis of rule-out melanoma—0.69, compared to 0.89 for patients with a diagnosis of suspected melanoma.

Although data are sparse, the sensitivity of a complete skin examination performed by a dermatologist is thought to be high. One of the studies in Table B-1 provided an indirect measure of sensitivity and specificity through registry data.[40] In this study, performed in the Netherlands, 1,551 of 1,763 participants who had negative screening examinations consented to be followed through two population-based cancer registries for 42 months. Similarly, 87 of 93 patients with positive tests were also followed. Fifteen patients with negative screening results (about 1 percent) appeared in at least one of the cancer registries to have skin cancer. Review of medical records revealed that 12 of the patients had new lesions, while 3 patients had documented lesions that had been misdiagnosed. One patient had a basal cell carcinoma on his back that had been diagnosed as a common nevus. A second patient had a squamous cell carcinoma on his wrist

TABLE B-1 Skin Cancer Screening Accuracy

Author, Year	Study Sample and Setting	Recruitment Focus	Patients (n)	Index Test	PCP or Derm	Definition of Suspicious Lesion
Screening for all skin cancer						
de Rooij, 1995; Rampen, 1995	Volunteers for skin cancer screening in the Netherlands	Patients with skin cancer risks	1,961	Lesion-specific exam or TSE	d	Skin cancer
Limpert, 1995	Free skin cancer-clinic at family physician's office	Not reported	247	TSE	p	Skin cancer
de Rooij, 1997	Volunteer melanoma screenings in the Netherlands following public campaign on melanoma and risk factors	Patients with melanoma risks	4,146	Lesion specific exam or TSE	d	Skin cancer
Jonna, 1998	Free skin cancer screening in San Diego for self-selected high risk	Patients with skin cancer risks	464	TSE	d	Skin cancer
Screening for melanoma						
Koh, 1996	Volunteer skin cancer education and screenings by the American Academy of Dermatology	Not targeted	282,555	Not reported	d	Suspected melanoma
Koh, 1996	Volunteer skin cancer education and screenings by the American Academy of Dermatology	Not targeted	282,555	Not reported	d	Rule out melanoma

NOTE: BCC = basal cell carcinoma; d = dermatologist; MM = malignant melanoma; p = primary care provider; PCP = primary care physician; SCC = squamous cell carcinoma; and TSE = total skin examination. The overall probability of cancer was calculated as the total number of cancers diagnosed divided by number of patients screened. For the first group of studies, all skin cancers are included in the numerator. For the Koh studies, only melanomas are included. Methods for calculating the high and low estimates of predictive value and likelihood ratios are described in the text.

[a]Proportion of patients referred for biopsy who actually had one.
[b]Method for estimating likelihood ration of a positive test is described in the text.

Suspicious Lesions		Probability of Cancer	BCC/ Skin Cancer (%)	MM/ Skin Cancer (%)	SCC/ Skin Cancer (%)	Positive Predictive Value		Biopsy Rate[a]	Likelihood Ratio[b]
n	%					Low	High		
93	4.7	0.031	85.1	12.8	2.1	0.51	0.54	0.935	37.32
51	20.6	0.057	92.9	7.1	0.0	0.27	0.42	0.647	12.26
173	4.2	0.011	73.5	26.5	0.0	0.28	0.30	0.912	37.95
132	28.4	0.060	85.2	11.1	3.7	0.21	0.58	0.364	21.80
763	0.3	0.001				0.17	0.19	0.890	183.57
3,695	1.3	0.001				0.06	0.09	0.690	78.33

that was recorded as a seborrheic keratosis. The third patient had a basal cell carcinoma on the forehead originally diagnosed as an actinic keratosis. Overall sensitivity of the initial examination was 0.940 and specificity was 0.975. For a patient with a negative initial skin examination, the probability of having no skin cancer on follow-up was 0.998.

While this follow-up study[40] provides the best available data on sensitivity and specificity in a screening setting, a caution should be raised about generalizing this study to screening in a primary care setting. The examiners were dermatologists. Additionally, it unclear how many lesions diagnosed as precursor lesions were, in fact, skin cancer. Patients with precursor lesions (n = 111) were excluded from the study.

Since positive predictive values are highly dependent on the probability of skin cancer in each study, positive likelihood ratios were computed. The positive LRs in Table B-1 ranged from 12 to 37 for patients screened for all types of skin cancer.[34,35,37,40,41] Thus, according to the conditional probability definition of LR, p(positive test| skin cancer)/p(positive test| no skin cancer), patients with suspicious lesions for any type of skin cancer were 12 to 38 times more likely to have skin cancer than to not have skin cancer. When screened specifically for melanoma, patients with a suspected melanoma diagnosis were 184 times more likely to have melanoma than to not have melanoma.[39] Patients with a rule-out melanoma diagnosis were 78 times more likely to have melanoma than to not have melanoma.

Most LR results shown in Table B-1 must be considered with caution. With the exception of one study,[40] the computation of LRs assumed that there were no false negative results. In this study, 3 of 50 skin cancer patients had false negative results, suggesting that skin exams have a false negative rate of 6 percent.[40] When the LR was recomputed in this study and the false negative rate was assumed to be 0 percent, the LR increased from 37.32 (using false negative rate of 6 percent) to 39.78 (0 percent false negative rate). Similarly, if the false negative rate was actually 10 percent, the LR for this study would be 35.84. If it were assumed to be 0 percent, the computed LR would be 39.78. Taken to an extreme, if the examiner missed one of every five patients with skin cancer (a false negative rate of 20 percent), the computed LR would be overestimated by 27 percent. However, if the false negative rate found in the follow-up study[40] can be generalized to the studies that did not identify false negatives,[34,37,39,41] the inflation may be approximately 6 percent.

In summary, estimates of accuracy are based on a handful of mass screening, cross-sectional studies. All studies suffer from work-up bias. However, one study[40] attempted to reduce this bias by following all patients with negative tests to determine how many patients with skin cancer were missed. Also, all studies except one[34] provide accuracy measures for dermatologists in mass screening settings but not for primary care physicians. Accuracy for dermatologists screening patients is thought to be high, with a sensitivity of 0.94 and a specificity of 0.975.[40]

Non-Screening Studies

Several studies have examined the accuracy of nondermatologists' assessments of photographs of skin lesions or of preselected patients with lesions, using the histologic diagnosis as the reference standard. One recent review summarized studies that used color slides (rather than actual patients) to test physicians' accuracy in predicting the histologic diagnosis (mostly NMSC).[42] When these studies were combined, dermatologists performed better (93 percent correct) than family medicine attending physicians (70 percent correct) and internal medicine attending physicians (52 percent correct). Another recent review found that in studies that used photographs or selected patients with known lesions, use of the ABCD(E) or seven-point checklist had a sensitivity of 50–97 percent and a specificity of 96–99 percent for the histologic diagnosis of skin cancer.[20] Nondermatologists' examinations were less sensitive than examinations performed by dermatologists. Many of these studies were small and used convenience samples of attending physicians at academic medical centers. More importantly, these studies did not examine the accuracy of a total-body skin examination or the ability of physicians to efficiently identify suspicious lesions in the setting of a screening program.

One well-designed prospective study of the accuracy of total-body skin examination found that skin cancer specialists' decisions about biopsy were more sensitive and much more specific than those of general practitioners (GPs).[43] Four skin cancer specialists and 63 randomly selected general practitioners in Australia performed total-body skin examinations on 109 selected patients, 43 of whom had suspicious pigmented lesions diagnosed previously by a skin specialist. The sensitivity of total-body skin examination for detecting suspicious lesions was 0.72 for the GPs, versus 0.97 for the four skin cancer specialists. The positive predictive value for the GPs was 0.39. Of the 43 patients with suspicious lesions, 12 (28 percent) had melanomas. While the GPs' diagnoses were highly sensitive for melanomas (0.97), they classified about 11 benign lesions as suspicious for each melanoma. For the four dermatologists, the ratio was 2.1 benign lesions to 1 melanoma. Because the proportion of patients who had suspicious lesions (and melanoma) was much higher in this study than would occur in unselected patients, the positive predictive value of primary care physicians' examinations would be lower in an actual screening study.

How accurate are risk-assessment tools as a screening test for skin cancer? (Arrow 1a, Q2)

Another screening strategy is to use a questionnaire or interview to identify a group of high-risk patients. In this strategy, only high-risk patients would have total-body skin examinations. Potentially, such a strategy could reduce the cost of screening because fewer total-body skin examinations and biopsies would be required to diagnose patients with skin cancer. The association of demographic, behavioral, and clinical factors with the risk of skin cancer has been well studied, and studies have established that physicians and patients can reliably measure some of these factors. As discussed below, however, the validity of formal risk assessment tools to screen unselected patients in primary care has not been established.

Risk Factors for Nonmelanoma Skin Cancer

A past history of skin cancer, or of actinic keratoses (AK), and white race are the strongest risk factors for nonmelanoma skin cancer. Among whites who have no prior history of skin cancer or AK, sun exposure is the most important risk factor for nonmelanoma skin cancer. Cumulative sun exposure and possibly intermittent intense sun exposure,[44] total time spent outdoors,[45] geographic area of residence,[46] and lifetime number of severe sunburns[46] have all been shown to be associated with higher risk of NMSC. Other risk factors include past history of NMSC, [47] light or red hair,[45,46] propensity to sunburn,[46,47] and family history of skin cancer.

Risk Factors for Melanoma

A high count of common moles larger than 2 mm and the presence of atypical moles are risk factors for melanoma.[48–51] In these studies, the risk of malignant melanoma was at least three times as high in patients who had 50–99 common moles as in patients with fewer than 10 moles. Similarly, the likelihood of melanoma increased several times (odds rate [OR] ranged 1.6–7.3) for patients with one to four atypical moles compared to patients with no atypical moles.

Other risk factors for melanoma are red or light hair (OR ranged 1.4–3.5); a few (OR 1.9) or many actinic lentigines (OR 3.5); very heavy sun exposure (OR 2.63); reported growth of a mole (OR 2.3); skin that does not tan easily (OR 1.98); a family history of melanoma (OR 1.81); light eye color (OR ranged 1.55–1.60); and light skin color, types 1 or 2 (OR ranged 1.40–1.42).[48–50,52,53] The validity of some risk factors, such as hair color and sun exposure, is lower in the elderly.[48,54]

The relation of sun exposure to melanoma is complex. Since the second edition of the U.S. Preventive Services Task Force's *Guide to Clinical Preventive Services* was published in 1996, a meta-analysis of case-control studies found that "intermittent" sun exposure was associated with increased risk of melanoma, while heavy occupational exposure was found to be slightly protective.[55] This meta-analysis included 23 case-control studies on "intermittent" sun exposure, 20 occupational sun exposure case-control studies, and 21 case-control studies on sunburn, all completed by 1992. Intermittent exposure was defined as recreational and vacation sun exposure. Patients with the highest level of intermittent exposure had nearly twice the risk of melanoma as those with the lowest "intermittent" exposure (OR 1.71; 95 percent confidence interval [CI] 1.54–1.90). Patients with heavy occupational exposure were at slightly decreased risk compared to those with low occupational exposure (OR 0.86; 95 percent CI 0.77–0.96). Patients with histories of sunburn (usually a result of intermittent sun exposure) were at increased risk for melanoma (OR 1.91) compared to those without sunburn history. Since the meta-analysis was published, an analysis of body site distribution among incident melanoma cases in British Columbia found that intermittent sun exposure was a risk factor for melanoma in individuals less than 50 years of age.[56] A recent case-control study also supported the hypothesis that intermittent ultraviolet exposure is a risk factor for melanoma in younger individuals who are susceptible to burning.[57]

Reliability of Measures of Risk

To be useful as practical tools for classifying patients into risk groups, risk factors must be reliably assessed by patients or physicians. As noted above, the two strongest risk factors for melanoma are the presence of atypical moles and a large number of common moles.

Several studies have examined the reliability of mole counts by patients, interviewers, and dermatologists. In these studies, having a trained interviewer or the patient count the moles on the arm was not useful as an indicator of total-body mole count,[58-60] but patients' counts of moles on the trunk or total body were more reliable.[59-61] In a large, population-based prospective study, 670 Swedish women completed a melanoma risk-assessment questionnaire twice (one to years apart). The test–retest reliability of a mole count by the patient was high (kappa = .52–.83).[59] In a work site screening study, 104 of 125 employees correctly placed themselves in high- or low-risk melanoma categories based on count of total-body moles larger than 5 mm.[61] Of 104 lower-risk patients (with fewer than six large moles), 92 correctly assessed themselves when compared to a dermatology fellow's assessment. However, only 12 of 21 high-risk patients (more than six large moles) assessed themselves correctly. This suggests that patients are able to screen themselves for large-mole-count risk with specificity of 0.88 and sensitivity of 0.57. Women tended to overcount moles and men tended to undercount them.

There is less information on the reliability of self-report of other risk factors. In the Swedish study described above,[59] response agreement was good for questions related to hair color (kappa = .77) and freckles (kappa = .83), but only fair for the number of raised nevi on the left arm (none, 1–3 or >3) (kappa = .40) and sunburn history (kappa = .54). In another study, the agreement between patients' self-appraisal of skin characteristics and clinical skin examinations by a physician was reflected in kappa values of .67 for freckles and .43 for atypical nevi.[62]

Use of Risk Assessment in Practice

The ideal study to measure the accuracy of risk assessment tools would assign risk levels for patients in a primary care setting, perform total-body skin examinations on patients classified as high and low risk, and then monitor the patients regularly to determine what proportion of incident melanomas occurred in the high-risk group. In fact, no longitudinal studies of the use of a risk assessment tool in primary care practice have been reported.

Although it was not done in a primary care setting, a large, prospective study validated the use of an initial count of atypical moles in predicting the incidence of melanoma over five years.[63] In that study, 3,889 employees a the Lawrence Livermore National Laboratory had total-body skin examinations performed by a dermatology fellow specializing in melanoma. Atypical moles were diagnosed clinically using previously defined criteria:[64] "ill-defined border; irregular border; irregularly distributed pigmentation; a diameter more than 5 mm; erythema (blanchable in lesion or at edge); and accentuated skin markings." Seven percent of the subjects were in the highest-risk category—that is, had few to many moles that met five or more of these criteria. This highest-risk group accounted for 56 percent (five of nine) of the subjects who developed melanoma over five years. By contrast, 64 percent of the patients were in the lowest-risk category—had no atypical moles. This lowest-risk group accounted for 11 percent (one out of nine) of the patients who developed melanoma.

Two recent cross-sectional studies have examined the reliability and practicality of classifying primary care patients into risk groups using a standardized, self-administered instrument.[60,62] One of these[62,65] applied a melanoma risk assessment questionnaire[66] in 16 randomly selected group practices in Cheshire, United Kingdom. Patients were asked about freckling propensity, number of moles, existence of large moles with irregular borders or colors, and history of sunburn. Their responses were compared with the results of a physical examination by a physician.

Although this study did not track the incidence of melanoma over time, it did provide data on the proportion of primary care patients who would be classified as high risk. A total of 3,105 patients completed the questionnaire. According to their responses, patients were then placed into the following risk groups: "marginally increased risk" (49.2 percent); "increased risk" (26.6 percent);

"very increased risk" (4.4 percent); and "worrying high risk" (4.3 percent). Most patients in the two highest-risk groups were not aware of their high-risk status.

In summary, several recent case-control studies confirm earlier evidence that patients with atypical moles and/or many (>50) common moles are at increased risk for melanoma. Evidence suggests that patients can count the number of moles 5 mm or larger in reasonable agreement with physicians. No prospective evidence is available linking risk assessment by limited physical examination with incidence of melanoma, but one well-done prospective study demonstrated that this strategy could identify a relatively small (<10 percent) group of primary care patients for more thorough evaluation.

Consequences of Screening

We examined the consequences of screening described in 24 recent reports of screening programs (Table B-2).[34,35,37,39-41,63,67-85] In these studies, we examined (1) how often skin cancer is suspected in individuals who are screened; (2) how often melanoma and nonmelanoma skin cancers are diagnosed; (3) how often referrals for follow-up and biopsies are performed; and (4) how the type of skin examination, examiner, and compliance affect the yield of screening. This information is summarized in Table B-2. We also examined the distribution of thickness and stage of lesions found through screening versus usual care (Table B-3) and the adverse effects of screening.

There are limitations in using data from these studies to draw conclusions about screening in a case-finding setting. The majority of recently published studies were in a mass-screening setting. To be effective in reducing morbidity and mortality, screening should reach those who are at high risk both for developing skin cancer and for presenting with thicker lesions in the absence of screening. People who attend mass screening are a self-selected group, tend to be more skin aware, and may come because they are worried about a lesion that they have already discovered and for which they would have sought medical attention anyway. While some mass screening programs tend to attract a relatively high-risk group,[68,69] others do not, and very high-risk individuals, particularly ill elderly individuals, may be underrepresented.[86,87]

How often does screening detect suspicious lesions? (Arrow 1b, Q1)

Rates of suspected melanoma in mass screening, case finding, and population-based screening ranged from 0 to 8 per 100 people screened, with the most common findings between 1 and 3 per 100. Most studies found from 2 to 10 suspected nonmelanoma skin cancers per 100 screened. In some populations, the rate of suspected basal or squamous cell carcinoma was much lower (4 per 10,000 in a Japanese study[67]) or higher (21 per 100 screened in surfers).[73] Studies did not report the prevalence of nonmelanoma skin cancer by age, and

TABLE B-2 Studies of Screening for Skin Cancer

Author, Year	Population/ Setting/ Recruitment	Screening Test, Examiner	Media Target; Reported Risk Factors	Referral Procedure (pt's PCP, pt's dermatologist, study PCP/derm, reminder, no reminder)	Referral (p)
Mass Screening					
Jonna, 1998	464 volunteers, hospital, US; 72% < 65, 94% white, 43% male	TSE, dermatologists	Targeted high risk	Pt's PCP or dermatologist, no reminder	
Limpert, 1995	247 volunteers, PCP clinic, US; mean age 53.5 (range 4–84), 100% white, 38% male	TSE, family physician	Not targeted	Pt's PCP, pt's dermatologist, or study PCP, reminder	
Rampen, 1995	1,961 volunteers, hospital, Netherlands	TSE or partial skin exam, dermatologists	Targeted high risk	Not specified	0.1
McGee, 1994	279 volunteers, New Zealand; 41% 40–59 y/o, 29% ≥ 60 y/o	Not specified, general medical practitioners	42% came because of a "worrying mark," 25% fair skin, 53% h/o severe sunburn, 22% fair or red hair, 8% personal h/o sc, 20% family h/o sc	Pt's PCP, no reminder	0.2
Koh, 1996	282,555 volunteers, hospitals, US	Not specified (need Koh, 90)	Not targeted	Pt's PCP or dermatologist, no reminder	
de Rooij, 1995	2,463 volunteers, hospital, Netherlands; 53% >50 y/o	Lesion specific TSE	Not targeted	Pt's PCP, no reminder	
de Rooij, 1997	4,146 volunteers, hospital, Netherlands, 34% >50 y/o	Lesion specific TSE	Targeted high risk	Pt's PCP, no reminder	0.12
Katris, 1996	3,379 volunteers, hospital and community, Australia; 35% ≥ 50 y/o, 16% ≥ 60 y/o	TSE	Targeted high risk	Not specified	
Katris, 1998	256 volunteers, hospital and community, Australia	TSE, nurses, and plastic surgeons	Target high risk	Not specified	
Rivers, 1995	1,681 volunteers, community, Canada; 16% ≥ 65 y/o	TSE partial skin exam lesion specific, dermatologists	Beachgoers; 33% had 2 or more risk factors (blond or red hair, blue or green eyes, propensity to sunburn)	Pt's PCP	

Results (p)

Suspected MM	Confirmed MM	Confirmed Melanoma in Situ	Suspected BCC/SCC	Suspected AK	Negative Screen	Biopsy	MM Biopsy Suspected MM only	MM Biopsy all Suspicious Lesions
0.08	0.002	0.002	0.21		0.42	0.21	0.15	0.04
	0.004				0.57	0.18		0.02
0.003	0.003	0.001	0.02		0.9			
0.03			0.08					
0.02	0.001	0.001					0.11	
0.01	0.003	0.001	0.04	0.06				
0.02	0.001	0.002	0.02	0.02		0.08	0.17	0.03
0.02	0.08	0.038	0.13		0.83		0.08	
0.05			Surgeon: .10 Nurse: .07	Nurse: .03	Surgeon: .70 Nurse: .60			
0.005								

Continued

TABLE B-2 *Continued*

Author, Year	Population/ Setting/ Recruitment	Screening Test, Examiner	Media Target; Reported Risk Factors	Referral Procedure (pt's PCP, pt's dermatologist, study PCP/derm, reminder, no reminder)	Referral (p)
Dozier, 1997	1) 49 volunteers, community, US; mean age 29.7 2) 53 volunteers, hospital, US; mean age 35.4	1) partial skin exam 2) TSE dermatologists	1) surfers 2) not targeted	1) Pt's PCP, reminder 2) Pt's PCP, no reminder	
Population Based Screening					
Harvey, 1995, 1996	560 random population sample, community, UK; 100% ≥ 60 y/o	Partial skin exam, dermatologists	NA	Pt's PCP, reminder	0.02
Ichihashi, 1995	4,736 consecutive attendees at regional health exam, Japan	Partial skin exam, dermatologists	NA	Study dermatologist, no reminder	
Tornberg, 1996	1,654 random sample, hospital, Sweden; 100% 40–54 y/o	Not specified, nurses, dermatologist, oncologist	NA	Study dermatologist, no reminder	0.05
Bergenmar, 1997	501 random sample, hospital, Sweden; 100% 40–54 y/o	NA	NA		
Casefinding					
Ruskiewicz 1998	1,000 consecutive patients, optometrist office, US; mean age 66.3 (range 35–96)	Partial skin exam, optometrist	NA; .096 had prior dx of SC or AK	Dermatologist	
Whited, 1997	190 consecutive patients, pcp and specialty clinic, US	Partial skin exam, dermatologists, internists, physician assistants	NA		
Worksite Screening					
Friedman, 1995	421 hospital employees, identified as high risk and invited, US; mean age 41 (SD 10.6)	Not specified, dermatologists	Targeted high risk	Pt's dermatologist or study dermatologist	0.32
Schneider	3,889 laboratory employees, 9% of 20–24 y/o employees, 56% of 70 y/o and older employees	Not specified, dermatologists	NA; participants classified according to no. of atypical moles: 64% none, 29% possible or probable, 7% clear pattern of marked atypical moles	Study dermatologist	

Results (p)

Suspected MM	Confirmed MM	Confirmed Melanoma in Situ	Suspected BCC/SCC	Suspected AK	Negative Screen	Biopsy	MM Biopsy Suspected MM only	MM Biopsy all Suspicious Lesions
1) 0.0 2) 0.0			1) .16 2) .02	1) .41 2) .15				
0.004			0.02	0.23	0.75			
0			0.0004	0.01				
0.09	0	0	0	0	0.91	0.04	0	
0			0.1	0.003	0.9			
						0.31		0
0.002			0.02	0.09				
	0.002							

Continued

TABLE B-2 *Continued*

Author, Year	Population/ Setting/ Recruitment	Screening Test, Examiner	Media Target; Reported Risk Factors	Referral Procedure (pt's PCP, pt's dermatologist, study PCP/derm, reminder, no reminder)	Referral (p)
Other					
Herd, 1995	421 patients with suspected MM, specialty clinic, UK	TSE, dermatologists	NA	Study dermatologist	
Marghoob, 1995	290 patients with BCC or SCC, dermatology practice, US	TSE (melanoma only), dermatologists	All had BCC and/or SCC	Study dermatologist	
Van der Spek-Keijser, 1997	Pathology study of all MM diagnosed from 1980 to1992 after regional preventive skin cancer campaign, Netherlands, 95% Caucasians	NA	NA	NA	
Veirod, 1997	Follow-up study of 50,759 participants in health screening from 1977–83, Norway, 16–56 y/o	NA	NA	NA	

NOTE: AK = actinic keratoses; BCC = basal cell carcinoma; d = dermatologist; MM = malignant melanoma; p = primary care provider; PCP = primary care physician; SCC = squamous cell carcinoma; and TSE = total skin examination.

Results (p)

Suspected MM	Confirmed MM	Confirmed Melanoma in Situ	Suspected BCC/SCC	Suspected AK	Negative Screen	Biopsy	MM Biopsy Suspected MM only	MM Biopsy all Suspicious Lesions
							0.036	
0.22	0.034						0.15	
0.002								

TABLE B-3 Thickness of Malignant Melanoma Lesions Found in Screening Studies

Study	N (p)							
	0.5 – 1 mm	1.0 – 1.5 mm	1.5 – 2 mm	2 – 2.5 mm	2.5 – 3 mm	3 – 3.5 mm	3.5 – 4 mm	>4 mm
De Rooij	12 (.92)			1 (.08)				
Herd	82 (.76)			26 (.24)				
Katris	4 (1.0)			0 (0)				
Jonna	1 (1.0)			0 (0)				
Schneider	9 (1.0)			0 (0)				
Koh	180 (.87)			22 (.11)				4 (.02)
Marghoob	10 (1.0)			0 (0)				
Van der Spek	1,451 (.67)			506 (.23)			206 (.10)	

we found no clear difference in prevalence between studies of mostly older individuals and studies in younger individuals.

Suspected actinic keratosis was generally the most frequent finding in these studies, but rates were variable. The highest rates were 41 per 100 screened in the surfers,[73] 23 per 100 in a population sample of people over age 59,[73-75] and 15 per 100 in a small mass-screening study.[73]

How often does screening result in a diagnosis of cancer? (Arrow 1b, Q2 and Q3)

Rates of confirmed melanoma and melanoma in situ were consistently in the range of 1 to 4 per 1,000 people screened, with two exceptions. An Australian study that targeted high-risk people[70] had a rate of eight confirmed melanomas per 100 people screened. The other, a population-based study in Sweden,[77] had no confirmed melanomas of 152 suspected melanomas in 1,654 people screened.

Eight studies in Table B-2 reported the number of histologically confirmed nonmelanoma skin cancers. The prevalence varied widely, from 0.05 of people screened to 0.0004, with most reporting between 0.01 and 0.05.

How often does screening lead to referral for follow-up and biopsy? (Arrow 1b, Q4)

Among all the studies that we reviewed, rates of referral for follow-up care of suspicious lesions ranged from 2 to 34 per 100 people screened. Two studies reported rates of compliance with a recommendation to see a physician for follow-up. In one mass-screening study,[41] 95 percent of people complied with recommended follow-up, and in a work site program,[81] 45 percent complied.

As for biopsies, five studies reported the number of biopsies performed as a result of screening.[34,37,41,77,80] In these studies, from 4 to 31 biopsies per 100 people screened were performed. Among patients with suspected melanoma, from 0 to 17 percent had a final diagnosis of melanoma. Among all patients who underwent a biopsy, 0 to 0.04 proved to have a melanoma.

How do characteristics of the screening program affect the yield of screening? (Arrow 1b, Q5)

Certain characteristics of a screening program could affect compliance with follow-up recommendations and, ultimately, with the yield of screening. We consider three such characteristics below: (1) the type of skin examination, (2) the recruitment strategy, and (3) the procedure for referring patients for follow-up.

Type of Skin Examination

Examiners conducted either total-body skin examination,[34,37,70,71,73,82,83] partial skin examination (e.g., only above the waist or on sun-exposed areas),[73–76,79,80] examination only of lesions the participant was worried about,[35,41] or some combination of these (see Table B-2). Overall, compared with partial skin examination or examination of lesions the patient was worried about, the use of total-body skin examination did not appear to increase the rate of confirmed melanomas. One study[88] specifically addressed the question, In self-selected patients who have noticed a skin lesion, does total-body skin examination increase the likelihood of finding skin cancers? In that study, 2,910 of 4,146 (70 percent) people screened complained of at least one skin lesion. When these lesions were examined, 13 melanomas and 44 nonmelanoma skin cancers were diagnosed on biopsy. For those patients who originally came in with specific lesions, an additional total-body skin examination was offered. For the 1,356 patients who went on for a total-body skin examination, no malignant melanomas and three basal cell carcinomas were identified. This finding raises doubts about the benefits of conducting total-body skin examinations on everyone rather than lesion-specific examinations.

Recruitment Strategy

In 12 papers, one of which reported on two studies, screening involved a media campaign to encourage individuals to seek a skin examination (mass screening) (see Table B-2); in seven of these programs, the media campaign targeted individuals with suspicious lesions on self-examination or risk factors for melanoma, while six were not targeted. We found no systematic relationship between these characteristics and the proportion of individuals eventually diagnosed with cancer. However, most studies did not report sufficient information to determine how well targeting succeeded in recruiting a high-risk population, and the descriptions of the study samples were not adequate to exclude differences in baseline risk factors between studies as the main reason for observed differences in results.

Procedure for Referring Patients for Follow-Up

In most studies the patient was instructed to see a primary care clinician or dermatologist for follow-up of suspicious lesions. In some studies, the patient's physician was contacted directly, or the patient was sent to a study dermatologist. Some studies used reminders such as letters to the patient.

Although not depicted in Table B-2, we collected information on compliance rates for screening, follow-up, and biopsy when possible. Three population-based studies invited a target group of people to be screened and reported response rates.[36,74,75,77,89] In these studies, between 60 and 70 percent of those invited attended screening. One work site screening program that identified and invited high-risk people reported a lower response rate of 19 percent.[80] The mean age of this sample was somewhat lower than that in the population-based studies.

Compared to usual care, how much earlier does screening detect skin cancers and precancerous lesions? (Arrow 1b, Q6)

Eight studies reported the thickness of melanoma lesions found through screening (Table B-3). In four studies,[37,63,70,83] all detected melanoma lesions were 1.0 mm or thinner, and in a fifth,[41] 92 percent were 1.0 mm or thinner. In three other studies that used 1.5 mm as the cutoff, the proportion of melanomas 1.5 mm or less was 67–87 percent.[39,82,84]

No study of screening directly followed an unscreened population to compare the distribution of thickness or stage of melanomas detected. Nonetheless, the proportion of thin melanomas is clearly higher in screening programs than in usual care. In an analysis of SEER data from 1992 to 1994, 57 percent of melanomas were thinner than 0.76 mm, 23 percent were 0.76–1.5 mm, 15 percent were 1.51–3.99 mm, and 5 percent were 4.0 mm or thicker.[39] The SEER registry routinely reports the TNM stage, but not the thickness, of melanomas at the time of diagnosis. From 1989 to 1994, 81 percent of melanomas detected through usual care were localized, 9 percent regional, 4 percent distant, and 6 percent unstaged. In population-based studies, moreover, the incidence of melanoma detected by screening is higher than base rates, and the increase is almost entirely attributable to thin melanomas.

What is the effect of screening on patients' skin knowledge and self-care behavior? (Arrow 1c)?

Advocates of screening note that having a total-body skin examination could improve morbidity and mortality indirectly by promoting skin awareness and sun protection measures. In a follow-up study to the American Academy of Dermatology's Melanoma/Skin Cancer Screening Programs (see reference to Koh, 1996, in Table B-1), 1,049 participants who had skin lesions were surveyed about their skin health behaviors two months after undergoing a total-body skin examination. Among the 643 respondents, the proportion of individuals who regularly checked their skin increased from 60 to 84 percent after screening.[90]

What are the adverse effects of screening? (Arrow 2)

Total-body skin examination is noninvasive. In one study of self-selected participants found by screening to have skin lesions, patient satisfaction was high (81 percent), and only a small proportion of patients reported embarrassment or discomfort as a result of screening (4.8 percent).[90]

False positive skin examination results might also be considered an adverse effect. In any screening program, most lesions referred for biopsy because of clinical suspicion of skin cancer are false positives. There are no studies by which to judge the extent of harm, if any, related to these tests.

Misdiagnosis is another potential adverse effect of screening. It is known to occur, but no studies have been done on its rate of occurrence. The diagnosis of melanoma has a serious emotional and financial impact, and even when the melanoma is very thin and has an excellent prognosis, obtaining insurance can be very difficult.[7] Critics worry that if screening becomes widespread, pathologists may set the threshold low for diagnosing borderline lesions as melanoma, since the risk to the patient and the potential legal cost to the pathologists for missing melanoma are overwhelming.[9] The effects on diagnostic criteria of widespread screening are hard to predict, but uncertainty about these effects should be considered in weighing a recommendation to screen.

Some experts consider diagnosis of common, nonmalignant skin lesions found incidentally in screening to be a costly adverse effect of screening. Screening detects large numbers of benign skin conditions, especially seborrheic keratoses, which are very common in the elderly. Detection of these lesions could be considered an "adverse effect" of screening if it leads to additional biopsies and unnecessary or expensive procedures. While this has been shown to occur in usual care,[91] none of the studies of screening examined the rate at which this occurred.

Is there direct evidence that screening for skin cancers leads to reduced morbidity and mortality? (Arrow 3)

No randomized trials or case-control studies of screening for skin cancer have been completed. Well-done, frequently cited observational studies of the relationship between early detection and mortality have been done,[92] but in such studies the effect of promoting primary prevention and self-examination cannot be distinguished from that of routine screening in patients seeing the physician for unrelated reasons.[86] The lack of data reflects the lack of population-based programs that focus on routine total-body skin examination by a physician.

The absence of randomized trials is also not surprising since melanoma is relatively rare in the general population. A recent review by J.M. Elwood examined the options for conducting a randomized trial of screening in detail.[31] Elwood calculated that to have a 90 percent chance of detecting a one-third reduction in mortality, a trial of screening with total-body skin examination in the general population aged 45–69 would require 400,000 subjects in each group.

Put differently, about 21,000 people would have to be screened to prevent one death.

An alternative would be to conduct a trial in patients classified as high risk by a risk assessment questionnaire. Using this approach, Elwood assumed that 7 percent of the population would be classified as high risk; 35 percent of all melanomas occur in this high-risk group; 60 percent of patients complete the questionnaire; and 80 percent of the high-risk patients would comply with total-body skin examination. He calculated that to have a 90 percent chance of detecting a one-third reduction in mortality, 6 million questionnaires would have to be administered to enroll 100,000 high-risk subjects in each group.

In fact, a trial involving 600,000 subjects has begun in Australia and is expected to require nine more years to complete.

Effectiveness of Early Treatment

Screening in a population is justified if there is evidence that early detection and treatment improve outcomes such as mortality and quality of life. Other issues to be considered include consequences of false negative and false positive tests, acceptability of the test, and the risks of screening and of treatment.

Does treatment of nonmelanoma skin cancer found by screening reduce morbidity and mortality? (Arrow 4a)

Early treatment of basal and squamous cell carcinoma might reduce morbidity and disfigurement, but no studies have evaluated whether screening improves the outcomes of these cancers. Basic information, such as the proportion of Medicare patients with nonmelanoma skin cancer who suffer disfigurement or death, is lacking. If we assume that 20 percent of squamous cell cancers in the elderly are either lethal or disfiguring, this assumes a prevalence of 0.025 for men and women combined and that screening would reduce this by half, about 400 patients would have to be screened to prevent one lethal or disfiguring case. These calculations, while theoretical, do suggest that screening is potentially beneficial and that a trial of early detection in the elderly should examine outcomes in nonmelanoma skin cancer rather than just melanoma.

Does treatment of melanoma found by screening reduce morbidity and mortality? (Arrow 4b)

Well-designed observational studies can provide persuasive information about the effect of early detection on mortality. For some cancers, notably colon cancer, observational studies make a convincing case for the effectiveness of early detection, even in the absence of randomized controlled trials. Such a conclusion must be based on data that link actions taken as a result of screening to health outcomes.

In the absence of randomized trials and case-control studies of screening or of early treatment, the inference that earlier treatment as a result of screening improves health outcomes must rely on three lines of indirect evidence: (1) a case-control study in which skin self-examination reduces the incidence of lethal melanoma; (2) comparison of the stages of cancers and mortality found in screening to those found in usual practice; and (3) evidence from studies of the consequences of delay in diagnosis. These are summarized below.

Case-Control Study of Self-Examination

While there are no case-control studies of screening, one case-control study has examined the effect of skin self-examination on mortality from melanoma.[49] In this study, 650 incident cases of melanoma in 1987–1989 were identified through the Connecticut Tumor Registry and compared with randomly selected, age- and sex-matched controls. After five years of follow-up, cases were classified as "lethal" if the individual died or had distant metastases.

A structured questionnaire was used to assess skin self-examination attitudes and behavior. The definition of skin self-examination used in this study was, "did you ever (in your life) carefully examine your own skin? By this I mean actually check surfaces of your skin deliberately and purposely?" Based on their responses to this and related questions, 13 percent of the cases and 17.5 percent of control subjects were classified as careful or rigorous examiners, and an additional 57.4 percent of cases and 66.7 percent of controls were classified as casual examiners. The questionnaire also assessed potential confounding factors, such as risk factors for skin cancer, but did not assess general health behaviors such as diet, exercise, and medical care-seeking behavior that might affect the risk of cancer and the likelihood of early detection.

The investigators performed two multivariate analyses: one for primary prevention and one for secondary prevention. In the first analysis, after adjustment for sun exposure, skin color, the number of nevi, and other risk factors, skin self-examination was negatively associated with incidence of melanoma (OR 0.66; CI 0.44–0.99).

In the second analysis, after adjustment for confounding risk factors, skin self-examination was associated with a reduced risk of lethal melanoma (OR 0.37; CI 0.16–0.84). Survival analysis comparing patients who practiced skin self-examination with those who did not suggested that after an average of 5.4 years, self-examination was associated with a lower probability of lethal melanoma. The authors noted that the shape of the survival curves—the curve for the self-examination group plateaus after three years, while survival continues to decrease up to five years in the patients who do not practice self-examination—ooffers some reassurance that the observed benefit is due to actual improvement offers some reassurance that the observed benefit is due to actual improvement in survival rather than to lead-time bias.

As noted by the authors, this case-control study provides suggestive, rather than definitive, evidence for the effectiveness of skin self-examination. More direct evidence is needed to link self-examination behaviors to specific actions that could reduce the incidence or lethality of melanoma. To prevent melanoma, self-examination on the part of the patient must lead to actions—such as identification of a suspicious lesion, self-referral to a physician, earlier treatment of precancerous lesions, and health behavior changes—to prevent the development of new melanomas. While the study indicates that patients who practiced self-examination had undergone more biopsies than those who had not, it does not report the frequency of these intermediate steps or whether their frequency was different enough from that of other patients to explain the observed differences in outcome.

Apart from concerns about the strength of the study design, how relevant is a study of skin self-examination to screening by primary care providers? If skin self-examination prevents death from melanoma, it may be more likely that examination by a physician could also prevent deaths, especially if examination by a physician promotes more accurate self-examination. In fact, case finding by a physician might be expected to be more effective because it reaches patients, especially elderly men, who are at high risk and are the least likely to practice self-examination effectively[87] or to respond to an invitation or health promotion campaign. However, self-examination occurs much more frequently (monthly, on average, in the case-control study) than screening by a physician and can note findings—in particular, changes in size, border, or color of lesions—that cannot be recognized easily by infrequent examinations. Nevertheless, this case-control study provides the strongest available evidence that early detection of melanoma reduces mortality.

Comparing Stages of Cancers and Mortality Found in Screening to Those Found in Usual Practice

Advocates cite the results of public information campaigns in Australia and the United Kingdom as evidence of the potential benefits of screening. In Australia, public information campaigns have promoted sun protection behaviors and early detection for more than 15 years. Melanoma mortality, which had increased for decades, reached a plateau in 1985 and, in recent years, has fallen slightly.[93] It is thought that this trend is related to skin health promotion activities, including primary prevention and self-examination, but because it is not a prominent feature of these campaigns, it is not possible to determine what role, if any, screening by physicians has played.

In the United Kingdom, registry data were used to compare rates of invasive melanoma before and after public information campaigns to promote early detection of skin cancers. In the West of Scotland, a community-based skin health promotion campaign compared melanoma thickness and mortality before and after implementing a public information campaign and rapid referral system in 1985.[92] The number and proportion of thin melanomas diagnosed yearly in the population increased immediately afterward. The response to the public information campaign was stronger in women than in men. In women, within 2 years, the rate of diagnosis of thick melanomas (>3.5 mm) began to decrease and, within 5 years, sustained decreases in thick melanomas and in melanoma mortality were observed. In men, the rate of diagnosis of thick melanomas did not change and the melanoma mortality rate rose. As in Australia, the role of screening by physicians in these results is not clear.

A subsequent implementation of a similar program in seven British districts failed to replicate these results.[82,94,95] The incidence rates of both thin and thick melanomas increased during the public information campaign (1987–1989) and have remained higher than before the program began.

In contrast to these health promotion efforts, mass-screening programs cannot be evaluated using population-based registries. Mass screening increases the proportion of melanomas detected in an "early" stage (see Table B-3), but the significance of this finding is unclear. Survival is strongly related to lesion thickness at the time of resection, but it is difficult to know the extent to which comparison of the distribution of the stage of cancers found by screening to those found in usual care is affected by lead-time bias or length bias. The natural history of melanoma, in particular the significance of the many additional thin melanomas found in screened populations, is another source of uncertainty.

Retrospective Studies of the Consequences of Delay in Diagnosis

The argument for screening would be strengthened if evidence pointed to a consistent relationship between delay of diagnosis and the thickness of melanoma. Nine case series examined the causes and consequences of apparent delay in the diagnosis of melanoma. The two largest studies, one from Scotland and one from Australia, found no relation between delay in diagnosis and tumor thickness.[18,82] The Australian study found that male sex, nodular melanoma, and location on the head and neck (but not delay) were associated with thick melanoma.

Five studies, which were performed in specialty clinics, observed patients with melanoma of the hand, foot, eye, penis, or nailbeds.[96–100] In these studies, misdiagnosis was a common cause of delay in treatment. Effects of delay on tumor thickness or survival were reported in three of the studies, and the results were inconsistent. In a study of 83 patients with acral melanomas, 17 of 33 subungual melanomas and 10 of 50 palmoplantar melanomas were clinically misdiagnosed by physicians.[96] Misdiagnosis caused a median delay of 12 months in the diagnosis of palmoplantar melanomas and 18 months in the diagnosis of subungual melanomas. Delay in diagnosis was associated with increased tumor thickness, more advanced stage at time of melanoma diagnosis, and a lower estimated five-year survival rate (15.4 percent versus 68.9 percent for palmoplantar; 68.5 percent versus 90.9 percent for subungual). In another series of 140 patients with melanoma of the foot, delay in diagnosis had no effect on clinical outcome.[100] Another series of 102 consecutive melanoma patients found no relationship between delay in diagnosis and tumor thickness.[101]

Two recent case series from specialized clinics in major referral centers reported that lesions detected by physicians were thinner than those detected by patients.[102,103] In one of these, 24 of 102 consecutive patients had physician-detected melanomas; the median thickness was 0.23 mm versus 0.9 mm in self-detected melanomas. Eleven of the 24 physician-detected melanomas were in situ. In the other study, 172 of 590 consecutive patients had physician-detected melanomas; these were significantly thinner, but the difference was not as striking (0.9 mm versus 1.3 mm).

The latter study[103] also carefully examined the relationship between melanoma thickness and delay, either to seek medical advice or after seeking medical care, and concluded that poor prognosis was due to rapidly growing tumors rather than delays. They examined four intervals: (1) the time patients first noticed a lesion and the time they considered it to be suspicious; (2) from then until they saw a physician; (3) from then until the physician proposed removal; and (4) from then until surgical resection. In the 418 patients who had self-detected cancers, the first, third, and fourth intervals were not associated with tumor thickness. Not surprisingly, once a lesion was recognized as being dangerous, patients with thicker lesions sought medical attention more quickly (i.e., for the second interval, thinner lesions had the longest delay). In a subgroup of 247 patients who reported a delay of less than 5 years between the time they noticed the lesion and the time they believed it to be dangerous, the time between noticing a lesion and considering it dangerous was longest for lesions 1.5–2.99 mm thick, but was shorter for lesions thicker and thinner than this.

Cost-Effectiveness Studies of Screening for Skin Cancer

A cost-effectiveness analysis of screening for malignant melanoma is currently in press.[104] The analysis found that the average projected discounted life expectancy was 15.0963 without screening versus 15.0975 with screening. This difference is equivalent to an increase of about nine hours per person screened or 337 days for each person with melanoma.

If a screening examination by a dermatologist is assumed to cost $30, the incremental cost-effectiveness (CE) ratio was $29,170 per year of life saved. The CE ratio was unexpectedly low because, in the model, savings from prevention of late-stage melanomas offset most of the costs of screening. Thus, the key assumptions in the model, affecting the calculation of both effectiveness and cost, were that the proportion of late-stage melanomas would decrease from 6.1 percent without screening to 1.1 percent with screening. Similarly, the model assumed that invasive cancers would decrease from 70.3 to 58.1 percent and melanomas thicker than 1.5 mm would decrease from 20.1 to 12.6 percent of invasive melanomas. These assumptions are based on comparison of cross-sectional data on the stages of melanoma in individuals who attended the American Academy of Dermatology's mass screening programs with data on usual care from the SEER registry.

SUMMARY

Table B-4 (see page 210) summarizes the literature review by describing the evidence for each link in the analytic framework (see Figures B-3 and B-4). The quality of the evidence at each link ranged from poor to fair and is explained in Table B-4.

The case for screening is based on the assumption that melanoma and other skin cancers have a long latency period during which they can be treated with a high rate of success. Another assumption is that early detection prevents progression of early-stage cancers to advanced, lethal stages. These assumptions are reasonable, but studies of early detection have not focused on screening and have not adequately linked it with reduced incidence of invasive disease.

Despite these information gaps, skin cancer screening, perhaps using a risk assessment technique to identify high-risk patients who are seeing the physician for other reasons, is the most promising strategy for addressing the excess burden of disease in older individuals. This group has substantial morbidity and mortality from skin cancer. By themselves, primary prevention efforts and promotion of self-examination seem unlikely to change these rates substantially. While the efficacy of screening has not been established, the screening procedures themselves are noninvasive, and the follow-up test, skin biopsy, has low morbidity.

In this situation, indirect evidence of efficacy might be sufficient to decide that the potential benefits of screening outweigh the potential harms. To better estimate the benefit of earlier detection, we need to know how much earlier, compared to usual care, screening will detect cancers that would eventually have become aggressive. Population-based studies using concurrent comparisons could provide better information about the consequences of delay and how much they can be reduced by screening. No studies of screening have measured these parameters.

Gaps in our knowledge of the progression to thick melanoma in the elderly should also be addressed. Better information about the natural history of thin melanomas and about the history and patterns of growth of melanoma in the elderly is particularly important, because there is little evidence from empirical studies that lethal tumors in this group are detectable when they are still in a curable stage.

Appendix B continues on page 212

TABLE B-4 Summary of Evidence for Screening for Skin Cancer

Linkage in Analytic Framework	Evidence Code	Quality of Evidence
1a. Accuracy of total body skin examination: evidence that total body skin examination can detect skin cancer.	II-2	Fair: The accuracy of a total body skin examination by primary care physicians in unselected patients may be low. Reliability of pathologic diagnosis in community practice in the U.S. is not clear.
1b. Accuracy of risk-assessment: evidence that a questionnaire or interview, followed by exam in selected patients, can detect skin cancer.	II-2	Fair: Mole counts and other factors predict elevated risk over time, but no study has determined the accuracy of risk stratification followed by total body skin examination in selected patients as a screening method.
2. Adverse effects of screening: evidence that screening causes significant harms.	III	Poor: most postulated adverse effects have not been evaluated in studies.
3. Effectiveness of early detection: evidence that persons detected through screening have better outcomes than those who are not screened.	II-3	Poor: There are no studies that directly link screening to lower mortality and morbidity. Most well-done population-based studies concern promotion of self-care behaviors such as self-examination rather than universal screening.

4a. Effectiveness of treatment of nonmelanoma skin cancer found by screening.	III	Poor: The hypothesis that early detection by screening could reduce mortality and morbidity is plausible but has not been examined in studies.
4b. Effectiveness of treatment of melanoma found by screening.	II-1, III	Fair: There are no controlled studies of treatment in patients found by screening to have thin melanomas, but epidemiologic studies, studies of skin health behaviors, and studies of factors associated with advanced melanoma suggest that elderly men are at high risk and are unlikely to benefit from health promotion efforts. Studies of delay in diagnosis have conflicting results, and the ability of screening to reach individuals at high risk and to find aggressive tumors while they are still curable have not been established.

*I = randomized controlled trial; II-1 = controlled trial without randomization; II-2 = cohort or case-control analytic studies; II-3 = multiple time series, dramatic uncontrolled experiments; II-1 = controlled trial without randomization; II-2 = cohort or case-control analytic studies; II-3 = multiple time series, dramatic uncontrolled experiments; and III opinions of respected authorities, descriptive epidemiology.

ADDENDUM B-1 STRATEGY FOR SKIN CANCER SEARCH

1. Skin neoplasms

2. Exp mass screening
    - genetic screening
    - mass chest x-ray
    - multiphasic screening
    - vision screening
    - mandatory screening

3. Screen$.tw. (Text word taken from title and abstract of article)

4. Exp physical examination
    - self-examination
    - skinfold thickness

5. Exp neoplasms metastasis
    - lymphatic metastasis
    - neoplasm circulating cells
    - neoplasm seeding
    - neoplasms, unknown primary

6. Neoplasm recurrence, local

7. Recurrence

8. Exp morbidity
    - incidence
    - prevalence

9. Exp sensitivity and specificity
    - predictive value of tests
    - ROC curve

10. 2 **or** 3 **or** 4 **or** 5 **or** 6 **or** 7 **or** 8 **or** 9

11. Skin neoplasms/mo (*mortality*)

12. Skin neoplasms/ep (*epidemiology*)

13. 10 **or** 11 **or** 12

14. 1 **and** 13

15. **Limit** 14 to human

16. **Limit** 15 to english language

17. *Looked at english* abstracts *for foreign language articles*

ADDENDUM B-2 SCREENING FOR SKIN CANCER: INCLUSION CRITERIA FOR EVIDENCE TABLES

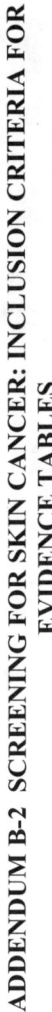

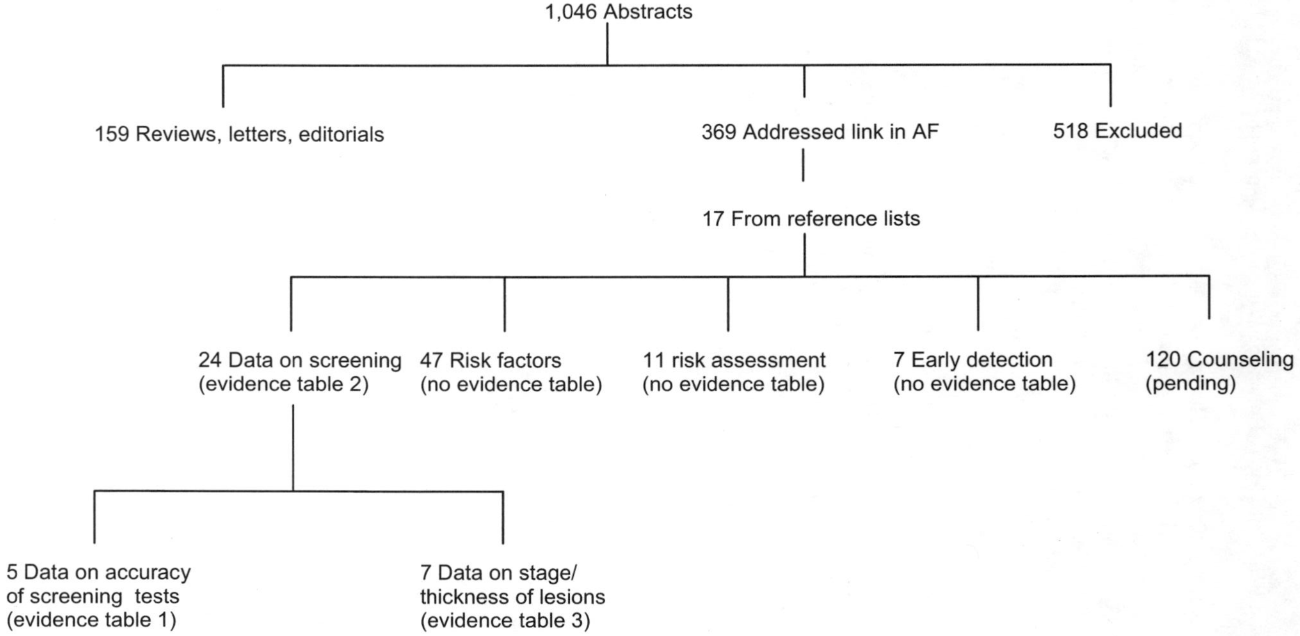

1,046 Abstracts

159 Reviews, letters, editorials

369 Addressed link in AF

518 Excluded

17 From reference lists

47 Risk factors (no evidence table)

11 risk assessment (no evidence table)

7 Early detection (no evidence table)

120 Counseling (pending)

24 Data on screening (evidence table 2)

5 Data on accuracy of screening tests (evidence table 1)

7 Data on stage/ thickness of lesions (evidence table 3)

REFERENCES

1. Landis SH, Murray T, Bolden S, Wingo PA. Cancer statistics, 1999. CA Cancer Jr Clin. 1999; 49:8.
2. Ries LAG, Kosary CL, Hankey BF, Miller BA, Edwards BK. SEER Cancer Statistics Review, 1973–95. Bethesda, MD: National Cancer Institute, 1998.
3. Jelfs P, Coates M, Giles G. Cancer in Australia 1989–1990 (with projections to 1995). Canberra, Australian Institute of Health and Welfare; 1996.
4. Kelly J. Melanoma in the elderly—A neglected public health challenge. Med J Aust 1998; 169:403–404.
5. Dennis LK. Analysis of the melanoma epidemic, both apparent and real: data from the 1973 through 1994 surveillance, epidemiology, and end results program registry. Arch Dermatol, 1999; 135:275–280.
6. Berwick M, Halpern A. Melanoma epidemiology. Curr Opin Oncol. 1997; 9:178–182.
7. Swerlick RA, Chen S. The melanoma epidemic: More apparent than real? Mayo Clin Proc 1997; 72:559–564.
8. Burton R, Armstrong B. Recent incidence trends imply a nonmetastasizing form of invasive melanoma. Melanoma Res 1994; 4:107–113.
9. Swerlick RA, Chen S. The melanoma epidemic. Is increased surveillance the solution or the problem? Arch Dermatol 1996; 132:881–884.
10. Burton R. An analysis of a melanoma epidemic. Int J Cancer 1995; 55:765–770.
11. Gallagher RP, Hill GB, Bajdik CD, et al. Sunlight exposure, pigmentation factors, and risk of nonmelanocytic skin cancer. II. Squamous cell carcinoma. Arch Dermatol 1995; 131:164–169.
12. Green A, Battistutta D, Hart V, Leslie D, Weedon D. Skin cancer in a subtropical Australian population: Incidence and lack of association with occupation. The Nambour Study Group. Am J Epidemiol 1996; 144:1034–1040.
13. Kricker A, English DR, Randell PL, et al. Skin cancer in Geraldton, Western Australia: A survey of incidence and prevalence. Med J Aust 1990; 152:399–407.
14. Chuang TY, Popescu A, Su WP, Chute CG. Basal cell carcinoma. A population-based incidence study in Rochester, Minnesota. J Am Acad Dermatol 1990; 22:413–417.
15. Chuang TY, Popescu NA, Su WP, Chute CG. Squamous cell carcinoma. A population-based incidence study in Rochester, Minnesota. Arch Dermatol 1990; 126:185–188.
16. Karagas MR, Greenberg ER, Spencer SK, Stukel TA, Mott LA. Increase in incidence rates of basal cell and squamous cell skin cancer in New Hampshire, USA. New Hampshire Skin Cancer Study Group. Int J Cancer 1999; 81:555–559.
17. McGovern V, Cochran A, Van der Esch E. The classification of malignant melanoma, its histological reporting and registration: Revision of the 1972 Syndey classification. Pathology 1986; 18:12–21.
18. Hersey P, Sillar RW, Howe CG, et al. Factors related to the presentation of patients with thick primary melanomas. Med J Aust 1991; 154:583–587.
19. Heenan PJ, Yu L, English DR. Melanoma in the elderly—A neglected public health challenge [letter]. Med J Aust 1999; 170:394–395.

20. Whited JD, Grichnik JM. Does this patient have a mole or a melanoma? *JAMA* 1998; 279:696–701.

21. Corona R, Mele A, Amini M, et al. Interobserver variability on the histopathologic diagnosis of cutaneous melanoma and other pigmented skin lesions. J Clin Oncol 1996; 14:1218–1223.

22. Farmer ER, Gonin R, Hanna MP. Discordance in the histopathologic diagnosis of melanoma and melanocytic nevi between expert pathologists. Hum Pathol 1996; 27:528–531.

23. Gershenwald JE, Buzaid AC, Ross MI. Classification and staging of melanoma. [Review] [114 refs]. Hematology—Oncology Clinics of North Am 1998; 12:737–765.

24. Breslow A. Thickness, cross-sectional areas and depth of invasion in the prognosis of cutaneous melanoma. Ann of Surg 1970; 172:902–908.

25. Preston DS, Stern RS. Nonmelanoma cancers of the skin. N Engl J Med 1992; 327:1649–1662.

26. Stern RS, Lunder EJ. Risk of squamous cell carcinoma and methoxsalen (psoralen) and UV-A radiation (PUVA). A meta-analysis. Arch Dermatol 1998; 134:1582–1585.

27. Osterlind A, Hjalgrim H, Kulinsky B, Frentz G. Skin cancer as a cause of death in Denmark. Br J Dermatol 1991; 125:580–582.

28. Screening for Skin Cancer (Including Counseling to Prevent Skin Cancer). DiGuiseppi C, Atkins D, Woolf SH, Kamerow DB, (eds.) Guide to Clinical Preventive Services, 2nd edition. Baltimore: Williams & Wilkins 1996:pp. 141–152.

29. Rigel DS, Friedman RJ, Kopf AW, et al. Importance of complete cutaneous examination for the detection of malignant melanoma. J Am Acad Dermatol 1986; 14:857–860.

30. Elwood JM. Screening for melanoma. Miller AB, (ed.) Advances in Cancer Screening. Boston: Kluwer Academic Publishers, 1996:pp. 129–146.

31. Elwood JM. Screening for melanoma and options for its evaluation. J Med Screen 1994; 1:22–38.

32. Sackett DL, Haynes RB, Guyatte GH, Tugwell P. Clinical Epidemiology, A Basic Science for Clinical Medicine, 2nd Edition Boston: Little, Brown and Company, 1991.

33. Sox HC, Blatt MA, Higgins MC, Marton KI. Medical Decision Making. Boston: Butterworth-Heinemann 1988.

34. Limpert GH. Skin-cancer screening: A three-year experience that paid for itself. J Fam Pract 1995; 40:471–475.

35. de Rooij MJ, Rampen FH, Schouten LJ, Neumann HA. Skin cancer screening focusing on melanoma yields more selective attendance. Arch Dermatol 1995; 131:422–425.

36. de Rooij MJ, Rampen FH, Schouten LJ, Neumann HA. Factors influencing participation among melanoma screening attenders. Acta Derm Venereol 1997; 77:467–470.

37. Jonna BP, Delfino RJ, Newman WG, Tope WD. Positive predictive value for presumptive diagnoses of skin cancer and compliance with follow-up among patients attending a community screening program. Prev Med 1998; 27:611–616.

38. Rampen RH. Point-counterpoint. Mass population skin cancer screening is not worthwhile. J Cutan Med Surg 1998; 2:128–129.

39. Koh HK, Norton LA, Geller AC, et al. Evaluation of the American Academy of Dermatology's National Skin Cancer Early Detection and Screening Program. J Am Acad Derm 1996; 34:971–978.

40. Rampen FH, Casparie-van Velsen JI, van Huystee BE, Kiemeney LA, Schouten LJ. False-negative findings in skin cancer and melanoma screening. J Am Acad Dermatol 1995; 33:59–63.

41. de Rooij MJ, Rampen FH, Schouten LJ, Neumann HA. Volunteer melanoma screenings. Follow-up, compliance, and outcome. Dermatol Surg 1997; 23:197–201.

42. Federman DG, Concato J, Kirsner RS. Comparison of dermatologic diagnoses by primary care practitioners and dermatologists. A review of the literature. Arch Fam Med 1999; 8:170–172.

43. Burton RC, Howe C, Adamson L, et al. General practitioner screening for melanoma: Sensitivity, specificity, and effect of training. J Med Screen 1998; 5:156–161.

44. Gallagher RP, Ma B, McLean DI, et al. Trends in basal cell carcinoma, squamous cell carcinoma, and melanoma of the skin from 1973 through 1987. J Am Acad Dermatol 1990; 23:413–421.

45. Gamble JF, Lerman SE, Holder WR, Nicolich MJ, Yarborough CM. Physician-based case-control study of non-melanoma skin cancer in Baytown, Texas. Occup Med 1996; 46:186–196.

46. Grodstein F, Speizer FE, Hunter DJ. A prospective study of incident squamous cell carcinoma of the skin in the Nurses' Health Study. J Natl Cancer Inst 1995; 87:1061–1066.

47. Kaldor J, Shugg D, Young B, Dwyer T, Wang YG. Non-melanoma skin cancer: Ten years of cancer-registry-based surveillance. Int J Cancer 1993; 53:886–891.

48. Bataille V, Bishop JA, Sasieni P, et al. Risk of cutaneous melanoma in relation to the numbers, types and sites of naevi: A case-control study. Br J Cancer 1996; 73:1605–1611.

49. Berwick M, Begg CB, Fine JA, Roush GC, Barnhill RL. Screening for cutaneous melanoma by skin self-examination. J Natl Cancer Inst 1996; 88:17–23.

50. Garbe C, Buttner P, Weiss J, et al. Risk factors for developing cutaneous melanoma and criteria for identifying persons at risk: Multicenter case-control study of the Central Malignant Melanoma Registry of the German Dermatological Society. J Invest Derm 1994; 102:695–699.

51. Tucker MA, Halpern A, Holly EA, et al. Clinically recognized dysplastic nevi. A central risk factor for cutaneous melanoma. JAMA 1997; 277:1439–1444.

52. English DR, Armstrong BK. Identifying people at high risk of cutaneous malignant melanoma: Results from a case-control study in Western Australia. Br Med J (Clin Res Ed) 1988; 296:1285–1288.

53. Marrett LD, King WD, Walter SD, From L. Use of host factors to identify people at high risk for cutaneous malignant melanoma. Can Med Assoc J 1992; 147:445–453.

54. Bliss JM, Ford D, Swerdlow AJ, et al. Risk of cutaneous melanoma associated with pigmentation characteristics and freckling: Systematic overview of 10 case-control studies. The International Melanoma Analysis Group (IMAGE). Int J Cancer 1995; 62:367–376.

55. Elwood JM, Jopson J. Melanoma and sun exposure: An overview of published studies. Int J Cancer 1997; 73:198–203.

56. Elwood JM, Gallagher RP. Body site distribution of cutaneous malignant melanoma in relationship to patterns of sun exposure. Int J Cancer 1998; 78:276–280.

57. Walter SD, King WD, Marrett LD. Association of cutaneous malignant melanoma with intermittent exposure to ultraviolet radiation: Results of a case-control study in Ontario, Canada. Int J Epidemiol 1999; 28:418–427.

58. Byles JE, Hennrikus D, Sanson-Fisher R, Hersey P. Reliability of naevus counts in identifying individuals at high risk of malignant melanoma. Br J Dermatol 1994; 130:51–56.

59. Westerdahl J, Anderson H, Olsson H, Ingvar C. Reproducibility of a self-administered questionnaire for assessment of melanoma risk. Int J Epidemiol 1996; 25:245–251.

60. Little P, Keefe M, White J. Self screening for risk of melanoma: Validity of self mole counting by patients in a single general practice. BMJ 1995; 310:912–916.

61. Lawson DD, Moore DH, 2nd, Schneider JS, Sagebiel RW. Nevus counting as a risk factor for melanoma: Comparison of self-count with count by physician. J Am Acad Dermatol 1994; 31:438–444.

62. Jackson A, Wilkinson C, Ranger M, Pill R, August P. Can primary prevention or selective screening for melanoma be more precisely targeted through general practice? A prospective study to validate a self administered risk score. BMJ 1998; 316:34–38; discussion 38–39.

63. Schneider J.S., Moore DH, 2nd, Sagebiel RW. Risk factors for melanoma incidence in prospective follow-up. The importance of atypical (dysplastic) nevi. Arch Dermatol 1994; 130:1002–1007.

64. Kelly JW, Crutcher WA, Sagebiel RW. Clinical diagnosis of dysplastic melanocytic nevi. A clinicopathologic correlation. J Am Acad Dermatol 1986; 14:1044–1052.

65. Jackson A, Wilkinson C, Pill R. Moles and melanomas—who's at risk, who knows, and who cares? A strategy to inform those at high risk. Br J Gen Pract 1999; 49:199–203.

66. MacKie RM, Freudenberger T, Aitchison TC. Personal risk-factor chart for cutaneous melanoma. Lancet 1989; 2:487–490.

67. Engelberg D, Gallagher RP, Rivers JK. Follow-up and evaluation of skin cancer screening in British Columbia. J Am Acad Dermatol 1999; 41:37–42.

68. McGee R, Elwood M, Williams S, Lowry F. Who comes to skin checks? NZ Med J 1994; 107:58–60.

69. Hourani LL, LaFleur B. Predictors of gender differences in sunscreen use and screening outcome among skin cancer screening participants. J Behav Med 1995; 18:461–477.

70. Katris P, Crock JG, Gray BN. Research note: The Lions Cancer Institute and the Western Australian Society of Plastic Surgeons skin cancer screening programme. Aust NZ J Surg 1996; 66:101–104.

71. Katris P, Donovan RJ, Gray BN. Nurses screening for skin cancer: An observation study. Aust NZ J Pub Health 1998; 22:381–383.

72. Rivers JK, Gallagher RP. Public education projects in skin cancer. Experience of the Canadian Dermatology Association. Cancer 1995; 75:661–666.

73. Dozier S, Wagner RF Jr, Black SA, Terracina J. Beachfront screening for skin cancer in Texas Gulf coast surfers. South Med J 1997; 90:55–58.

74. Harvey I, Frankel S, Marks R, Shalom D, Nolan-Farrell M. Non-melanoma skin cancer and solar keratoses. I. Methods and descriptive results of the South Wales Skin Cancer Study. Br J Cancer 1996; 74:1302–1307.

75. Harvey I, Frankel S, Marks R, Shalom D, Nolan-Farrell M. Non-melanoma skin cancer and solar keratoses II Analytical results of the South Wales Skin Cancer Study. Br J Cancer 1996; 74:1308–1312.

76. Ichihashi M, Naruse K, Harada S, et al. Trends in nonmelanoma skin cancer in Japan. Recent Results Cancer Res 1995; 139:263–273.

77. Tornberg S, Mansson-Brahme E, Linden D, et al. Screening for cutaneous malignant melanoma: A feasibility study. J Med Screen 1996; 3:211–215.

78. Bergenmar M, Tornberg S, Brandberg Y. Factors related to non-attendance in a population based melanoma screening program. Psycho-Oncology 1997; 6:218–226.

79. Ruskiewicz J. Skin cancer and actinic keratoses. J Am Optom Assoc 1998; 69:229–235.

80. Whited JD, Hall RP, Simel DL, Horner RD. Primary care clinicians' performance for detecting actinic keratoses and skin cancer. Arch Int Med 1997; 157:985–990.

81. Friedman LC, Webb JA, Bruce S, Weinberg AD, Cooper HP. Skin cancer prevention and early detection intentions and behavior. Am J Prev Med 1995; 11:59–65.

82. Herd RM, Cooper EJ, Hunter JA, et al. Cutaneous malignant melanoma. Publicity, screening clinics and survival—The Edinburgh experience 1982–90. Br J Dermatol 1995; 132:563–570.

83. Marghoob AA, Slade J, Salopek TG, Kopf AW, Bart RS, Rigel DS. Basal cell and squamous cell carcinomas are important risk factors for cutaneous malignant melanoma. Screening implications. Cancer 1995; 75:707–714.

84. van der Spek-Keijser LM, van der Rhee HJ, Toth G, Van Westering R, Bruijn JA, Coebergh JW. Site, histological type, and thickness of primary cutaneous malignant melanoma in western Netherlands since 1980. Br J Dermatol 1997; 136:565–571.

85. Veierod MB, Thelle DS, Laake P. Diet and risk of cutaneous malignant melanoma: A prospective study of 50,757 Norwegian men and women. Int J Cancer 1997; 71:600–604.

86. Koh HK, Geller AC. Public health interventions for melanoma. Prevention, early detection, and education. Hematol Oncol Clin North Am 1998; 12:903–928.

87. Hanrahan PF, Hersey P, D'Este CA. Factors involved in presentation of older people with thick melanoma. Med J Aust 1998; 169:410–414.

88. De Rooij MJ, Rampen FH, Schouten LJ, Neumann HA. Total skin examination during screening for malignant melanoma does not increase the detection rate. Br J Dermatol 1996; 135:42–45.

89. Dhir A, Orengo I, Bruce S, Kolbusz RV, Alford E, Goldberg L. Basal cell carcinoma on the scalp of an Indian patient. Dermatol Surg 1995; 21:247–250.

90. Geller AC, Halpern AC, Sun T, et al. Participant satisfaction and value in American Academy of Dermatology and American Cancer Society skin cancer screening programs in Massachusetts. J Am Acad Dermatol 1999; 40:563–566.

91. Stern RS, Boudreaux C, Arndt KA. Diagnostic accuracy and appropriateness of care for seborrheic keratoses. A pilot study of an approach to quality assurance for cutaneous surgery. JAMA 1991; 265:74–77.

92. MacKie RM, Hole D. Audit of public education campaign to encourage earlier detection of malignant melanoma. BMJ 1992; 304:1012–1015.
93. Giles GG, Armstrong BK, Burton RC, Staples MP, Thursfield VJ. Has mortality from melanoma stopped rising in Australia? Analysis of trends between 1931 and 1994. BMJ 1996; 312:1121–1125.
94. Melia J, Cooper EJ, Frost T, et al. Cancer Research Campaign health education programme to promote the early detection of cutaneous malignant melanoma. II. Characteristics and incidence of melanoma. Br J Dermatol 1995; 132:414–421.
95. Melia J. Early detection of cutaneous malignant melanoma in Britain. Int J Epidemiol 1995; 24:S39–44.
96. Metzger S, Ellwanger U, Stroebel W, Schiebel U, Rassner G, Fierlbeck G. Extent and consequences of physician delay in the diagnosis of acral melanoma. Melanoma Res 1998; 8:181–186.
97. Warso M, Gray T, Gonzalez M. Melanoma of the hand. J Hand Surg 1997; 22:354–360.
98. Larsson K, Shaw H, Thompson J, Harman R, McCarthy W. Primary mucosal and glans penis melanomas: The Sydney Melanoma Unit experience. Aust NZ J Surg 1999; 69:121–126.
99. Holden R, Damato B. Preventable delays in the treatment of intraocular melanoma in the UK. Eye 1996; 10:127–129.
100. Bennett DR, Wasson D, MacArthur JD, McMillen MA. The effect of misdiagnosis and delay in diagnosis on clinical outcome in melanomas of the foot. J Am Coll Surg 1994; 179:279–284.
101. Baccard M, Chevret S, Chemaly P, Morel P. Delay in diagnosing melanoma. A prospective study in 102 patients. Annal Dermatol Venereol 1997; 124:601–606.
102. Epstein DS, Lange JR, Gruber SB, Mofid M, Koch SE. Is physician detection associated with thinner melanomas? JAMA 1999; 281:640–643.
103. Richard MA, Grob JJ, Avril MF, et al. Melanoma and tumor thickness: Challenges of early diagnosis. Arch Dermatol 1999; 135:269–274.
104. Freedberg K. Screening for melanoma: A cost-effectiveness analysis. J Am Acad Dermatol 1999; 41:738–745.

APPENDIX C

Medically Necessary Dental Services

B. Alex White, D.D.S., Dr.P.H., Lauren L. Patton, D.D.S.,
William G. Kohn, D.D.S., and James A. Lipton, D.D.S., Ph.D.

OVERVIEW

The Balanced Budget Act of 1997 directed the Secretary of Health and Human Services to request the National Academy of Sciences to analyze "the short- and long-term benefits, and costs to Medicare" of extending Medicare coverage for certain preventive and other services. Congress directed that the report include specific findings with respect to coverage of a number of services, including medically necessary dental services.

The purpose of this background paper is to present scientific evidence related to medically necessary dental services for selected medical conditions or in conjunction with certain medical procedures. This review is not intended to make specific recommendations about the clinical management of oral conditions or the prevention of oral complications or to address the entire range of diseases, conditions, or procedures for which medically necessary dental services may be indicated. Rather the intent is to review the evidence about certain oral health interventions in preventing or reducing morbidity and/or mortality for selected medical conditions. For a very limited set of medical diagnoses or under very specific clinical conditions, dental services are covered under Medicare. Evidence on the effectiveness of dental services in these circumstances is not covered in this review, although some information may be included for clar-

---

Senior Investigator, Center for Health Research, Kaiser Permanente Northwest Division; Associate Professor, Department of Dental Ecology, University of North Carolina at Chapel Hill; Associate Director for Science, Division of Oral Health, Centers for Disease Control and Prevention; Assistant Director for Training and Career Development, Division of Extramural Research, National Institute of Dental and Craniofacial Research, National Institutes of Health.

ity. The primary focus is on the effectiveness of dental services not currently covered by Medicare.

What Are Medically Necessary Dental Services?

Several definitions of medically necessary dental services have been proposed. In 1995, the National Alliance for Oral Health held a consensus conference on medically necessary dental services and proposed the following definition: "that care that is a direct result of, or has a direct impact on, an underlying medical condition and/or its resulting therapy" (Consensus Conference, 1995). The consensus conference also noted that such care was integral to comprehensive treatment to ensure optimum health outcomes and could potentially reduce health care expenditures for treatment of complications.

In 1990, the American Dental Association's House of Delegates adopted the following comprehensive definition of medically necessary dental services:

> the reasonable and appropriate diagnosis, treatment, and follow-up care (including supplies, appliances, and devices) as determined and prescribed by qualified, appropriate health care providers in treating any condition, illness, disease, injury, or birth developmental malformations. Care is medically necessary for the purpose of controlling or eliminating infection, pain, and disease; and restoring facial disfiguration, or function necessary for speech, swallowing, or chewing.

Several important points are implied by these definitions, which are illustrated in Figure C-1. First, medically necessary dental services can be provided across a continuum of underlying diseases or conditions. Medically necessary dental services may be provided to prevent the onset of a disease

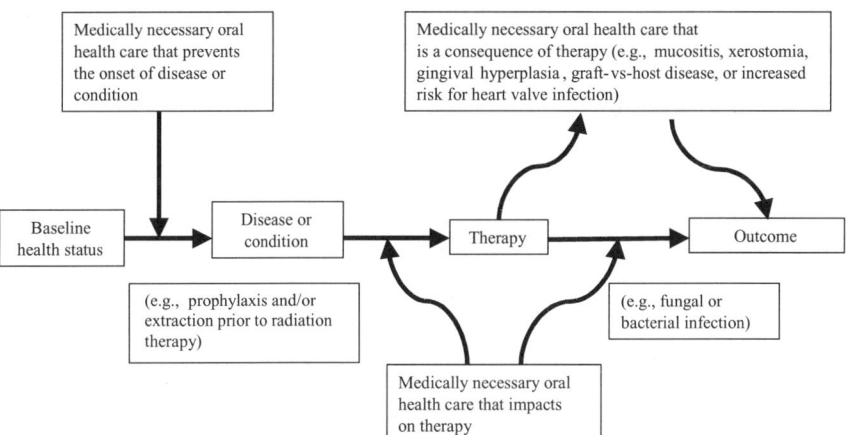

FIGURE C-1 A model of medically necessary dental services.

or condition, to manage oral conditions that can impact medical care (e.g., fungal or bacterial infections from oral sources), or to manage the oral manifestations of treatment (e.g., xerostomia secondary to radiation therapy). Medically necessary dental services are not restricted to or defined by an established set of medical diseases or conditions. Rather, it is the potential impact of oral health on medical outcomes, including the onset of certain diseases and the effect of medical treatment on oral health, that defines medically necessary dental services. Second, medically necessary dental services include preventive, diagnostic, and treatment services and are not limited only to diagnosis or selected procedures. Identification of potential oral sources of infection through an oral examination alone, for example, will not eliminate the infection. Additional treatment will be necessary to improve health outcomes. Finally, medically necessary dental services should have a measurable impact on morbidity and/or mortality and improve physiological, clinical, and/or behavioral outcomes of care for the defined medical disease or condition.

Selected Clinical Conditions Under Consideration

Numerous medical diseases and conditions may require medically necessary dental services to improve health outcomes, including developmental and acquired maxillofacial defects, developmental disabilities, diabetes, hemophilia, orphaned diseases (e.g., ectodermal dysplasia), and anesthesia for uncooperative pediatric and other patients. Time and resource constraints required that only a limited number of diseases and conditions be considered. Consequently, this background paper focuses on these five diseases or conditions: head and neck cancer, leukemia, lymphoma, organ transplantation, and repair or replacement of heart valve defects. The five conditions are a subset of a much larger set of diseases and conditions for which medically necessary dental services may be indicated. These were selected based in part on their prevalence and on the level of evidence for clinical management. The potential oral complications associated with these conditions are shown in Table C-1.

Currently Covered Dental Services Under Medicare

With certain exceptions, Medicare does not cover dental services. Figure C-2 illustrates current Medicare coverage policy for dental services. First, Medicare does not cover any services that are beyond the scope of the dental practice. Each state determines which services fall within and outside the scope of dental practice. Reimbursement for dental services under Medicare cannot go beyond what is allowed in each state.

TABLE C-1 Selected Medical Diseases and Conditions and Potential Oral Complications Associated with Treatment

Clinical Condition	Potential Complication(s)
Head and neck neoplasms	Secondary to radiotherapy: xerostomia, rampant dental caries, mucositis, osteoradionecrosis, infection Secondary to surgery: hard- and soft-tissue defects
Leukemia and lymphoma	Stomatotoxicity of chemotherapy and total-body irradiation; early septicemia from oral organisms; possibility of acute and chronic graft-versus-host disease (for bone marrow transplantation); hemorrhage
Organ transplantation	Infection from oral organisms secondary to immunosuppression; gingival hyperplasia secondary to immunosuppressive drugs
Heart valve repair or replacement	Valvular infection from oral organisms

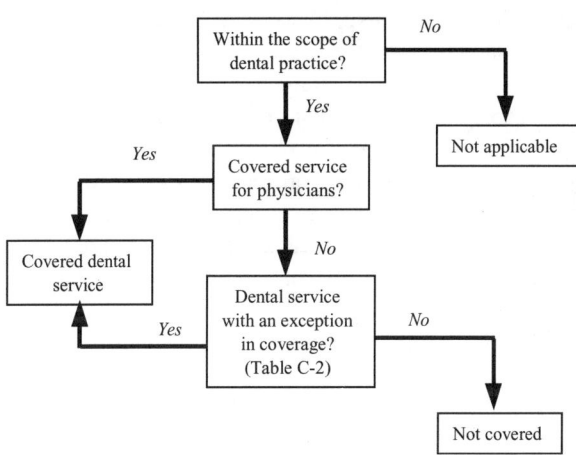

FIGURE C-2 Overview of current Medicare coverage policy for dental services.

Given the scope of dental practice, services that are covered for physicians are also covered for dentists. The term "physician," when used in connection with the performance of any function or action, includes a doctor of dental surgery or of dental medicine who is legally authorized to practice dentistry by the state in which he or she performs such function and who is acting within the scope of his or her license when performing such functions (section 1861(r)(2) of the Social Security Act (42 USC 1395x)). Such services include any otherwise covered service that may legally and alternatively be performed by doctors of medicine, osteopathy, and dentistry (e.g., dental examinations to detect infections prior to certain surgical procedures; treatment of oral infections, hemorrhage, and mucositis; and interpretations of diagnostic x-ray examinations in connection with covered services).

Specific dental services that are usually provided only by dentists are not covered. Under current Medicare statute, no payment can be made under Part A (hospital) or Part B (physician) for any expenses incurred for items or services:

> where such expenses are for services in connection with the care, treatment, filling, removal, or replacement of teeth or structures directly supporting the teeth, except that payment may be made under Part A in the case of inpatient hospital services in connection with the provision of dental services if the individual, because of his/her underlying medical condition and clinical status or because of the severity of the dental procedure, requires hospitalization in connection with the provision of such services. (Section 1862(a)(12) of the Social Security Act (42 USC 1395y))

The coverage or exclusion of any given dental service is not affected by the professional designation of the physician rendering the services (i.e., an excluded dental service remains excluded and a covered dental service is still covered whether furnished by a dentist or a doctor of medicine or osteopathy).

The limited exceptions to coverage for dental services under Medicare are summarized in Table C-2. Under Part B (physician services), if an otherwise noncovered procedure or service (e.g., removal of teeth) is performed by a dentist as "incident to" and as an integral part of a covered procedure or service performed by the same dentist (e.g., surgery of the jaw), the total service performed by the dentist on such an occasion is covered. For example, the reconstruction of a ridge performed primarily to prepare the mouth for dentures is a noncovered procedure. However, when the reconstruction of a ridge is performed as a result of, and at the same time as, the surgical removal of a tumor (for other than dental purposes), the totality of surgical procedures is a covered service. Likewise, the wiring of teeth is a covered service when it is done in connection with the reduction of a jaw fracture if the reduction and wiring are performed by the same practitioner.

Second, tooth extractions to prepare the jaw for radiation treatment of neoplastic disease are covered services. This is an exception to the requirement that to be covered, a noncovered procedure or service performed by a dentist must be incident to and an integral part of a covered procedure or service *performed by him or her*. Ordinarily, the dentist extracts the patient's teeth, but another physician (e.g., a radiation oncologist) administers the radiation treatments.

TABLE C-2 Current Medicare Coverage for Dental Services

Clinical Condition	Covered Service	Part A (hospital)	Part B (physician)
Underlying medical condition and clinical status require hospitalization for dental care	Inpatient hospital services only	X	
Severity of dental procedure requires hospitalization for dental care	Inpatient hospital services only	X	
Any oral condition for which nondental services are covered	All dental services if incident to and an integral part of covered procedure or service		X
Neoplastic jaw disease	Extractions prior to radiation		X
Renal transplant surgery	Oral or dental examination on an inpatient basis	X[a]	X[b]

[a] If the dentist is on staff at the hospital where the service is provided.
[b] Outpatient payment for physicians only.

Finally, an oral or dental examination performed on an inpatient basis as part of a comprehensive workup prior to renal transplant surgery is a covered service. The purpose of the examination is not for the care of the teeth or structures directly supporting the teeth. Rather, the examination is for the identification, prior to a complex surgical procedure, of existing medical problems where the increased possibility of infection would not only reduce the chances for successful surgery but also expose the patient to additional risks in undergoing such surgery. Such a dental or oral examination would be covered under Part A of the program if performed by a dentist on the hospital's staff or under Part B if performed by a physician. (When performing a dental or oral examination, a dentist is not recognized as a physician under section 1861(r) of the law; see *Carriers Manual* section 2020.3.)

Whether such services as the administration of anesthesia, diagnostic x-rays, and other related procedures are covered depends on whether the primary procedure being performed by the dentist is itself covered. Thus, an x-ray taken in connection with the reduction of a fracture of the jaw or facial bone is covered. However, a single x-ray or x-ray survey taken in connection with the care or treatment of teeth or the periodontium is not covered.

Based on current statute, regulations, and the *Coverage Issues* and *Carriers Manuals,* it appears that an oral examination would be a covered service for a person with certain oral conditions if (1) the management of the condition included a covered service and (2) the person providing the covered service also performed the oral examination. For example, individuals with a fractured mandible would require an oral examination as an integral part of the management of the fracture. The oral examination would be covered for the dentist if that dentist is also treating the fracture. Another example might include crowns on teeth for individuals requiring an obturator following head and neck surgery if the crowns are a necessary part of obturator placement. Likewise, for persons with neoplastic jaw disease, oral examination would be covered *if* they required extractions prior to radiation. For persons with neoplastic jaw disease who were edentulous or who did not require an extraction, the examination would not be covered. For the five medical conditions considered here, currently covered and noncovered services are shown in Table C-3.

The information presented here on coverage for dental services is contained within current statute, regulations, and coverage manuals. Certain Medicare fiscal intermediaries have made exceptions for coverage of certain procedures such as examinations for persons with head and neck neoplasms regardless of whether the person had an extraction. Given the lack of clarity and variability among carriers, this information is not included here.

Increasing Number of Persons 65 and Above Who Are Retaining Natural Teeth

During the next 10 years, the number of persons 65 years of age and over who are eligible for Medicare will increase from an estimated 34.5 million in 1999 to about 39.4 million in 2010 (Figure C-3) (U.S. Bureau of the Census Statistics, www.census.gov/population/www/index.html).

By 2010, individuals 65 years of age and older will represent about 13.2% of the U.S. population, up from about 12.7% in 1999. Not only will the number of persons 65 and above increase, the proportion maintaining some or all of their natural dentition will also increase, as suggested by epidemiological data spanning the past 35 years. The first National Health Examination Survey, conducted in 1960–1962, found that about 45.1% of men and 53.0% of women aged 65–74 years were edentulous (without teeth) (NCHS, 1973). For 75- to 79-year-old men, the percentage edentulous was 55.7%; for 75- to 79-year-old women, the percentage edentulous was 65.6%.

The National Health and Nutrition Examination Survey, conducted between 1971 and 1974, found that the edentulism prevalence declined to about 45.5% among persons 65 to 74 years of age, 43.6% among men and 47.0% among women (NCHS, 1981). An epidemiological study conducted by the National Institute of Dental Research in 1985–1986 found that among persons 65 years old and over attending senior centers, 41.1% were edentulous (NIDR, 1987).

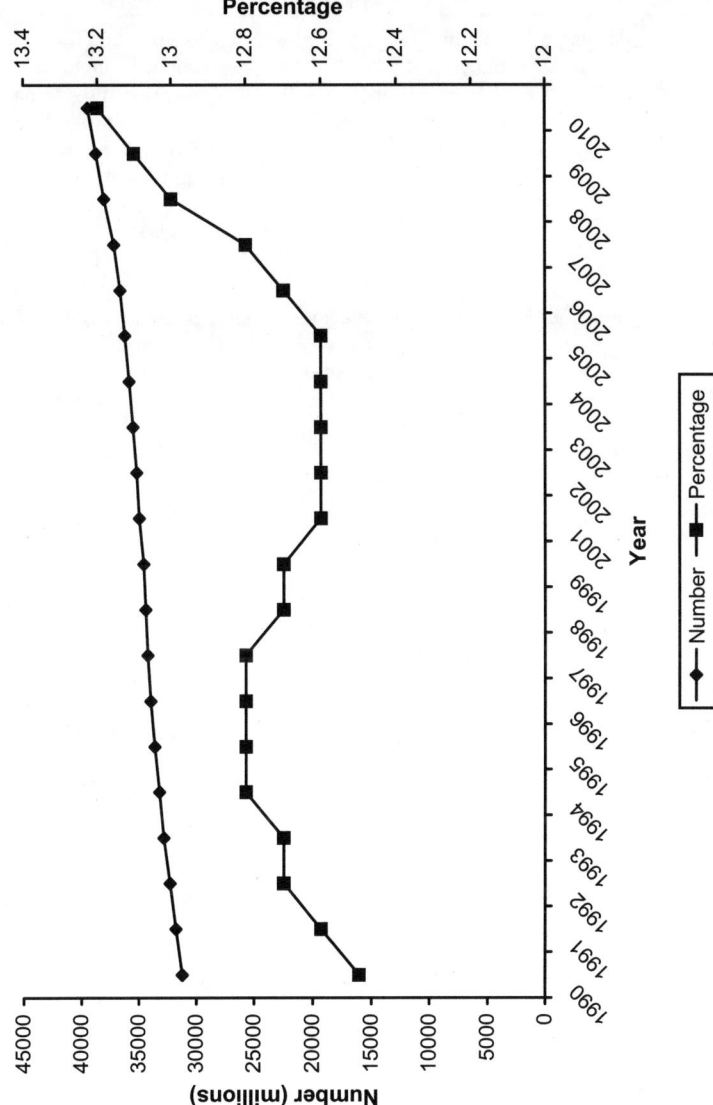

FIGURE C-3 Number and percentage of persons 65 years of age and above, United States, 1990–2010.

TABLE C-3 Summary of Dental Services Currently Covered and not
Covered Under Medicare for Selected Diseases or Conditions

Disease or Condition	Dental Services Currently Covered Under Medicare	Dental Services not Currently Covered Under Medicare
Head and neck neoplasms	Extraction of teeth prior to radiation Oral examination if extractions are to be performed	Oral examination if no extractions are to be done prior to radiation Preventive care to reduce risk of radiation caries (e.g., fluoride trays, supplemental topical fluoride) Treatment of radiation caries
Leukemia and lymphoma	Management of mucositis, hemorrhage, and related side effects of underlying disease	Oral examination prior to treatment Dental treatment to reduce risk of infection or eliminate infection prior to or following treatment
Organ transplantation	Management of infection following transplantation Oral examination prior to renal transplant surgery on an inpatient basis	Oral examination for transplants other than kidney Oral examination for renal transplants on an outpatient basis Dental treatment to reduce risk of infection or eliminate infection for any transplantation prior to or following transplant
Heart valve repair or replacement	None	Oral examination prior to repair or replacement Dental treatment to reduce risk of infection or eliminate infection prior to or following repair or replacement of valve

The 1989 National Health Interview Survey found that self-reported edentulism had declined to about 28.4% among persons 65 to 74 years of age and
43.0% among persons 75 years of age and over (Bloom et al., 1992). The Third
National Health and Nutrition Examination Survey, Phase I, conducted between
1988 and 1991, reported an edentulism rate of 26.0% among persons 65 to 69

years of age, 31.1% among persons 70 to 74 years of age, and 43.9% among persons 75 years of age and older (Marcus et al., 1996). Most recently, data from the 46 states that participated in the oral health module of the 1995–1997 Behavioral Risk Factor Surveillance System (BRFSS) indicated that about 22.9% of persons 65–74 years of age and 26.7% of persons 75 years of age or over were edentulous (MMWR, 1999). Given this trend, one would hypothesize that the proportion of Medicare-eligible persons 65 years of age or over who may require medically necessary dental services will increase.

Decision Framework for Medically Necessary Dental Services

Figure C-4 illustrates a generic decision model for medically necessary dental services that applies to each of the five diseases and conditions under consideration here and serves as a framework for the literature review and synthesis. As noted earlier, medically necessary dental services can occur in the context of a disease or condition.

Among persons with selected diseases or conditions, following the diagnosis and prior to initiation of medical therapy, a pretreatment oral assessment may or may not be provided. An explicit decision is required to provide the care, which is represented by the filled square in Figure C-4. This assessment may include a clinical examination and radiographs. Some of those assessed will have potential oral sources of infection or other complications. Dental care prior

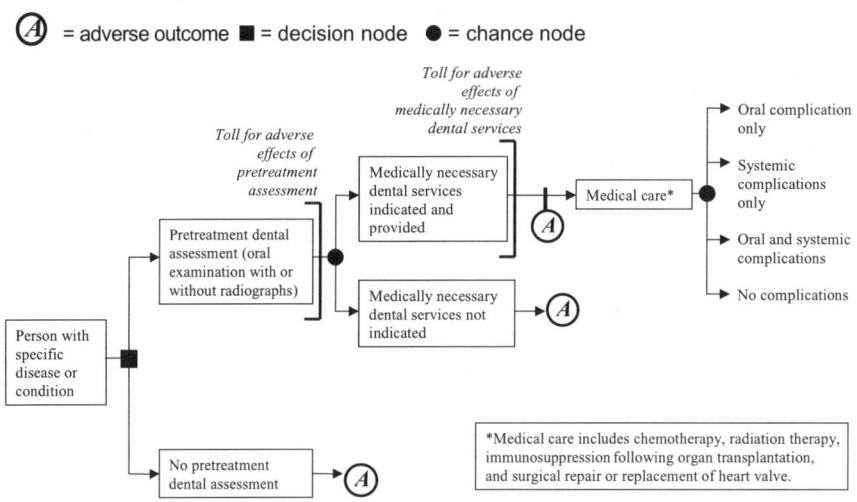

FIGURE C-4 Decision model for medically necessary dental services.

to medical treatment may be indicated and provided. The chance nature of this event is represented by the filled circle in Figure C-4. In conjunction with, or as a consequence of, medical therapy, individuals may develop oral complications associated with the medical treatment (e.g., mucositis or xerostomia), systemic complications from oral sources (e.g., infection or hemorrhage), or some combination thereof. Each of these can adversely affect the outcome of medical therapy by increasing morbidity, mortality, and cost. The purpose of this background paper is to review and assess the literature to determine the extent to which medically necessary dental services can reduce the likelihood of these complications or lessen their effect.

Decision Analytical Framework

Specific analytic questions guided our literature search and synthesis efforts. For each of the conditions under consideration, we initially sought to address the following question: *Is there direct evidence that medically necessary dental care—including screening, diagnostic and preventive services, and treatment—provided to persons with a defined medical diagnosis prior to or during acute therapy for that diagnosis improves health outcomes?* Direct evidence is evidence that relates a diagnostic strategy or therapeutic intervention to the occurrence of a principal health outcome (Eddy et al., 1992). Outcomes by definition are multidimensional. In this context, principal health outcomes refer to those outcomes that are of most interest to the patient, such as symptoms, functional status, morbidity, and death (Fleming and DeMets, 1996). Our goal, then, was to identify studies that related a specific dental intervention—oral examination and treatment prior to organ transplantation, for example—to an outcome—improved quality-of-life and decreased mortality, for example.

When direct evidence was not identified, we sought to identify indirect evidence that related to medically necessary dental services for each of the conditions being considered. Indirect evidence requires two or more bodies of evidence to relate the diagnostic strategy, exposure, or therapeutic intervention to the principal health outcome (Eddy, et al., 1992). For example, one study may demonstrate that a screening and treatment protocol for patients prior to heart valve replacement eliminates potential sources of oral infection. A second study may demonstrate that oral sources of infection are important contributors to valve failure. Neither study alone provides direct evidence that screening and treatment prior to heart valve replacement reduce morbidity or mortality; together, the two studies provide indirect evidence that screening and treatment to eliminate oral sources of infection prior to heart valve replacement improve principal health outcomes.

A number of questions guided our efforts to survey and synthesize indirect evidence to support medically necessary dental services. These questions reflect the various components of the decision framework illustrated in Figure C-4.

• The first question related to the effectiveness of pretreatment assessment prior to initiation of therapy to reduce risks of adverse outcomes such as postoperative infection or osteoradionecrosis. Assessment procedures are not without risk, and adverse effects can occur (represented by a toll).

• During assessment, the clinician may identify oral conditions that require dental care prior to medical treatment, including extractions and selected periodontal procedures. Such procedures may result in adverse effects (represented by a toll).

• In the third phase, during which medical therapy occurs, oral complications may arise from the therapy (e.g., mucositis), systemic complications may arise from oral sources (e.g., infection), some combination of oral and systemic complications may arise, or no complications may arise.

• In the final phase, following medical therapy, oral complications may impact on principal health outcomes such as osteoradionecrosis secondary to radiation-induced xerostomia, graft-versus-host disease in bone marrow transplant recipients, or infection in an immunosuppressed individual.

General Analytic Approach

Evidence of the effectiveness of dental services for the five diseases and conditions under consideration was obtained from the published literature. We conducted a comprehensive search of the literature from 1980 through 1999 to obtain relevant references using the following search terms: dentistry, dental care, oral surgical procedures, periodontal diseases, head and neck neoplasms, leukemia, lymphoma, organ transplantation, and heart valve diseases. We further limited the search results to human studies published in English. Results from these searches were provided to each author, who reviewed this information and conducted additional searches as indicated, including additional search terms, additional years, or both.

CONDITION 1: HEAD AND NECK CANCER

Introduction

Head and neck cancers represent about 4% of all cancers diagnosed in males and 2% of cancers diagnosed in females (USDHHS, 1991). The American Cancer Society's (ACS's) Department of Epidemiology and Surveillance Research estimates that 29,800 new oral cavity and pharynx cancers and 10,600 new larynx cancers will occur in the United States in 1999 (Landis et al., 1999). Incidence in the 65 years and over age group has been relatively stable over time. The estimated annual change in incidence from 1973 to 1996 was -0.4% for cancers of the oral cavity and pharynx and +0.4% for cancers of the larynx (Ries et al., 1999). The National Cancer Institute's (NCI's) Surveillance, Epidemiology, and End Results (SEER) Program regional treatment data suggest that 44.7% of oral cavity and pharynx cancer patients and 49.2% of larynx cancer patients are 65 years or older (SEER, 1993). If these estimates are applied to the ACS U.S. case estimates, this age group accounts for about 13,220 new oral cavity and pharynx and 5,215 new larynx cancer cases. Largely due to failure of early detection, the majority of oral cancer cases are diagnosed after regional or distant spread, resulting in an overall five-year survival rate for oral cavity and pharynx cancers of 55% among U.S. whites and 32% among African Americans (Landis et al., 1999).

Radiation and/or surgery are the primary treatment methods for new cases of head and neck cancers, with a lesser role played by chemotherapy (Shaha and Strong, 1995). Recently described organ-preserving protocols using neoadjuvant chemotherapy with cisplatin and fluorouracil followed by radiation therapy are gaining acceptance for larynx cancer and can be expected to result in increasing oral morbidity (Shah et al., 1997; Spaulding et al., 1994). SEER estimates that for patients diagnosed with cancer of the oral cavity and pharynx from 1988 to 1993, 53.8% of all ages and 49.7% of those age 65 and above received radiation therapy alone or in combination with other modalities as treatment for their cancer (SEER, 1993). For cancer of the larynx over this same time period, SEER estimates that 73.9% of all ages and 74.2% of those age 65 and above received radiation therapy alone or in combination with other modalities as treatment for their cancer (SEER, 1993). Radiation delivered in therapeutic doses to the head and neck region results in a number of acute and chronic complications (Beumer et al., 1979a,b).

The purpose of this systematic review is to evaluate the evidence base for expanding Medicare coverage in the arena of medically necessary dental services for the head and neck cancer patient treated with radiation therapy. The emphasis is on dental services that may be necessary in the course of radiation therapy because radiation therapy may have a poor outcome if the appropriate dental services are not included. Current Medicare Part B coverage for dental services for beneficiaries with head and neck neoplasms is limited to "extraction of teeth to prepare the jaw for radiation treatment of neoplastic disease" (Table C-3).

Methods

This review is based on a search of the literature from the MEDLINE database from 1966 to March 1999, including studies identified from reference lists in core articles obtained in the search. In addition to the search terms used for all topics in this appendix, as described in the section on general analytic approaches, separate searches were conducted specifically on the head and neck topic with key words as follows: (1) (head and neck cancer and radiation and oral complications).ti,ab.rw,sh; (2) (oral cancer and radiation and dental).ti,ab.rw,sh; (3) (radiotherapy and head and neck neoplasms).ti,ab.rw,sh;

(4) (head and neck cancer and radiation therapy and dental).ti,ab.rw,sh; and (5) (quality of life and radiotherapy and mouth neoplasms/or tongue neoplasms/or mandibular neoplasms/or oral cancer).ti,ab.rw,sh. The literature search resulted in 60 original papers from the selected search terms and 55 additional articles from the core paper reference lists. Inclusion criteria for papers accepted for closer review were the following: the study was identified as a randomized clinical trial, a case-control study, a cross-sectional observational cohort study, or a controlled follow-up study. Case reports and smaller case series (less than 50 cases) were excluded from further review. Only studies involving subjects over 18 years of age were accepted.

General Observations from the Literature Search

The systematic review of the literature revealed that our knowledge in this area is based primarily on multicase series from academic health centers reporting oral complication rates and the influence of dental factors on complications among radiated patients involved in prospective observational studies or retrospective cohort analyses. Few randomized clinical trials have evaluated the impact of oral health interventions on treatment outcome (Dreizen et al., 1977; Horiot et al., 1983; Marx et al., 1985). One group is currently conducting a multicenter international study to validate its recently proposed model to guide preradiation dental treatment decisionmaking in patients with head and neck cancer (Bruins et al., 1998).

The number of comparative multicase cohort studies of the efficacy of different treatment protocols is limited. The efficacy of various preradiation dental assessment and treatment approaches (e.g., aggressive dental extraction versus dental preservation) is determined largely through time cohort comparisons of outcomes (Bedwinek et al., 1976; Keys and McCasland, 1976; Murray et al., 1980a,b). It became evident that large, well-designed, case-control prospective studies are urgently needed in this important area. Current management recommendations are based on limited clinical studies supplemented by expert opinion and consensus as discussed at the National Institutes of Health Consensus Development Conference on Oral Complications of Cancer Therapies: Diagnosis, Prevention and Treatment, held in Bethesda, Maryland, in April 1989 (NIH, 1989).

Acute and Chronic Complications of Radiation Therapy to the Head and Neck Region

Orofacial complications are unfortunately common with all modalities of treatment for head and neck malignancy (Dreizen, 1990). High-dose radiation therapy delivered by external beam, implant devices (brachytherapy), or both may be required to manage more than half of head and neck neoplasms (SEER,

1993). Of the early or acute orofacial complications requiring consideration and management solely during the course of therapy, oral mucositis is one of the most common and distressing. Mucositis decreases the quality of life by causing pain and interfering with nutritional intake and may require cessation of radiation until some healing occurs. Mucositis surveillance and management commonly occur in conjunction with radiation treatments and are already covered by Medicare; hence, these are not a focus of this review.

Chronic or longer-term orofacial complications of radiation to the head and neck region include xerostomia and consequent dental demineralization or "radiation" caries (when salivary glands are radiated), trismus (when muscles of mastication are radiated), and osteoradionecrosis (ORN) (Beumer et al., 1979a,b; Dreizen, 1990). Salivary gland tissue is highly susceptible to radiation damage at both the acinar cell and the vascular levels, resulting in reduction in resting or basal and stimulated salivary flow (Liu et al., 1990; Valdez et al., 1992). The extent and permanency of xerostomia depend on the total radiation dose delivered and the volume and type of salivary gland tissue in the field of radiation (Liu et al., 1990; Valdez et al., 1992). With conventional bilateral external beam radiotherapy doses of 60–70 Gy to the parotid glands, saliva production decreases rapidly, with eventual 95% reduction and limited recovery (Dreizen et al., 1977). Partially radiated glands (e.g., mantle field or unilateral field) have less diminution in flow, 30–40% and 50–60%, respectively (Liu et al., 1990). Detrimental changes in salivary constituents also occur, such as lowered pH and lowered bicarbonate concentration resulting in decreased buffering capacity (Funegard et al., 1994). As a consequence of xerostomia, tooth demineralization and cavitation can occur at a rapid rate and involve atypical "radiation caries" patterns of decay on the incisal or cuspal tips and the cervical regions of teeth (Makkonen, 1987; Markitziu et al., 1992).

The most serious, although uncommon, orofacial complication is ORN. Radiation to the bone results in endarteritis obliterans, with small-vessel thrombosis and a slow protracted loss of osteocytes and osteoblasts with a consequent slow bone remodeling that leads to the risk of bone necrosis and subsequent infection (Dreizen, 1990). The mandible is at greater risk with its more compact bone of higher density and poorer blood supply than the maxilla. Higher radiation dose, fraction size, and number of fractions increase the risk as do continued tobacco and alcohol abuse, poor nutritional status or oral hygiene, and immune defects (Kluth et al., 1988). Although ORN may occur spontaneously, trauma is a significant precipitating event, with dental extractions being a common traumatic event. Trauma from tooth extraction and periodontal disease contributes to the three times higher ORN incidence in dentate than edentulous patients (Murray et al., 1980a,b). The highest incidence of ORN occurs when extractions immediately proceed or follow radiation therapy (Epstein et al., 1987). Figure C-5 shows a proposed mechanism for the consequences of radia-

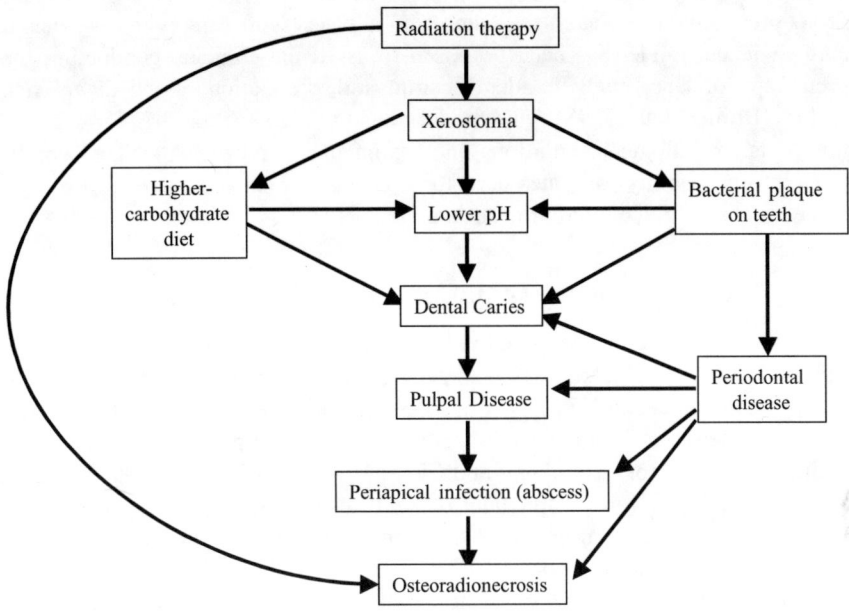

FIGURE C-5 Proposed mechanism for the interaction of radiation and oral cavity dental processes leading to pathology of radiation injury. SOURCE: Modified from Keys and McCasland, 1976.

tion therapy in the oral cavity, including the potential for necrotic breakdown of the mandible or maxilla.

Pretreatment Dental Assessment

Expert opinion and professional consensus suggest that to be effective, pretreatment dental assessment should be conducted by knowledgeable dental professionals in collaboration with the radiation oncologist and head and neck cancer surgeon. Oral health care interventions and long-term maintenance should be implemented with education and motivation programs to enhance patient understanding and compliance (Wright, 1990). The goals of pretreatment assessment include identification of possible sources and sites of ORN, presurgical assessment for prosthetic rehabilitation, and initiation of a preventive protocol for radiation-induced caries (Sonis et al., 1990). Comprehensive oral evaluation includes clinical, radiographic, and adjunctive components (Sonis et al., 1990). Teeth with compromised long-term prognosis due to pulpal or periodontal infection in the poorly compliant patient should be extracted prior to radiation, while intact teeth can be preserved under certain circumstances in the highly motivated patient who is able to maintain ideal oral hygiene, can adhere to rigorous preventive oral health regimens, and has access to comprehensive dental care. A recent model has been proposed to assist the clinician conducting the pretherapy oral screening in identification and elimination of the dental risk factors (Bruins et al., 1998). This model transforms clinical criteria for evaluating dental pathological conditions and malignancy- and patient-related conditions into probability estimates used to determine the choice between restoring and extracting a given tooth prior to radiation.

Prevalence of Dental Disease in the At-Risk Population

The oral health status of individuals diagnosed with new head and neck cancers has been evaluated by oral screening prior to radiation therapy in several cancer treatment centers (Brown et al., 1990; Lockhart and Clark, 1994; Roos et al., 1996). Between 33 and 43% of head and neck cancer patients are edentulous at the time of diagnosis (Lockhart and Clark, 1994; Niewald et al., 1996; Roos et al., 1996). While a full complement of adult teeth is 32, 75 upper- to middle-class dentate preradiation patients with a mean age of 60 years had—on average—10 teeth remaining in one U.S. observational study by Lockhart and Clark (1994). On oral screening, 94% of these patients had some plaque and calculus, 66% had significant bone loss, and 71% had decay in one or more teeth. Consistent with this was an observational cohort of oral cancer patients in Germany with a mean age of 55.5 years reporting dental findings obtained on 126 patients prior to radiation that indicated a mean of 11 teeth remaining (Niewald et al., 1996). This German population had an average of 2.4 carious, 1.0 necrotic, 2.4 loose, and 0.7 destroyed teeth. One case-control study indicated that 100 dentate patients with head and neck squamous cell carcinoma examined prior to radiation had greater extent of tartar buildup (53% versus 35%), greater extent of moderate to severe gingival inflammation (63% versus 42%), and more decayed teeth (59% versus 39%) than 214 tumor-free controls (Maier et al., 1993).

Preventive Dental Treatment Needs

Baseline dental treatment needs for the dentate population of preradiation patients have been identified in observational studies. Both dentate and edentulous patients undergoing any comprehensive pretreatment oral assessment would be evaluated by comprehensive oral examination and dental or panoramic radiographs. The percentage of dentate patients requiring specific preventive or therapeutic dental services is as follows: dental prophylaxis or scaling, 20–95%; dental restorations, 55–64% (mean five teeth); extractions, 44–75% (mean six teeth); and endodontic therapy, 0–7% (Brown et al., 1990; Epstein et al., 1999; Lockhart and Clark, 1994; Niewald et al., 1996; Roos et al., 1996; Toljanic et al., 1998).

Efficacy of Pretreatment Care: Aggressive Extraction—
No Prevention Versus Dental Preservation Approach

Perhaps the most significant impact dental care can have on improving the clinical outcome of radiation treatment for the head and neck cancer patient is the ability of adequate pretreatment care to reduce the risk for ORN of the jaws. A paradigm shift occurred in the early 1970s to a dental preservation approach from the approach of routine whole-mouth extractions or at least extraction of all teeth in the field of radiation, regardless of dental status, in an attempt to prevent ORN. The earlier aggressive extraction approach was not coupled with dental caries preventive measures, so postradiation extractions frequently became necessary for teeth that had not been removed prior to radiation. Keys and McCasland (1976) compared outcomes of two time cohorts of patients with cancer of the head and neck (excluding larynx) treated at the Walter Reed Army Medical Center using fairly constant radiation techniques, dose levels, and treatment policy. A preservation-oriented comprehensive dental care program (DCP) was instituted in 1969 with the following objectives: to reduce radiation caries incidence, to preserve as many useful teeth as possible for optimal dental function while avoiding edentulous arches for which prosthodontic alternatives are limited, to prevent significant ORN, and to provide a mechanism for continuing maintenance of optimal dental health during and after cancer therapy. The comprehensive program involved three phases: (1) before radiation, (2) during radiation, and (3) after radiation. Phase I consisted of an oral evaluation and a caries control program including prophylaxis, oral hygiene instructions, daily fluoride gel application, restoration of active decayed teeth, and needed extractions. Phase II consisted of oral hygiene reinforcement. Phase III consisted of all subsequent definitive dental and prosthetic care.

Results comparing 115 radiation patients treated under the DCP between 1970 and 1974 with the last 74 patients radiated prior to the program's institution revealed that all aspects of the dental condition were improved under the DCP (Keys and McCasland, 1976). Full-mouth extraction cases were reduced from 36% of pre-1970 patients to 6% in 1970–1974 under the DCP. Additional results of the DCP protocol revealed increases in teeth saved (from 50 to 78%) and decreases in teeth extracted postradiation (14 to 2%), reduced need for restorations postradiation (37 to 10%), lower caries incidence (46 to 12%), and fewer edentulous arches (49 to 43%). Although no cost analysis was available, some data on dental effort were reported. Of 1,113 teeth involved before 1970, 49% were extracted and 1% restored prior to radiation versus 22 and 10%, respectively, of 1,915 teeth cared for under the DCP. Postradiation dental effort included extractions of 7% of teeth, restoration of 16%, and other care (includes prosthetic and endodontic care) of 6% before the DCP versus 2% extraction, 8% restoration, and 4% other under the DCP. Patients managed prior to the DCP had—on average—six more dental visits (23.1 versus 17.3) than those managed under the DCP, with reduction in average number of pretreatment visits per patient from 9.4 to 8.0 and posttreatment visits from 13.7 to 9.3. Incidence of ORN was historically low at Walter Reed, with only 13 patients exhibiting this problem from 1950 to 1970. One case of ORN developed during the DCP protocol (1970–1974). Hence, no conclusions can be drawn with regard to the DCP's influencing ORN rates.

One of the mainstays of the dental preservation approach in the radiation-induced xerostomic patient is the use of daily topical fluoride to prevent tooth decay. The earliest randomized, placebo-controlled prospective clinical study of the efficacy of topical fluoride to prevent caries in 42 xerostomic, irradiated patients was conducted at one of the leading U.S. cancer centers, M.D. Anderson Hospital and Tumor Institute in Texas, by Dreizen and coworkers (1977). Dental prophylaxis, oral hygiene instructions, and dental restorations preceded randomization. Patients ($n = 13$) on the regimen of oral hygiene, 1% sodium fluoride (NaF) gel in plastic carriers, and unrestricted diet had significantly ($p < .001$) lower caries incidence (3.23 versus 22.21 mean decayed, missing, and filled tooth surfaces—DMFS) than the group ($n = 14$) on the oral hygiene-placebo gel-unrestricted diet regimen. The nine patients who began in the placebo gel group and were crossed over to the fluoride gel group due to a postradiation caries upsurge evident on a three-month interval exam also had significantly ($p < .001$) lower caries incidence (3.67 versus 22.21 mean DMFS) than the group on the oral hygiene-placebo gel-unrestricted diet regimen. Restriction of sucrose in the diet added to the NaF gel regimen ($n = 11$) further reduced the mean DMFS to 0.55. In this study, patients were reexamined every 3 months, for an average of 9 months for the placebo gel group, 26 months for the NaF gel group, 22 months for the crossover group, and 13 months for the NaF gel and sucrose restriction group.

Subsequently, several clinical trials have been conducted to compare the efficacy of different fluoride regimens where no fluoride-free control groups were used. Horiot and coworkers (1983) enrolled 222 irradiated patients in a prospective randomized protocol to compare daily applications of topical NaF gel with high-content fluoride toothpaste (1,350 parts per million [ppm] F⁻). At 12–36 months' follow-up, dental caries were observed in 3% of gel patients versus 11% ($p = .1$) of toothpaste patients. Al-Joburi and coworkers (1991) enrolled 184 dentate postradiation patients (mean dose 57 Gy) in a clinical trial of the efficacy of two fluoride systems to prevent radiation caries. One-year reexamination of 143 patients for coronal and root surface caries revealed significantly higher decay rates for the noncompliant patients ($p < .05$) compared to either the group using daily brushed-on 0.4% stannous fluoride (SnF) gel or the group using 1.1% NaF gel applications for the first three months followed by twice daily remineralizing mouthwash for the last nine months. Comparison of the fluoride treatments indicated that continual daily use of SnF brush-on gel was superior to three-month NaF gel or nine-month remineralizing mouth rinse in preventing root caries. Pochanugool and coworkers (1994) reported on a small, single-center clinical trial involving 73 postradiation patients, where the dental effects of three topical fluoride regimens were compared by simple sampling. The three regimens were: (1) 1% NaF gel applied daily in a plastic tray, (2) 1% NaF oral solution used five minutes a day, and (3) combined gel and oral solution use. A dental care program involving preradiation screening, restoration, and extraction of condemned teeth was in effect at the time of this trial. Groups were comparable in follow-up time and age, with total radiation dose of 45–76 Gy (mode 70 Gy) for all patients. The need for further restorations varied by treatment group from 68.2% using the NaF solution, to 65.5% on NaF gel, to 54.4% using both. Need for further extractions varied from a low of 6.9% for the NaF gel group to a high of 22.7% for the NaF solution group, suggesting some increased ability to preserve teeth for the NaF gel users. Obtaining adequate patient compliance with daily fluoride gel applications in custom carriers remains a challenge, necessitating regular dental follow-up (Epstein et al., 1995, 1996).

Expert opinion suggests that to maximize the impact of pretreatment assessment, it should occur at least two weeks prior to therapy initiation to allow adequate time for recommended treatment and healing (Keys and McCasland, 1976; Sonis et al., 1990). When the urgency of radiation precludes ideal timing of oral screening and treatment, the initial dental evaluation should be conducted as soon as possible to form the basis of a preventive dental treatment plan for reducing complication risks. Comprehensive protocols for the prevention of oral sequelae resulting from head and neck radiation therapy have been presented (Jansma et al., 1992).

Influence of Paradigm Shift to Dental Preservation on Incidence of Osteoradionecrosis

The incidence of ORN declined in the 1970s and after, with changes in the approach to oral preparation for radiation therapy presumably playing a major role in this decline (Table C-4). One of the earliest demonstrations of the potential for dental conservation to reduce the incidence of the most morbid radiation complication, ORN, was conducted at M.D. Anderson (Bedwinek et al., 1976). Bedwinek and coworkers (1976) compared two periods of dental management for patients treated with definitive radiation to the oral structures with respect to incidence and precipitating factors for ORN. During a period of elective dental extraction (1/1/66–6/30/69), 203 patients (19.7%) developed ORN, with precipitating factors assigned as follows: dental extraction (11.8%), denture irritation (2.5%), and spontaneous (5.4%). In contrast, during the subsequent period of dental conservation (7/1/69–6/30/71), 178 patients (7.9%) developed ORN, with precipitating factors assigned as follows: dental extraction (2.3%), denture

TABLE C-4 Osteoradionecrosis Incidence in Studies of 100 or More Cases

Year	Author(s)	Radiation Years	Location	No. of Subjects	No. ORN	% ORN	Dental Preservation Program in Place?
1966	Grant and Fletcher	1954–1962	M.D. Anderson (TX)	176	66	37.5	No
1967	Rahn and Drone	1960–1962	M.D. Anderson (TX)	120	53	44	No
1971	Rankow and Weissman	1965–1968	Columbia (NY)	176	12	6.3	No
1972	Beumer et al.	1961–1969	UCSF (CA)	354	10	3.6	Unknown
1972	Wang	1959–1968	Mass General (MA)	262	15	6	Unknown
1974	Marciani and Plezia	Not reported	Allen Park VA (MI)	220	23	10.5	No
1976	Bedwinek et al.	1966–1969	M.D. Anderson (TX)	203	40	19.7	No
		1969–1971		178	14	7.9	
1981	Horiot et al.	1972–1979	Ctr. Leclerc (France)	208	4	2	Yes
1986	Marciani et al.	1976–1984	Lexington VA (KY)	109	3	3	Yes
1987	Epstein et al.	1977–1984	UBC (Canada)	1,000	27	2.7	Yes
1987	Makkonen et al.	1974–1977	U. Turku (Finland)	224	0	0	Unknown
1987	Schweiger	1979–1983	Mem Sloan-Ket (NY)	324	6	1.8	Unknown
1989	Widmark et al.	1974–1979	U. Goteborg (Sweden)	431	19	4.4	Unknown
1992	Kumar et al.	1980–1988	Med Col Bikaner (India)	1,104	14	1.2	Yes
1996	Niewald et al.	1988–1992	U. Saarland (Germany)	116	10	8.6	Yes
1998	Toljanic et al.	1986–1993	U. Chicago (IL)	193	9	4.7	Yes

irritation (1.1%), and spontaneous (4.5%). Dental conservation at M.D. Anderson involved restorative dental procedures, regular oral prophylaxis, and daily fluoride applications.

Murray and coworkers (1980a,b) extended the analysis on the M.D. Anderson cohort by comparing 404 subjects in an even later dental conservation period (7/1/71–12/31/75) with 249 subjects managed by elective dental extraction in the original 1/1/66–6/30/69 time period. ORN rates were reduced from 24.5% in the first period to 19.1% in the second period ($p = .06$) (Murray et al., 1980a). This study included more subjects and a longer observation time than the previous report of Bedwinek and coworkers (1976). Using multivariate logistic regression, Murray and coworkers (1980a;b) identified several ORN risk factors: a 5-fold higher risk for tumors near the mandible; tumor doses above 80 Gy created a 2.9-fold higher risk than doses below 50 Gy; and the dentate had a 2.6-fold higher risk than the edentulous. In reviewing incidence of necrosis by cause, in the elective extraction period, etiology was assigned to extractions prior to radiation for 32.4% ORN cases and to postradiation extractions in 2.9%, compared to 5.2 and 6.5%, respectively, in the dental conservation period. Spontaneous or unknown cause of ORN rose from 38.2% of cases to 74.0% of cases over these time periods. In a further evaluation of dental factors, Murray and coworkers (1980b) showed that ORN is most likely in the first 3–12 months following radiation, although the risk persists indefinitely. Timing of extractions influenced necrosis risk, with significantly higher necrosis rate among postradiation extraction patients than the rest of the dentate ($p = .004$) and those whose extractions occurred prior to radiation.

Kluth and coworkers (1988) at West Virginia University conducted a small case-control study of factors contributing to the development of ORN among patients receiving radiation for head and neck malignancies between July 1973 and June 1983. This study revealed an ORN rate of 10.3% during this period among patients followed for 18 months or until death. This resulted in 14 ORN cases among 135 radiated patients. Controls were 28 of the remaining 121 non-ORN patients matched for age, sex, general medical condition, tumor location, and stage (to some extent). Tumor stage among the ORN cases was slightly more advanced (85% Stage III, IV, or recurrent cancer among cases versus 64% of controls), although the control group received slightly higher radiation doses (50–70 Gy for 57% cases and 79% controls). ORN occurred in 4 of 14 patients receiving less than 50 Gy. Although the majority of patients in both groups had moderate to severe xerostomia, the dentate ORN cases (6/8) were more likely to have poor oral hygiene than controls (0/19). Inadequacy of preradiation dental care was apparent among 5 of 14 cases and 0 of 28 controls. Two patients in each group received inade-quate postradiation dental follow-up. Among ORN cases, five of nine with teeth had extractions before radiation, and two had extractions during or after radiation. In the control group, 6 of 19 patients with teeth had preradiation extractions and 3 had postradiation. Continued heavy tobacco and alcohol use were also more common among cases than controls (10 of 14 cases versus 0 of 28 controls).

Additional studies using cohorts of ORN patients have reported on dental factors identified as precipitating events. Beumer and coworkers (1984) analyzed risk factors for 83 episodes of ORN at the University of California at Los Angeles over an 11-year period ending July 1982. The most common precipitating factors were postradiation extractions (22 of 83; 26.5%), periodontal disease (19 of 83; 22.8%), and preradiation extractions (17 of 83; 20.4%). A recent analysis by Curi and Dib (1997) of necrosis risk factors among 104 cases of ORN of the jaws treated from 1972 to 1992 revealed that 89.4% resulted from induced trauma and 10.6% were spontaneous necrosis. More individuals with ORN had no preradiation oral care (57.7%) than had oral care (42.3%). Two peaks of ORN incidence were evident: the first peak less than 12 months from completion of radiation, with 16% resulting from oral or dental infections, and the second peak from 24 to 60 months after radiation, with 60% resulting from oral or dental factors, largely trauma from dental extractions. Breakdown of extraction sites has become a well-accepted causal event for ORN, suggesting that dental treatment planning aimed at limiting extractions to unsalvageable teeth is the most prudent approach to preparing the patient's mouth for the effects of radiation. Evidence is accumulating to support the paradigm shift toward dental preservation and away from radical preradiation extractions, which is the approach that current Medicare coverage supports.

Is There a Role for Prophylactic Hyperbaric Oxygen Therapy in the Prevention of Osteoradionecrosis from Postradiation Extractions?

Marx et al. (1985) have proposed a role for prophylactic hyperbaric oxygen (HBO) therapy in facilitating head and neck surgical wound healing and thus preventing ORN resulting from postradiation surgical trauma induced by extractions. HBO stimulates angiogenesis, with increased neovascularization and optimization of cellular levels of oxygen for osteoblast and fibroblast proliferation, collagen formation, and support of in-growing blood vessels, thus improving the healing capacity of hypoxic radiated tissue (Myers and Marx, 1990). Marx and coworkers (1985) at the University of Miami reported the use of a prophylactic regimen of HBO delivered prior to traumatic dental surgery in the postradiation patient treated with 60 Gy or higher dose. This randomized prospective multicenter clinical trial indicated a reduction of ORN from 29.9% among 37 patients (31 of 137 socket wounds) covered with penicillin during and after extractions to 5.4% among 37 patients (4 of 156 socket wounds) who underwent 20 sessions of preoperative and 10 sessions of postoperative HBO (Marx et al., 1985). Using a cost analysis, the $8,000 average total cost of their HBO–ORN preventive protocol with its 94.6% prevention rate stood up favorably against the average total cost (normalized to 1984 dollars) of $30,000 to $69,000 for ORN treatment (Marx et al., 1985).

Given the high cost and limited availability of prophylactic HBO, its use has remained controversial (Clayman, 1997; Lambert et al., 1997; Maxymiw et al., 1991). Maxymiw and coworkers (1991) in a single-technique 72-patient case series at Princess Margaret Hospital in Toronto reported no ORN resulted from postradiation extractions where 196 teeth were in the direct field of radiation (median dose of 50 Gy) by using prophylactic penicillin, low-dose or no vasoconstrictor-containing local anesthesia, atraumatic surgical technique, and largely single-tooth extractions. Similarly, Lambert and coworkers (1997) reported no ORN among 47 patients followed on average 2.9 years after receiving prophylactic HBO using the Marx protocol prior to postradiation multiple extractions. HBO may have the greatest prophylactic benefit when multiple adjacent teeth in the direct field of radiation require extraction. This need occurs most commonly when radiation patients have no or inadequate preradiation dental evaluation and treatment or when they fail preventive measures.

What Treatment Is Required to Manage Osteoradionecrosis of the Jaws?

Conservative measures are used initially following the development of bone necrosis in almost all cases. These consist of oral saline or antiseptic (e.g., chlorhexidine) rinses, oral antibiotics (e.g., metronidazole, clindamycin, amoxicillin) during times of acute infection episodes, and/or significant pain and gentle sequestrectomy. In the study of Beumer and coworkers (1984) at the University of California, Los Angeles, conservative measures healed 30 of 83 (36.1%) episodes, with greatest success with ORN induced by denture irritation or preradiation extractions and least success with bone exposures occurring spontaneously or in direct association with remaining dentition. Treatment beyond conservative management was required in the remaining 53 episodes as follows: surgical sequestrectomy, 18 (21.7%); radical jaw resection, 13 (15.7%); HBO alone, 6 (7.2%); HBO and surgical sequestrectomy, 6 (7.2%); and HBO with mandibular resection, 10 (12%). Radical mandibular resection was reserved for patients whose necrosis proceeded to intractable pain and/or pathological fracture usually accompanied by orocutaneous fistula. In a British study examining 22 ORN cases that were severe enough to require jaw resection identified among 2,853 radiated patients, dental extractions pre-, during, and postradiation were found to be causative in 10 cases (Coffin, 1983).

In recent years, HBO has gained an important role in treating radiation complications for head and neck cancer patients (Myers and Marx, 1990), often in conjunction with surgical management. A study of 29 patients treated with HBO for ORN of the mandible from 1984 to 1992 revealed that nearly all patients also underwent sequestrectomy (16 of 29 subjects; 55%) or mandibular resection (11 of 29 subjects; 38%) (van Merkesteyn et al., 1995). In a long-term follow-up study of 20 cases of ORN treated with HBO between 1975 and 1989, Epstein and coworkers (1997) reported that the majority (60%) remained resolved. Recurrences presented in 2 patients, suggesting that postradiation patients remain at risk of ORN indefinitely. HBO treatment of ORN is now covered by Medicare.

What Is the Quality of Life Impact of Head and Neck Cancer Treatment?

Oral complications following radiation therapy for oropharyngeal carcinoma adversely affect quality of life (Bundgaard et al., 1993; De Graff et al., 1999; Epstein et al., 1999; Teichgraeber et al., 1985). A recent survey of 65 postradiation patients using the general quality-of-life survey (the European Organization for Research and Treatment of Cancer [EORTC] Quality of Life Questionnaire QLQ-C30), with added oral symptom and function scales, revealed the following: 91.8% had dry mouth; 75.4%, changes in taste; 63.1%, dysphagia; 50.8%, altered speech; 48.5%, difficulty with dentures; 43%, difficulty chewing or eating; and 38.5%, increased tooth decay (Epstein et al., 1999). Pain, which was present in 58.4%, interfered with daily activities in 30.8%. The frequency of oral side effects correlated with radiation treatment fields and dose.

Responses of 188 posttherapeutic subjects with upper aerodigestive tract cancers to the same health-related quality-of-life (HRQL) instrument were analyzed to investigate the hypothesis that dental status is a predictor of HRQL (Allison et al., 1999). Two multivariate models containing age, gender, employment status, cancer site, and disease stage, plus a dental status category, were developed. Significantly worse HRQL was identified among those who were partially dentate with no prostheses. This group reported significantly more "problems with their teeth," more "trouble eating," and more "trouble enjoying their meals." The dental status category of edentulous patients with prostheses predicted a significantly better HRQL. Hence, a full complement of either healthy natural teeth or functional prosthetic teeth is valued by the postradiation patient.

Summary

This systematic review of the literature, focused on dental services that may be medically necessary in the context of radiation therapy to the jaws, has indicated that radiation results in poorer patient outcomes in the absence of a dental preservation program to maintain oral health. Adverse outcomes include increased incidence of radiation-induced dental caries often necessitating postradiation dental extractions and subsequent increased frequency of the most debilitating outcome of radiation to the jaws, ORN of the jaws. Prior to the 1970s a relatively aggressive extraction approach, often full-mouth extractions, coupled with no preventive services, was the treatment of choice. Preradiation extractions were found to be a risk factor for ORN, supporting a paradigm shift toward extraction of only the unsalvageable teeth while preserving the functional teeth with needed restorations, periodontal care, and caries-preventive daily fluoride treatments. It would appear that expanding Medicare coverage to include preradiation preventive dental care and routine postradiation preventive services for the head and neck cancer patient would effectively promote better clinical outcomes and would be consonant with the current standard of care for managing these individuals.

Based on data from several studies described above, Figure C-6 illustrates the clinical effectiveness of a dental preservation approach that may reduce the incidence of ORN by an average of 78%, or 8 percentage points—from 10.2% to 2.25%—largely due to reducing the both preradiation and postradiation oral surgical intervention. Under the aggressive extraction approach, most cases of ORN attributable to dental factors are attributable to preradiation extractions.

CONDITIONS 2 AND 3: LEUKEMIA AND LYMPHOMA

Introduction

Leukemia, an abnormal proliferation of white blood cells, and lymphoma, a disease affecting the lymphoid tissue, are distinct but related conditions. Treatment for these diseases is similar, involving high-dose chemotherapy and/or radiation therapy, resulting in profound immunosuppression. With both leukemia and lymphoma, the rationale for medically necessary dental services is to reduce or eliminate the risk of infection during treatment and to manage any complications that may occur, either during or following treatment. Consequently, background information and evidence for medically necessary dental services are presented together.

Methods

This review identified all publications from 1985 to 1999 that examined (1) the prevention and treatment of oral complications of leukemia and lymphoma caused by chemotherapy and bone marrow transplantation, and (2) oral side effects of various modalities of chemotherapy for leukemia and lymphomas. These publications were identified through MEDLINE.

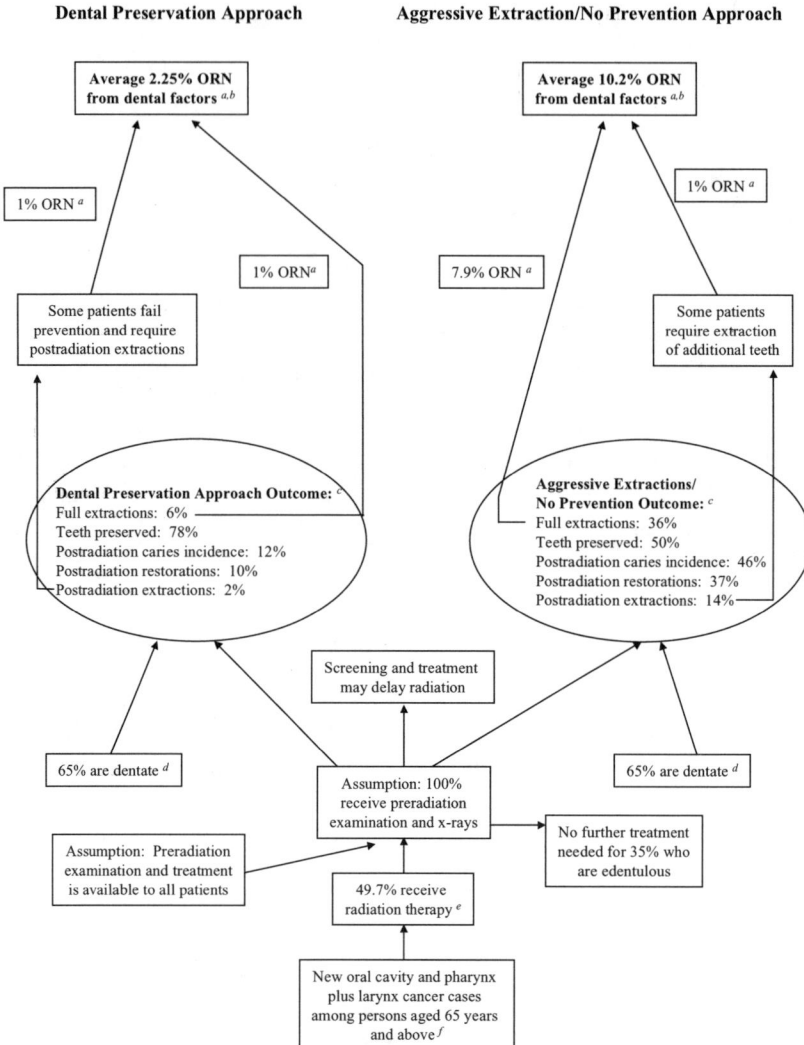

FIGURE C-6 Clinical effectiveness of dental preservation approach in reducing osteo-radionecrosis (ORN) as adverse medical outcome. Estimated net reduction of 78% ORN cases with preservation approach. SOURCES: a: Murray et al. (1980a,b); b: Bedwinek et al. (1976); c: Keys and McCasland (1976); d: Lockhart and Clark (1994), Niewal et al. (1996), and Roos et al. (1996); e: SEER (1993); and f: Landis et al. (1999).

Leukemia

The term leukemia signifies a heterogeneous group of neoplasms arising from malignant transformation of hematopoietic cells. Leukemic cells proliferate primarily in the bone marrow and lymphoid tissues, where they interfere with normal blood formation and immunity, and ultimately migrate into the peripheral blood, thereby infiltrating other tissues. Leukemias are classified according to the predominant cell type and as either acute or chronic, based on their natural history, with the former having a rapid clinical course. Causes of most leukemias are unknown, but various forms show association with certain genetic abnormalities, excessive exposure to ionizing radiation or certain chemicals, or retroviruses.

Patients with leukemia often present with fatigue, paleness, unexplained weight loss, repeated infections, bruising, and nosebleeds or other hemorrhages. In children, these signs can appear suddenly. Chronic leukemia can progress slowly with few symptoms. The various forms strike both sexes and all ages. Because the symptoms and signs are common to a variety of less serious conditions, early detection is often difficult. Diagnosis is made using blood tests and bone marrow biopsy.

Leukemia Incidence and Burden

An estimated 30,200 new cases of leukemia are anticipated in 1999, about evenly divided between acute leukemia and chronic leukemia (ACS, 1999; Ries et al., 1999). Leukemia is expected to strike many more adults (27,900) than children (2,300) this year. Acute lymphocytic leukemia accounts for about 1,500 (65%) of the cases of leukemia among children. In adults, the most common types are acute myeloid (about 10,100 cases) and chronic lymphocytic (about 7,800 cases). The incidence of leukemias in general is greatest among those individuals 65 years of age and older, with 0.051% of the population (or 51.4 per 100,000) newly affected each year. An estimated 22,100 deaths are anticipated from leukemia in 1999 (ACS, 1999; Ries et al., 1999).

The one-year relative survival rate for patients with leukemia is 63%. Survival drops to 43% at five years after diagnosis, due primarily to the poor survival of patients with some types of leukemia such as acute myelocytic. Survival for patients with acute lymphocytic leukemia has improved dramatically—from a five-year relative survival rate of 38% in the mid-1970s to 55% in the late 1980s. Survival rates for children increased from 53 to 78% over the same time period.

Five-year survival rates are lowest among the 65-year and older population for the acute myeloid and acute lymphocytic leukemias. Relatively slight differences are found among males and females for five-year survival rates for all leukemias except the chronic myeloid variety.

Leukemia—Clinical Oral Aspects

About 89% of patients with undiagnosed acute lymphocytic leukemia have oral problems associated with disease onset; 22% of these cite these problems as their reason for seeking medical care. Almost two-thirds of patients with other forms of acute leukemia demonstrate oral changes during the early, undiagnosed stages of disease. One-third of these seek medical evaluation for oral changes such as gingival oozing or bleeding, petechiae, hematoma or ecchymosis formation, oral ulceration, pharyngitis, gingival infection, or gingival hyperplasia (Sonis et al., 1995).

Intensive cancer chemotherapy and ionizing radiation result in oral mucositis in 36–100% of patients. Erythema and edema progress to ulceration and often mucosal bleeding accompanied by mild burning to severe pain. Mastication and deglutition may be intolerable. These clinical changes have important systemic implications for myelosuppressed patients who have had bone marrow transplantation (BMT), including risk of microbial invasion with serious regional or systemic infections. Despite many different approaches to palliation, there has been little substantive improvement in the ability to prevent or treat therapy-induced oral mucositis in patients with cancer. Most clinicians recommend dental treatment in patients undergoing BMT before it is started.

Lymphoma

The term lymphoma signifies neoplasms primarily of the lymphoid tissues. The two major variants of malignant lymphoma are non-Hodgkin's lymphoma and Hodgkin's disease. Although both tumors infiltrate reticuloendothelial organs, they differ from each other in both biological and clinical behavior, and are generally regarded as different diseases.

Patients with lymphoma present with enlarged lymph nodes, itching, fever, night sweats, anemia, and unexplained weight loss; fever may be intermittent for periods of several days or weeks. Risk factors are largely unknown, but partially involve reduced immune function and exposure to certain infectious agents. Persons with organ transplants are at higher risk from altered immune function. HIV and human T-cell leukemia/lymphoma virus-I (HTLV-I) are associated with increased risk of non-Hodgkin's lymphoma. In Africa, the Epstein-Barr virus is implicated in Burkitt's lymphoma. Other possible risk factors include occupational exposure to herbicides and perhaps other chemicals.

Lymphoma Incidence and Burden

An estimated 64,000 new cases of lymphoma are projected in 1999, including 7,200 cases of Hodgkin's disease and 56,800 cases of non-Hodgkin's lymphoma (ACS, 1999; Ries et al., 1999). Since the early 1970s, incidence rates for non-Hodgkin's lymphoma have nearly doubled; during the 1990s, the rate of increase appeared to be slowing. Incidence rates for Hodgkin's disease have declined over the past two decades, especially among the elderly. About 27,000 deaths in 1999 (non-Hodgkin's lymphoma, 25,700; Hodgkin's disease, 1,300) are anticipated.

Non-Hodgkin's disease has an incidence rate among the population 65 years of age or older that is eight times greater than among those under 65 years and is far more common among males than females. About 0.075% of the population, or 75.5 per 100,000 people, age 65 years and older develop non-Hodgkin's lymphoma each year. Among the population over 65 years old, males are about 1.5 times more likely than females to develop both Hodgkin's disease and non-Hodgkin's lymphoma.

Survival rates vary widely by cell type and stage of disease. The one-year relative survival rates for Hodgkin's and non-Hodgkin's lymphoma are 93 and 70%, respectively; the five-year rates are 82 and 51%. Ten years after diagnosis, the relative survival rates for Hodgkin's and non-Hodgkin's disease decline to 77 and 44%, and the 15-year survival rates to 66 and 36%, respectively.

The five-year survival rate for all types of lymphomas is less than 50% for individuals 65 years of age and older. No difference in survival is apparent among those over 65 years of age for either of the two types of lymphomas.

Lymphoma—Clinical Oral Aspects

Oral manifestations of Hodgkin's disease are limited. Patients usually present complaining of increasing unilateral painless swelling of the neck (Sonis et al., 1995). If the disease is widespread, patients may complain of difficulty with breathing and shortness of breath due to involvement of the mediastinal nodes.

Non-Hodgkin's lymphoma may appear in the mouth as a primary tumor or as a secondary manifestation of a tumor elsewhere. Most commonly, this lymphoma is manifest as a nonhealing painless ulceration with a pebbly, uneven surface that appears to glisten, with ill-defined borders, that undermines surrounding mucosa. The gingiva, palate, and tonsillar areas are most frequently affected. For the most part, the oral aspects of the lymphomas and leukemias are related to treatment.

Oral Complications of Treatment for Leukemia and Lymphoma: Chemotherapy and Bone Marrow Transplantation

Chemotherapy is the major clinical approach used for overall treatment of leukemia and is a key component of the management approach for lymphomas (Sonis et al., 1995). About 40% of all patients receiving chemotherapy develop oral side effects. In general, hematologic malignancies, such as leukemia and lymphoma, tend to be associated with the highest frequency of oral complications. Side effects tend to be directly related to the specific antineoplastic agent used, the drug dose administered at a given time, the timing of administration (single dose versus spread over time), and whether radiotherapy is administered at the same time. Oral side effects of chemotherapy are potentiated by radiotherapy.

Oral complications of cancer chemotherapy may be direct or indirect (Sonis et al., 1995). Direct problems result from a drug's direct effect on oral tissues. The most common direct oral effects are mucositis and ulceration, usually occurring within five to seven days after drug administration. Oral mucosal ulceration complicating bone marrow transplantation interferes with patients' comfort and nutrition and may lead to systemic infection derived from the mouth. The mucosal injury results from epithelial damage due to the cytotoxic effects of chemotherapy and radiation conditioning as well as from superficial oropharyngeal infection (Weisdorf et al., 1989). Other direct oral effects include xerostomia and neurotoxicity, most frequently affecting the mandibular molars. Indirect effects include infection (e.g., bacterial, fungal, or viral) or oral bleeding secondary to thrombocytopenia.

Bone marrow transplantation is being employed increasingly to treat types of cancer such as leukemia. The most common forms of BMT are allogeneic (in which marrow is transferred from a genetically matched donor to the recipient) and autologous (in which marrow is harvested from the patient, treated, preserved, and then reinfused after the patient receives chemotherapy). Patients receiving allogenic transplants are at risk not only for the direct and indirect effects of chemotherapy but also for graft-versus-host disease. Oral complications are the most frequent side effect of this disease and include lichen planus-like lesions, producing significant discomfort and xerostomia.

New treatment protocols using highly specific monoclonal antibodies directed at lymphoma cells and high-dose chemotherapy with BMT are now under investigation in selected patients who relapse after standard treatment.

Tables C-5 and C-6 present the dental and oral management considerations and manifestations as they relate to systemic aspects of Hodgkin's disease (Table C-5) and non-Hodgkin's lymphoma (Table C-6).

Oral Sources of Septicemia in Patients with Hematologic or Lymphatic Malignancies

Many potentially pathogenic microbial species inhabit the oral cavity. Oral microorganisms are normally harmless, leading to relatively minor, low-grade dental infections in the individual with a competent immune system. When leukemia, chemotherapy, or bone marrow transplantation compromise the immune system by producing dramatic declines in neutrophil (white blood cells, which hold the bacteria at bay) counts, however, these normal oral species may be dangerous if they gain access to the blood circulation (Wingard, 1990). Dental plaque, dental caries, and periodontal infections harbor bacteria that may result in hematogenous seeding (blood-borne infection) and septicemia. Seeding may occur through areas of oral mucositis or ulceration, through sites of gingival inflammation, with professional dental treatments, and with activities such as normal chewing and brushing (reviewed in Lockhart and Schmidke, 1994).

TABLE C-5 General Dental and Oral Considerations in Hodgkin's Disease

Systemic Aspect	Related Dental and Oral Management Consideration
Functionally immunosuppressed, at risk for infection	Chronic oral infections may become acute. Sources of oral infection should be eliminated
Effects of radiotherapy, especially mantle or supradiaphragmatic radiation, which involves the neck and inferior border of the mandible	Xerostomia as a consequence of radiation to the submandibular and sublingual salivary glands. Radiation caries can be frequent and troublesome. Oral therapy includes frequent prophylaxis, low-sucrose diet, salivary flow stimulation, and routine use of topical fluorides
Chemotherapy, which may cause myelosuppression	Oral infection and hemorrhage

SOURCE: Adapted from Sonis et al., 1995, pp. 270–271.

Dreizen and coworkers (1986) at M.D. Anderson Hospital in Texas reported on oral complications of antileukemia chemotherapy in 1,500 patients from 17 to 82 years of age. Daily oral exams and the culturing of suspicious oral lesions at least twice made it unlikely that contamination occurred during their hospitalizations. Oral infections, either single or polymicrobial, were documented in 513 (34.2%) patients. *Candida* and other fungi were causative in 20.7%, herpes simplex virus in 8.8%, gram-negative aerobic bacilli (*Pseudomonas, Klebsiella, Escherichia, Enterobacter, Serratia, Proteus*) in 8.1% and gram-positive cocci (*Staphylococcus, Streptococcus*) in 4.3%. Drug-induced mucositis and oral hemorrhages occurred in 16.3 and 13.6% of the population, respectively.

Bergmann (1989) determined the prevalence of acute oral infections and estimated their role as a possible cause of 78 episodes of fever in 46 immunocompromised patients with hematologic malignancies monitored with daily clinical and microbiological investigations. Overall acute infections were present in 92% of febrile episodes, with oral infections (largely acute candidiasis and infected mucosal ulcers) during 78% and extraoral infections (largely septicemia and pneumonia) during 73%. Acute oral infections were a probable cause of fever in 14% of febrile episodes and a possible or contributing cause of fever in a further 26%. Bergman (1988) further examined 19 septicemic episodes in this study population and, by comparing blood and oral surveillance cultures, found a probable oral focus of septicemia in two cases (10.5%), with an additional probable or possible source in six cases (31.6%). He suggests that prevention and elimination of oral infection may reduce the morbidity and perhaps mortality in these patients.

Overholser and coworkers (1982) followed 22 newly diagnosed hospitalized patients with acute nonlymphocytic leukemia from the initiation of chemo-

therapy until remission. Of interest were acute exacerbations, during myelosuppressive chemotherapy, of asymptomatic periodontal disease present at admission. In these 22 patients, 47 acute exacerbations developed, including 13 of
periodontal origin, with all but 3 of these 13 occurring during pronounced neutropenia (<100 neutrophils per microliter).

Heimdahl et al. (1989) reported on the clinical, pathological, and laboratory
features of oral infections in 181 consecutive patients treated with BMT at the
Karolinska Institute in Sweden between 1975 and 1987. Indication for BMT in
this study was leukemia in 131 (77%) subjects who had a mean age of 28 years
(range 1–54); 53 patients (29%) had dental infections that needed treatment (41
underwent extractions) before BMT. BMT was postponed because of oral infection in 10 (6%) patients. Four patients were medically unstable for dental treatment and underwent BMT with existing periapical infection; one of these four
turned into an acute phase during treatment and required systemically administered antibiotics and surgery. In 59 patients, microbiologically confirmed septicemia was observed during the neutropenic phase, which resulted in death in 12
patients. Septicemia was caused by oral organisms (alpha streptococci) in 24 of
59 (41%) patients, and this was associated with increased frequency of oral ulceration, particularly when methotrexate was used. Antiviral prophylaxis appeared to be protective. No attempt was made in this study to directly associate
alpha streptococci with specific oral sites.

In a cohort study of 49 patients with hematologic malignancy on high-dose
chemotherapy examined weekly by a dentist who obtained bacterial cultures
from saliva samples, Richard and coworkers (1995) found that 7 of 49 (14%)
developed a *viridans* streptococcal bacteremia during the study. *Viridans* strep-

TABLE C-6 General Dental and Oral Considerations in Non-Hodgkin's
Lymphomas

Systemic Aspect	Related Dental and Oral Management Consideration
May appear in mouth as a primary tumor or as a secondary manifestation of a tumor elsewhere	Most commonly found as a nonhealing, painless ulceration with a pebbly, un-even surface that appears to glisten. Borders of ulcer are not well defined and may undermine surrounding mu-cosa. The gingivae, palate, and tonsil-lar areas are most frequently affected
Treatment relies on multiagent chemo-therapy and radiotherapy	High frequency of oral complications associated with chemotherapy

SOURCE: Adapted from Sonis et al., 1995, pp. 271–272.

tococci with the same ribotype as the strain responsible for the bacteremia were recovered from the mouths of all bacteremic patients before the onset of bacteremia, with no shared ribotypes among patients. They concluded that their results support the idea that the oral mucosa was the portal of entry for *Streptococcus viridans* that caused bacteremia in their patients, and they advocate the use of first-line antibiotic regimens aimed at gram-positive organisms for high-risk patients repeatedly exposed to aggressive chemotherapy. While recognizing that there are ubiquitous oral reservoirs of *viridans* streptococci and only selective bacterial seeding occurs, suggesting unknown determinants of organism virulence, these authors also concluded that local oral prophylaxis or cleaning could be cost-effective for the prevention of streptococcal infections.

Greenberg et al. (1982) conducted a two-phase study of the role of oral flora in septicemia among patients with acute leukemia. In the first phase, nine patients aged 24–66 with acute nonlymphocytic leukemia who were admitted to the Oncology Unit at the Hospital of the University of Pennsylvania were followed. Each had a fever of 101°F or higher for eight or more hours. Blood, stool, sputum, urine, throat, oral mucosa, gingival sulcus, and oral ulcer cultures were obtained. Following a febrile episode, the investigators categorized infections as either oral site, likely oral site, likely extraoral site, extraoral site, or unknown. Six oral infections (three pericoronitis, one periapical, one infected oral ulcer, and one endodontic–periodontic lesion) were identified. Four of these met the associated-with-septicemia criteria, which included localized oral signs and symptoms, absence of other signs and symptoms, culture of the same organism from the oral infection and from blood in moderate to heavy amounts, and absence of the organism in cultures from other body sites. Septicemic oral organisms included *Klebsiella* (two), *Enterobacter* (one), and S*taphylococcus epidermidis* (one).

Role of Prechemotherapy Dental Treatment in Reducing Septicemias

In Phase 2 of the Greenberg et al. (1982) study, dental screening and selected preventive intervention were undertaken prior to chemotherapy on 24 medically able patients ages 20–74. This was in contrast to Phase 1, when treatment was delayed until the onset of a febrile episode. Dental treatment was required by nine patients prior to chemotherapy: periodontal therapy only in three cases, extractions only in three cases, and periodontal therapy and extractions in three cases. These 24 patients experienced 55 febrile episodes. Six septicemias occurred, but no definitive source was identified using the previous criteria. The source for three was suspected to be periodontal or gingival, but patients had no localized symptoms in two cases (*Enterococcus* and *Klebsiella*) and gingival symptoms only in one case (*Klebsiella*). These three patients did not receive prechemotherapy periodontal treatment due to the severe complications of their leukemia on admission.

Peterson et al. (1990) included some original data from a small study at the University of Maryland Cancer Center of 33 newly diagnosed patients with acute nonlymphocytic leukemia who were randomized to receive either limited or thorough mechanical oral hygiene (OH) prior to remission induction: 18 underwent limited OH and 15 underwent thorough mechanical OH (e.g., dental scaling) prior to induction chemotherapy. The limited OH group had five acute systemic infections clinically documented as periodontal in origin versus only one such infection in the thorough OH group. Each group also had four acute oral nonperiodontal infections, and seven (limited OH) and nine (thorough OH) patients had acute esophageal, pulmonary, or pharyngeal infections. This trend suggests that thorough dental scaling prior to chemotherapy would be of benefit in reducing subsequent risk of acute periodontal infection during neutropenia.

Toljanic et al. (1999) reported a prospective study of 48 consecutively entered patients with hematologic (90% leukemia) or solid malignant neoplasms (6% lymphoma) admitted for treatment at the University of Chicago Hospitals between 1993 and 1995. Prechemotherapy dental examination resulted in scoring dental lesions as mild to moderate versus severe, and acute versus chronic. Patients with acute dental pathology associated with nonsalvageable teeth ($n = 3$) underwent prechemotherapy dental treatment (extractions) to remove the source of infection. Patients diagnosed with chronic dental pathology only ($n = 38$) received no prechemotherapy dental treatment regardless of the severity of the score for this pathology. Each patient experienced at least one episode of severe neutropenia (absolute neutrophil count below 500 cells per microliter) lasting several days. Severe chronic pathology judged to be at risk of acute exacerbation under immune suppression was diagnosed in 21 patients. Of these 21 higher-dental-risk patients, 2 had intertherapy febrile episodes resulting from odontogenic sources. The authors recommend that a comprehensive exam be completed prior to chemotherapy to identify acute presentations of dental disease that require aggressive pretherapy treatment to prevent local exacerbation or systemic spread of ongoing infection. However, routine prechemotherapy treatment of chronic dental disease, especially disease of mild to moderate risk, may not be warranted.

Although the problem of infections of oral origin during hematologic malignancy, chemotherapy, or BMT-induced immune suppression is well documented and various preventive oral health and pretreatment dental protocols have been advocated (Epstein, 1990; Meurman et al., 1997; Peterson, 1990); they are based largely on clinical experience, expert opinion, and indirect evidence from small clinical or observational cohort studies, rather than large multicenter controlled clinical trials. There is limited direct evidence that eradication of dental infection prior to immunosuppressive chemotherapy improves the prognosis of patients with leukemia.

Oral Mucositis Treatment

Oral mucositis is the major toxic oral side effect of chemotherapy and bone marrow transplantation for leukemia and lymphoma. It thus has the greatest potential to interfere with medical care for these diseases. The randomized clinical trials have indicated that potentially effective treatments for reducing the severity or incidence, or at least providing palliation, of oral mucositis include the following:

- Acyclovir (Bergmann et al., 1995)
- Topical oral G-CSF (filgrastin) mouth rinses (Karthaus et al., 1998)
- Propantheline (Ahmed et al., 1993)
- Glutamine (Anderson et al., 1998)
- Helium–neon lasers (Barasch et al., 1995; Cowen et al., 1997)
- "Intensive oral health care" (Borowski et al., 1994)
- Patient-controlled analgesia with morphine (Coda et al., 1997; Hill et al., 1990; Pilliteri and Clark, 1998)
- Tretinoin topical cream (Cohen et al., 1997)
- Chlorhexidine mouth rinse (Ferretti et al., 1988)
- Vitamin E (Lopez et al., 1994)
- Relaxation and imagery training (Syrjala et al., 1995)

Lack of effect was found for the following approaches:

- Chlorhexidine mouth rinse (Epstein et al., 1992; Weisdorf et al., 1989)
- Prostaglandin E_2 (PGE_2) (Labar et al., 1993)

For dental and gingival conditions associated with chemotherapy for lymphoma, the following was found effective for prevention and treatment: twice-daily rinsing with an amine fluoride–stannous fluoride mouthwash (Laine et al., 1993; Meurman et al., 1991).

Ineffective procedures for dental and gingival conditions included chlorhexidine mouth rinse (Wahlin, 1989). It should be noted that the efficacy of chlorhexidine mouth rinse for gingival and dental conditions in these patients has been controversial.

CONDITION 4: ORGAN TRANSPLANTATION

Introduction

This review evaluates the evidence for expanding Medicare coverage of medically necessary dental care in solid organ transplant patients. Only a small number (470 of 20,935 total solid organ transplants in 1997) of liver, lung, heart, or pancreas transplants are provided to Medicare-eligible recipients (UNOS,

1999) (Table C-7). In 1972, the Social Security Act was amended to cover the medical costs associated with end-stage renal disease (ESRD) for eligible patients under Medicare. Currently, the vast majority of renal transplants are covered under Medicare or the Veterans Administration. Most oral complications, however, are similar across various organ transplants and are related primarily to a transplant recipient's net state of immunosuppression and the drug therapies utilized. Current Medicare Part B coverage for dental services for beneficiaries receiving a solid organ transplant is limited to "oral or dental examination performed on an in-patient basis as part of a comprehensive work-up prior to renal transplant surgery" (Table C-2).

Solid organ transplantation has become an accepted part of standard medical therapy for irreversible failure of a variety of organs. More than 20,000 organ transplants were performed in 1998 (Table C-8), and an estimated 75,000 transplant recipients are alive today.

The waiting list (Table C-9) and waiting time to transplant continue to grow, however, and numerous individuals die each year awaiting transplant.

Despite a recent increase in the number of living donors not only for kidneys but also for other organs such as lung, liver, and pancreas, organ donor shortage is at the forefront of problems in this field. Given these factors, the importance of maximizing the potential for success of each transplant is critical. Chronic rejection and infection are the most important factors leading to transplant failure. Transplant teams strive to eliminate potential sources of infection prior to transplantation and to minimize the effects of the drug-induced chronic immunosuppression that is required for long-term graft success.

The mouth is a potential source of local and systemic infection. Medical and dental references typically cite the need for a comprehensive oral examination and elimination of potential oral sources of infection prior to transplant surgery. This section examines the evidence that the provision of oral health care, pre- and/or posttransplant, affects short- or long-term graft survival, affects patient survival, or reduces postoperative complications.

TABLE C-7 Number of Transplant Recipients Aged 65 Years and Above, United States, 1997

Kidney: 12,357[*]	Heart: 165
Liver: 264	Lung: 40
Pancreas: 1	Heart–lung: 0

[*]Includes all renal transplants since most are covered under Medicare through the ESRD program.

SOURCE: UNOS, 1999.

TABLE C-8 Number of Transplants Performed in the United States in 1998

Type of Transplant	Number
Kidney alone (3,172 living donors)	11,990
Kidney–pancreas	965
Pancreas alone	253
Liver	4,450
Heart	2,340
Heart–lung	45
Lung	849
Intestine	69
Total	20,961

NOTE: Data subject to change due to future data submission or correction. Double kidney, double lung, and heart–lung transplants are counted as one transplant.

SOURCE: Based on UNOS Scientific Registry data as of April 14, 1999.

TABLE C-9 UNOS National Patient Waiting List for Organ Transplants (as of May 12, 1999)

Type of Transplant	Registrations for Transplants	Patients Waiting for Transplants
Kidney	43,734	41,833
Liver	13,181	12,987
Pancreas	453	442
Pancreas islet cell	118	118
Kidney–pancreas	1,915	1,847
Intestine	120	120
Heart	4,267	4,248
Heart–lung	248	244
Lung	3,299	3,250
Totals	67,335	63,219*

NOTE: UNOS policies allow patients to be listed with more than one transplant center (multiple listing); thus the number of registrations is greater than the actual number of patients.

*Some patients are waiting for more than one organ, therefore the total number of patients is less than the sum of patients waiting for each organ.

Methods

This material is based on evidence gathered from a MEDLINE (Ovid) search of the biomedical scientific literature from 1984 to April 1999, studies identified from reference lists in core articles obtained in the MEDLINE search, and personal communications with transplant center clinicians. Initial search inclusion criteria included randomized clinical trials, case-control studies, cross-sectional observational cohort studies, or controlled follow-up studies. Search terms included organ transplantation and oral; dentistry, dental; mouth; stomatitis; complications. Separate searches were also conducted with each type of organ transplant and the dental-related key words.

This systematic review of the literature revealed that our knowledge in this area is based primarily on case reports from individual transplant centers reporting oral complications posttransplant and indirect evidence of biological plausibility based on the potential for local and systemic infection from oral sources in immunosuppressed individuals. Numerous articles in the literature from experienced clinicians at academic research centers cite the need to provide oral health care to immunosuppressed patients and suggest protocols for their care. This review suggests that much of the relevant information is derived empirically; nevertheless, it is the standard of medical care in a large number of organ transplant centers. A well-documented adverse oral consequence related to receiving transplant therapy, gingival enlargement from the use of cyclosporine and nifedipine (and other calcium-channel blockers), is also reviewed.

Infections

A basic tenet is that all infections should be eliminated before transplantation (Fishman and Rubin, 1998). Infection is a contraindication to transplantation because the immunosuppressive therapy required postoperatively can lead to a fulminant infection. Improvements in immunosuppressive protocols have resulted in reduced graft rejection even in poorly matched donor–receptors. Unfortunately, immunosuppressive drugs also suppress host defenses against bacterial, viral, and fungal infections (Ruskin et al., 1992). Infection is a major cause of death in renal transplant patients and most often occurs in the first six months following transplant, when immunosuppressive therapy is at its peak (Naylor et al., 1988). About two-thirds of solid organ transplant recipients will experience infectious complications in the first year after transplantation. Most transplant recipients will require some level of lifelong immunosuppressive therapy, making infection a lifetime concern.

Early infections range from common cystitis in 40–50% of patients, surgical wound infection, transfusion-related infection before or during organ transplantation (especially hepatitis C transmission), dialysis-related sepsis, urinary tract infection, and aspiration pneumonia. Delayed infections most often occur due to virus (herpes simplex [HSV], cytomegalovirus [CMV], Epstein-Barr virus [EBV]), fungus (*Candida albicans*), or other opportunistic organisms (Finberg and Fingeroth, 1998; Kusne and Manez, 1997; Muzyka and Glick, 1995). Since the advent of cyclosporine therapy, opportunistic infections have become less common; yet infections with *Pneumocystis* organisms, CMV, EBV, HSV, herpes zoster, and *Cryptococcus* still occur (Fischel et al., 1991; Hanto, 1998; Schweitzer et al., 1991).

Immunosuppressed organ transplant patients are more susceptible to oral infections, especially those of fungal or viral origin. The oral cavity is also a source of gram-negative enterococcal infections (*Pseudomonas, Proteus, Klebsiella*). Oral fungal infections have been reported to occur in 6 to 42% of liver transplant patients (Colonna et al., 1988; Kusne, 1988). Candidiasis is the most frequently implicated fungal infection, although *Mucor* and *Aspergillus* have also been reported. No evidence could be found that these intraoral fungal infections spread systemically. Additionally, medications routinely taken by transplant recipients such as immunosuppressants, antifungals, antibiotics, aminoglycosides, steroids, and narcotics may mask the signs and symptoms of oral infection.

CMV and HSV commonly infect humans, with serological evidence in 40–80% of adults (Berry et al., 1988). In the vast majority of people, these infections are asymptomatic. More than 75% of organ transplant patients are seropositive for CMV (Rubin and Tolkoff-Rubin, 1988). CMV and HSV infections manifesting as nonspecific oral ulcers are frequently found in the first six months posttransplant. These ulcers may occur anywhere along the gastrointestinal tract, and prophylactic screening and preemptive treatment protocols are followed at most transplant centers. CMV is a major cause of graft rejection infections. The mouth is a frequent site of nonspecific ulcers that often harbor CMV, and CMV has also been isolated from areas of gingival hyperplasia. The diagnosis of CMV may be difficult to make in a transplant patient; therefore the patient should be examined regularly for this disease. In the mouth, a biopsy of a lesion can be immunohistochemically stained to confirm the presence of CMV (Epstein et al., 1993). HSV infections are also common in transplant recipients, and the mouth is a frequent site of ulcers. Oral lesions suggestive of infection should be evaluated by cytological examination, culture, and/or biopsy when indicated (MacPhail et al., 1995; Rees, 1998; Samaranayake et al., 1986).

Increased susceptibility to infections has implications for dental care because transient, usually asymptomatic, bacteremias occur from chewing, brushing, and a wide variety of dental manipulations, particularly those involving the mucous membranes (Haffajee and Socransky, 1994; Okabe et al., 1995; Strom et al., 1998; van der Meer et al., 1992). Certain bacteremias may cause serious complications in these already compromised patients. Life-threatening systemic infections with common oral pathogens such as *Streptococcus viridans, Lacto-*

bacillus, and *Candida albicans* have been reported (Antony et al., 1996; Reyna et al., 1982).

Longer-term posttransplant, more than 80% of patients have a good result from transplantation and are maintained on minimal long-term immunosuppressive therapy with good function. Their infectious disease problems are similar to those of the general community and are primarily respiratory (Fishman and Rubin, 1998).

Immunosuppression Therapy

Appropriate immune suppression is critical for long-term graft survival. Immunosuppressive therapy is usually provided by various combinations of glucocorticoids, azathioprine, cyclosporine, tacrolimus, monoclonal antibody OKT 3, or antilymphocyte globulin. Almost all renal transplant immunosuppressive regimens include cyclosporine or tacrolimus, and appropriate serum levels are essential to prevent graft rejection. Higher serum levels are associated with more severe adverse side effects. Serum levels can be increased unintentionally by simultaneous intake of various drugs; thus, the prescription of any drug for patients receiving immunosuppressive drugs should be preceded by medical consultation (McCauley, 1997; Naylor and Fredericks, 1996).

Cyclosporine is an excellent immunosuppressant drug that is often prescribed following organ transplantation because it selectively suppresses cell-mediated immunity. Cyclosporine appears to block the formation and release of interleukin-2 and thus prevents the amplification of the T-cell response to a foreign body. Unlike most other immunosuppressants, it does not interfere with bone marrow function. It is most often used in combination with low doses of glucocorticoids, usually prednisone, and /or azathioprine.

Complications of the drug include nephrotoxicity, renal vasculopathy, hypertension, chronic renal interstitial fibrosis (which is also common in heart transplantation), neurotoxicity, gingival overgrowth, and increased susceptibility to malignancies, including B-cell lymphoma; squamous cell carcinoma of the skin, lip, or oral mucosa; or Kaposi's sarcoma. Malignancy may be transmitted from the donor or develop de novo after transplantation (Gruber et al., 1994; Jonas et al., 1997; Lipkowitz and Madden, 1994; Sheil et al., 1993); oral malignancies have been reported within sites of cyclosporine-induced gingival overgrowth (Rees, 1998; Varga et al., 1998). Cyclosporine-induced perioral dermatitis has been described, characterized by red papules, pustules, and scaling of the chin, upper lip, and nasolabial fold (Cohen, 1994).

Oral hairy leukoplakia may occur in HIV-negative individuals taking cyclosporine, and gingival overgrowth is a well-recognized occurrence. An incidence of about 30% or more has been observed in several studies (Seymour et al., 1997). Newer immunosuppressant drugs such as tacrolimus, sirolimus, and mycophenalate mofetil are now available as cyclosporine substitutes when appropriate. These agents appear to induce fewer side effects, and no gingival over-growth has been reported to date.

Pre-Transplant Oral Considerations

Although liver, heart, lung, or pancreas transplant patients will present with their own unique and complex medical problems that may have other oral mani-festations, their oral concerns relative to the immunosuppressive and transplant therapies will be quite similar to renal transplant recipients. Pre- and posttrans-plant screening, diagnosis, treatment, counseling, and follow-up considerations are similar. This discussion of the oral manifestations of renal transplant patients and considerations for the pre- and posttransplant care of this group will serve to illustrate the available evidence for the medical necessity of providing such care across all transplantation organ groups.

Most renal transplant candidates will be in some stage of renal failure that will present unique oral problems requiring the dental provider's careful atten-tion and special considerations. An increase in salivary calculus has been de-scribed. Conversely, caries incidence is reduced, possibly from plaque inhibition related to increased levels of salivary urea (DeRossi and Glick, 1996). Uremic stomatitis appears as dry, burning, painful oral tissues covered by a gray exudate or by mucosal ulcerations. Xerostomia may be common and may be accompa-nied by parotid enlargement or parotid infection. Enamel hypoplasia and discol-oration of the teeth may be present in children along with pulpal narrowing. Candidal overgrowth may be common, and bacterial and viral infections may occur. Secondary hypoparaythyroidism may lead to bony changes, including loss of density, loose teeth, jaw enlargement, and pain. Spontaneous gingival hemorrhage, ulcerations, and petechial lesions are common (Cohen, 1994; DeR-ossi and Glick, 1996; Ferguson and Whyman, 1998; Rose and Kaye, 1990; Zic-cardi et al., 1992) as is periodontal inflammation.

One recent study found that 100% of 45 renal dialysis patients had perio-dontal disease (Naugle et al., 1998). This is not surprising, given that national adult oral health data indicating that about 85% of all adults have some form of periodontal disease, with 7–13% having more severe forms (NHANES III, 1996). In addition, recent analysis of data from the Third National Health and Nutrition Examination Survey (NHANES III) indicates that about 30% of adults in all age groups have at least one untreated carious lesion (CDC, unpublished data). Even though oral health and disease have not been documented in a sys-tematized manner in this particular patient population, there is no reason to sug-gest that this group would have better-than-average oral health. On the contrary, surveys of other medically compromised patient groups suggest that these indi-viduals suffer poor oral health (Maier et al., 1993). Additionally, diabetes was the primary diagnosis among 44% of new renal transplant recipients in 1998. Diabetic patients have been demonstrated to have a higher prevalence of more severe periodontal disease (Genco and Löe, 1993; Löe, 1993; Oliver and Tervonen, 1994).

In many transplant centers, an individual is not cleared for transplantation if oral infection exists. This may result in a potential recipient losing an opportunity if an appropriately matched organ becomes available during a period of serious dental infection and an increased wait time, causing increased risk of morbidity and mortality (Naugle et al., 1998). Cadaver kidneys must be transplanted within about 48 hours from the time they are removed from the donor. Liver, heart, and lungs are viable for only a matter of hours. However, although it has been long surmised that any active oral disease such as periodontal disease or active periapical lesions may compromise the success of a transplant, specific evidence of this fact is lacking.

What Type of Dental Services Could Be Considered Medically Necessary?

Numerous authors have asserted that the dentist should participate in treatment planning and provide necessary pretreatment for transplant patients. Also, under ideal circumstances, all potential oral foci of infection should be eliminated prior to transplant placement (Cohen, 1994; Kusne and Manez, 1997; Naylor et al., 1988; Rees 1998; Rose and Kaye, 1990). A basic tenet of transplant therapy is to prevent infection, and dental screening tests should identify likely sources of oral infection. Because many areas of oral pathology are intrabony and not readily apparent from the visual or tactile basic clinical dental examination, a radiographic survey is an important part of a pretransplant screening. A full mouth series of periapical and bitewing x-rays and a panoramic x-ray will typically provide a complete view of potential dental disease. Supplemental films can be ordered as required.

Early Detection of Dental Problems

Does early detection of potential dental problems improve the long-term outcome of the organ transplant? Does early detection improve the likelihood of a favorable outcome compared to waiting to see if a problem develops?

Direct evidence is not available to answer these questions. Indirect evidence, however, suggests that eliminating potential dental infections will prevent transplant delay for some individuals and posttransplant infections in others. Identification and treatment of severe dental problems prior to transplantation should decrease the chance of an untoward infection during the postoperative period of most intense immunosuppression. Peritransplant prophylactic antibacterial, antifungal, and antiviral strategies developed for nonoral infections are likely to control potential oral infections as well. No descriptive studies of overall dental disease status in transplant patients were found. Given the relatively high dental disease rates among U.S. adults, however, the probability of oral infections occurring in the population of transplant recipients is high.

Posttransplant Considerations

Patients remain at some level of immunosuppression for the rest of their lives and will be at higher risk of infection. Dentists need to be cognizant of this and be vigilant for signs of dental infection. A renal patient's dental problems can compromise his or her general health in more ways than just loss of function, esthetics, and comfort. However, no evidence could be found for levels of dental disease higher than in the normal population or for effects of dental disease on the potential for chronic graft rejection, the most common cause of graft failure.

About 30% of dentate renal transplant patients medicated with cyclosporine alone experience significant gingival overgrowth that requires surgical excision (Thomason et al., 1994). This figure increases to 40% when patients are medicated with both cyclosporine and nifedipine. Gingival hyperplasia may preclude one from eating and maintaining proper nutrition (Svirsky and Saravia, 1989). Several studies have shown that the development and severity of gingival overgrowth is related to the levels of oral hygiene and gingival inflammation, although these results are not always consistent (King et al., 1993; Thomason et al., 1993). The development of gingival hyperplasia is also frequent in those with pretransplant periodontitis or hyperplasia (Varga et al., 1998). Nephrotoxicity and neurotoxicity may be more severe in patients immunosuppressed with tacrolimus, although gingival enlargement has not been identified in association with this drug (Adams and Famili, 1991).

The true incidence of cyclosporine-induced gingival enlargement is difficult to determine since the drug is often used for organ transplant patients in combination with antihypertensive drugs such as the calcium channel blocking agent nifedipine, which is also associated with gingival overgrowth (Thomason et al., 1996, Wilson et al., 1998). Studies have indicated that both the incidence and the severity of gingival overgrowth are increased when patients are medicated with both cyclosporine and nifedipine (Thomason et al., 1993). Recent reports indicate that nifedipine-induced gingival overgrowth can be reversed by using alternative calcium channel blocking drugs such as amlodipine or isradipine (Jorgensen, 1997; Westbrook et al., 1997). Other calcium channel blockers, however, may induce increased plasma levels of cyclosporine, while nifedipine does not. This may explain the frequent use of nifedipine in postrenal transplant patients (Sakurai et al., 1995).

Treatment for drug-induced gingival overgrowth includes establishment of effective oral hygiene and discontinuance or reduction in dosage of the causative drug when possible. The pathogenesis of this untoward effect is uncertain, and the expression of gingival overgrowth and various periodontal and pharmacological variables remains a contentious issue. Clinical measures to prevent the occurrence of either cyclosporine- or nifedipine-induced gingival overgrowth are not reliable.

Cyclosporine-induced gingival overgrowth may affect all parts of the gingiva, but it has been suggested that the gingival changes are more pronounced in the anterior regions (Bartold, 1987; Rateitschak-Pluss et al., 1983; Wondimu et al., 1993). Surgical removal of enlarged gingiva is often necessary to facilitate patient function, oral hygiene measures, and aesthetics. It has been estimated that about 50% of individuals who develop gingival hyperplasia will require surgery.

Other Oral Lesions in Transplant Recipients

Only two studies were found that examined the prevalence of oral lesions in transplant recipients (King et al., 1994; Thomason et al., 1997). One study examined 159 renal transplant recipients and 160 matched controls. In this population, the prevalence of hairy leukoplakia (HL) and leukoplakia was 11.3 and 10.7%, respectively, compared with 0 and 5% in the controls. In HIV-infected individuals, HL is regarded as a marker for progression to AIDS (Katz et al., 1992). Hairy leukoplakia is thought to be caused by the EBV, but the clinical significance of HL in transplant patients has not been determined. In organ transplant patients, it may be regarded as an indication of severe immunosuppression. It remains to be seen whether the occurrence of HL is related to graft survival (Seymour et al., 1997). In this same study, oral candidiasis was observed in 9.4% of renal transplant recipients compared with 2.5% of controls; 3.8% of renal transplant recipients exhibited erythematous candidiasis, but this was not seen in the controls. The candidal infections and HL also have a well-established association with the immune suppression that accompanies HIV infection. In this study, the prevalence of oral lesions was 54.7% in renal transplant recipients and 19.4% in controls (King et al., 1994). Oral malignancies, particularly skin and lip cancers and Kaposi's sarcoma (Jacobs et al., 1981), have been found with higher prevalence in immunosuppressed organ transplant patients.

Summary

Fewer than 15,000 organ transplants performed in the United States in 1997 were among Medicare beneficiaries. Most of these were kidney transplant patients covered under the ESRD provision of the Social Security Act.

Currently, only a pretransplant dental screening performed on an inpatient basis is allowed under Medicare Part B. Transplant recipients are highly motivated to maintain their recovered health status and are generally compliant with pharmacotherapy and medical follow-up. In addition to routine blood tests and monitoring of immunosuppressive drug levels, recipients require immunization updates, screening for malignancy, hypertension, hyperlipidemia, and ophthalmological and dental complications. Little information is available about the consistent implementation of any of these health maintenance strategies, but dental care is desired by transplant patients and recommended by most medical authorities. In one small survey of 60 liver transplant patients, 75% sought annual dental examination (Zeldin et al., 1998). This number is slightly higher than the 62% of the U.S. population that typically seeks dental care annually. A study of 160 renal transplant recipients in London also showed slightly more transplant patients visiting a dentist annually than a matched control group (57.9% to 51.3%); 45.6% visited a hospital dental facility versus 7% of controls (King and Thornhill, 1996).

The major question is whether dental care provided pre- and/or posttransplant improves the outcome of medical transplant care. No controlled clinical studies have examined morbidity and mortality in transplant recipients relative to the provision of oral health care pre- or posttransplant. Nor have there been studies that demonstrate improved quality of life or less frequent complications. Anecdotal and some case reports indicate that oral infections can delay transplantation or severely complicate the postoperative course. Although most oral medicine textbooks and reviews advise that restoration to good oral health is a prerequisite for any patient who is immunosuppressed or about to undergo immunosuppressive therapy such as organ transplantation, this advice is primarily a result of tradition and collective medical experience rather than rigorous study. In addition, this broad category of patients represents a tremendous diversity of medical complication. It is difficult even within one organ category to standardize what a "typical" patient would be and to limit necessary care to only a particular segment of that population. There is great variation in the characteristics of patients, coexisting conditions, and other such factors. Given the enormous number of procedures and the individual circumstances of patients, limiting insurance coverage to a host of separately validated and specifically described procedures is impractical.

There are two cardinal therapeutic rules to be followed by clinicians in dealing with infections in transplant patients: (1) prevention is better than treatment; and (2) when treatment is required, the major determinant of the success of therapy is the rapidity with which the diagnosis is made and effective therapy is initiated. Oral disease is present and is a potential source of active infection in these medically compromised individuals. Although limited studies have been conducted on the oral health status of these individuals, some do suggest a high rate of periodontal infection and dental decay.

Dental management is complicated because of the oral disease and medical problems seen in this population. These patients survive under narrowly controlled conditions of intake and activity as well as under great physiological and psychological stress, with medications, diet, intensive treatments, limited lifestyle, and dependence on others. Dental treatment, even minor procedures, can present major problems for the clinician. Because of transplant patients' immunosuppressed condition, additional precautions are often necessary, including hospitalization, which can add significantly to the costs of care. Most medically controlled renal failure and transplant patients, however, can be safely and adequately treated in the private dental office.

The importance of pretransplantation workup and continued follow-up posttransplantation to eliminate any oral source of infection is emphasized. Hyperplasia from cyclosporine and/or nifedipine can be minimized with excellent oral hygiene. Persistent candidiasis and opportunistic infections also occur in patients that are immunosuppressed. Marked advances in immunosuppressive therapies, improved medical and surgical techniques, increased numbers of candidate patients, particularly in the pediatric population, and greater insurance recognition will mean that dentists will have an increasingly greater role in the management of organ transplant patients.

Although direct evidence of benefit from clinical trials is not available, this has been a neglected area of clinical research, and practices have been governed by experience. Dental examination and elimination of sources of oral infection appear to be the de facto standard of care at most transplant centers, and extending Medicare coverage to these individuals would be consistent with the current standard.

CONDITION 5: HEART VALVE REPAIR OR REPLACEMENT

Introduction

Valvular heart disease refers to one of several abnormalities of heart valve thickness and movement responsible for stenosis (pathological narrowing of the orifice of the valve) and regurgitation (backward flow of blood through the valve). Abnormalities may include mitral or aortic valve stenosis or regurgitation, tricuspid and pulmonary valve diseases, and congenital abnormalities. Treatment of valvular heart disease may involve medications or surgical repair or replacement. Surgical repair or replacement of a heart valve increases a person's likelihood of endocarditis, an inflammation of the endocardium. Endocarditis may be acute (usually caused by pyogenic organisms such as hemolytic streptococci or staphylococci) or subacute (usually caused by *Streptococcus viridans* or *S. faecalis*). Surgical repair or replacement with a prosthetic heart valve creates opportunities for bacteria to adhere to the valve and/or endocardium. The bacteria form vegetations that may enter the bloodstream and spread the infection to other parts of the body. Treatment of such infections requires long-term antibiotic therapy (four to six weeks) and may require valve replacement. Oral flora, particularly streptococcus, are implicated in approximately 40 percent of infective endocarditis cases (Roberts, 1999; Strom et al, 1998; van der Meer et al, 1992).

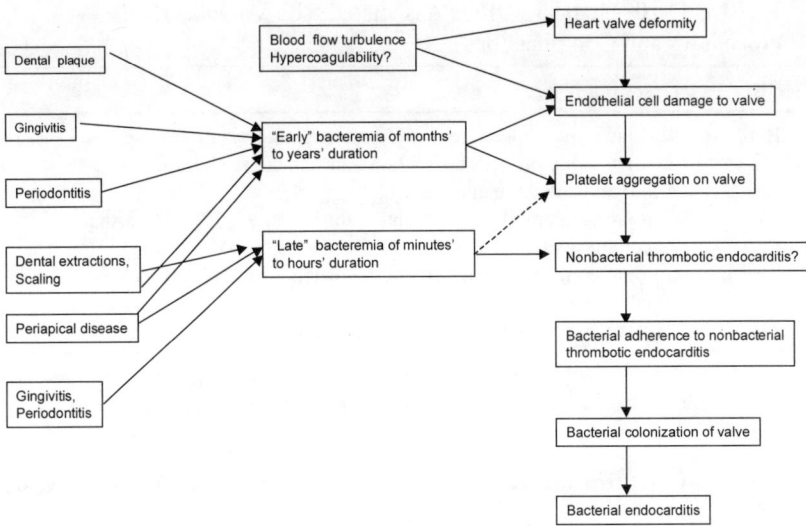

FIGURE C-7 Proposed causal model of dental-associated endocarditis. SOURCE: Drangsholt, 1998.

This review focuses specifically on medically necessary oral health care that is provided prior to surgical repair or replacement. Antibiotic prophylaxis prior to dental care for at-risk persons—with either valvular heart disease or a prosthetic heart valve—is not considered here.

One suggested model for the association between oral diseases and endocarditis is shown in Figure C-7 (Drangsholt, 1998). Dental plaque (accumulation of mainly oral microorganisms and their products that adheres to the teeth), gingivitis (inflammation of the gingiva as a response to bacterial plaque), periodontitis (inflammation of the periodontium or the supporting structures of the teeth), and certain dental procedures, such as scaling and root planing and dental extractions, may result in early bacteremias of months or years duration. In the presence of heart valve deformity or endothelial cell damage to the valve, platelets may adhere to the valve and result in nonbacterial thrombotic endocarditis (NBTE). Bacteria may adhere to the NBTE, colonize, and result in acute or subacute endocarditis, depending on the organism. Gingivitis, periodontitis, certain dental procedures, and periapical diseases (infections around the apex of the root of a tooth) may result in late bacteremias of minutes to hours duration and follow a similar cascade of events.

TABLE C-10 Medicare DRGs Associated with Valvular Heart
Procedures and Complications

DRG	Description
104	Cardiac valve procedures with cardiac catheterization
105	Cardiac valve procedures without cardiac catheterization
126	Acute and subacute endocarditis
135	Cardiac congenital and valvular disorders age > 17 with cardiac catheterization
136	Cardiac congenital and valvular disorders age > 17 without cardiac catheterization
137	Cardiac congenital and valvular disorders age 0–17

SOURCE: Health Care Financing Administration, Medicare Provider Analysis and
Review file: www.hcfa.gov/stats/medpar.htm (last updated December 15, 1998).

Medicare Utilization and Reimbursement of Valvular Heart Disease

Estimates of the number of discharges and Medicare reimbursements for
valvular heart diseases were obtained from the Health Care Financing Administration Medicare Provider Analysis and Review (MEDPAR) file (http://www.
hcfa.gov/stats/medpar.htm). Six diagnosis-related groups (DRGs) were included
and are shown in Table C-10.

The number of discharges for valvular heart diseases among Medicare beneficiaries is increasing. Between 1990 and 1995, the number of discharges increased from about 42,700 to 58,800 (Figure C-8). Of these, acute and subacute
endocarditis accounted for about 3,900 in 1990 and 4,950 in 1995.

Total inpatient days for valvular heart procedures between 1990 and 1995 are
shown in Figure C-9. For all DRGs, the total number of inpatient days declined
over the six-year period. Acute and subacute endocarditis declined from about
14% of inpatient days to about 10% of inpatient days during the period.

Medicare reimbursement for valvular heart disease procedures increased
over the six-year period (Figure C-10). In 1990, Medicare reimbursed about
$1.05 billion for these six DRGs. By 1995, this amount had increased to about
$1.61 billion. Reimbursements for acute and subacute endocarditis represented
between 4 and 5% of the total reimbursement.

Methods

This review is based on a literature search of the MEDLINE database from
1980 through March 1999. Search terms included dentistry, dental care, endocarditis, and heart valve diseases. Studies identified as a randomized clinical
trial, a case-control study, a cross-sectional observational cohort study, or a
controlled follow-up study were included in the review. Case reports and smaller

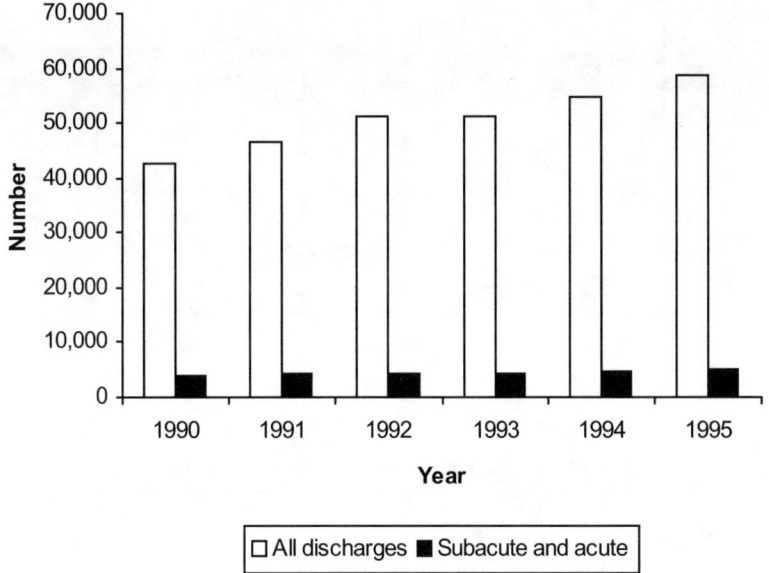

FIGURE C-8 Number of Medicare discharges for valvular heart repair or replacement, 1990–1995. SOURCE: Health Care Financing Administration, Medicare Provider Analysis and Review file: www.hcfa.gov/stats/medpar.htm (last updated December 15, 1998).

case series (less than 50 cases) were excluded from further review. Only studies involving patients over 18 years of age were accepted. Studies reporting on the risk of bacterial endocarditis associated with dental care and the need for antibiotic premedication were excluded.

Only studies that assessed risk reduction associated with elimination of dental disease and potential oral sources of infection were included, since this analysis focuses on dental disease, rather than its treatment, as a risk factor for endocarditis.

Results

No studies were identified that met the inclusion criteria addressing the efficacy or effectiveness of medically necessary oral health care in reducing pre-, peri-, or postoperative valvular repair or replacement complications.

One study (Terezhalmy et al., 1998) reported the findings of a comprehensive clinical and radiographic regional examination on 156 consecutive patients with valvular heart disease requiring mechanical or bioprosthetic valve implan-tation in 1993 at the Cleveland Clinic Foundation. These patients were referred by the Department of Thoracic and Cardiovascular Surgery to the Section on Oral Medicine, Department of Dentistry. About 38% were women, and the mean age was 62.8 years (median 66 years, range 26 to 87 years).

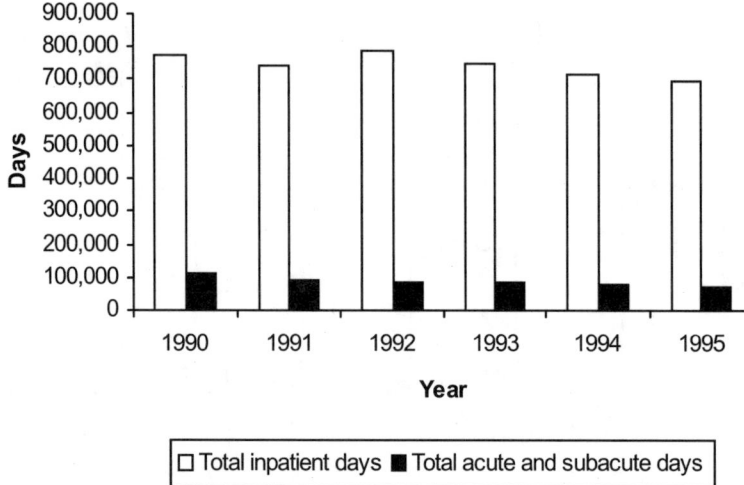

FIGURE C-9 Total inpatient days for all admissions, and acute and subacute days, among Medicare beneficiaries, 1990–1995. SOURCE: Health Care Financing Administration, Medicare Provider Analysis and Review file: www.hcfa.gov/stats/medpar.htm (last updated December 15, 1998).

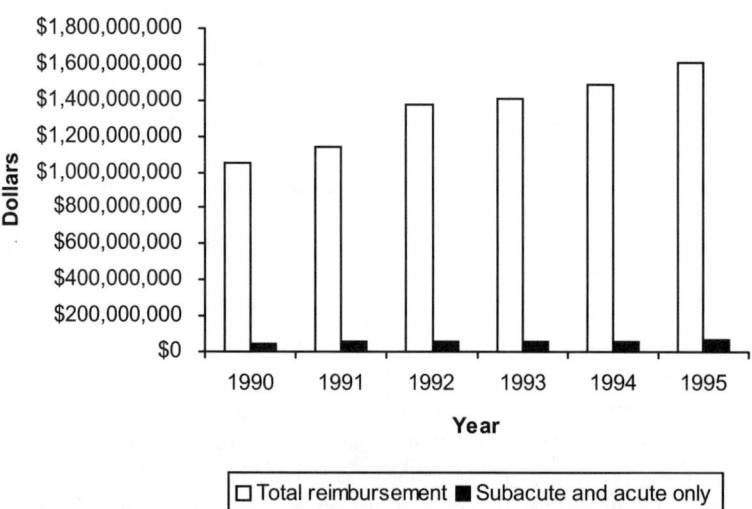

FIGURE C-10 Medicare reimbursement for valvular heart disease. SOURCE: Health Care Financing Administration, Medicare Provider Analysis and Review file: www.hcfa. gov/stats/medpar.htm (last updated December 15, 1998).

TABLE C-11 Selected Clinical and Radiographic Findings Among 156
Patients Undergoing Mechanical or Bioprosthetic Valve Implantation, 1993

Clinical Variable	No. or %
Mean number of teeth	19.3
Mean number of decayed teeth	1.1
Mean number of decayed tooth surfaces	2.5
Percentage of patients with at least one periapical abscess associated with a decayed or restored tooth	15.4%
Percentage of patients with evidence of past root canal treatment	30.8%
Percentage distribution of patients by level of periodontal disease	
Type I: Gingivitis	4.5%
Inflammation of the gingiva characterized clinically by changes in color, gingival form, position, surface appearance, and presence of bleeding and/or exudate)	
Type II: Early periodontitis	50.0%
Progression of the gingival inflammation into the deeper periodontal structures and alveolar bone crest, with slight bone loss. The usual periodontal probing depth is 3–4 mm with slight loss of connective tissue attachment and slight loss of alveolar bone	
Type III: Moderate periodontitis	26.9%
A more advanced stage of the above condition, with increased destruction of periodontal structures with noticeable loss of bone support possibly accompanied by an increase in tooth mobility. There may be furcation involvement in multirooted teeth	
Type IV: Advanced periodontitis	16.7%
Further progression of periodontitis with major loss of alveolar bone support usually accompanied by increased tooth mobility. Furcation involvement in multirooted teeth is likely	

Selected oral health findings from this study are shown in Table C-11. No comparison group was identified, so one cannot determine whether the disease burden in this group is higher than in other groups. The extent of medically necessary oral health care provided to these patients prior to surgery and subsequent outcomes were not reported.

ACKNOWLEDGMENTS

In response to questions raised at the Committee's public workshop on Medically Necessary Dental Care (May 19–20, 1999, see also Appendix A), Dr. James Lipton and Dr. Jane Atkinson of the National Institute for Dental and Craniofacial Research contacted a group of experts throughout the country to get information about the accepted dental procedures and associated costs for patients with lymphoma, leukemia, and head and neck cancer. The responses were very helpful in developing this background information and the Medicare cost estimates. In addition to Drs. Lipton and Atkinson, the assistance of the following individuals is gratefully acknowledged: Mark Schubert, D.D.S., M.S.D., Fred Hutchinson Cancer Research Center and University of Washington School of Dentistry; Douglas E. Peterson, D.M.D., Ph.D., School of Dental Medicine, University of Connecticut Health Center; Peter B. Lockhart, D.D.S., Department of Oral Medicine, Carolinas Medical Center; J. B. Epstein, D.M.D., M.S.D, Department of Dentistry, British Columbia Cancer Agency; Stephen Sonis, D.M.D., D.M.S., Brigham and Women's Hospital and Department of Oral Medicine and Diagnostic Sciences, Harvard School of Dental Medicine; Sook-Bin Woo, D.M.D., D.M.S., Division of Dentistry, Brigham and Women's Hospital; Spencer Redding, D.D.S., University of Texas Health Sciences, San Antonio; Bruce Barker, D.D.S., Department of Oral Pathology, University of Missouri Kansas City; Gerry Barker, R.D.H., M.Sc., Dental Oncology Support Services, Univiversity of Missouri Kansas City.

REFERENCES

Overview

Bloom B, Gift HC, Jack SS. *Dental Services and Oral Health: United States 1989.* National Center for Health Statistics. Vital Health Statistics 1992; 10(183).

Consensus Conference on Medically Necessary Oral Health Care. Final Recommendations. National Alliance for Oral Health. *Special Care in Dentistry* 1995; 15(5):201–202.

Eddy DM, Hasselblad V, Shachter R. *Meta-Analysis by the Confidence Profile Method: The Statistical Synthesis of Evidence.* San Diego: Academic Press, 1992.

Fleming TR, DeMets DL. Surrogate end points in clinical trials: Are we being misled? *Annals of Internal Medicine* 1996; 125:605–613.

Marcus SE, Drury TF, Brown LJ, Zion GR. Tooth retention and tooth loss in the permanent dentition of adults: United States, 1988–1991. *Journal of Dental Research* 1996; 75(Special Issue):684–695.

Morbidity and Mortality Weekly Report (MMWR). Total tooth loss among persons aged greater than or equal to 65 years—selected states, 1995–1997. *MMWR* 1999; 48(10):206–210.

National Center for Health Statistics (NCHS). Vital and Health Statistics. Series 11, Number 27. *Loss of Teeth in Adults, United States—1960–1962.* DHEW Publication Number (HRA) 74–1280. August 1973.

National Center for Health Statistics (NCHS). Vital and Health Statistics. Series 11, Number 223. *Decayed, Missing, and Filled Teeth Among Persons 1–74 Years, United States.* DHHS Publication Number (PHS) 81–1673. August 1981.

National Institute for Dental Research (NIDR). *The National Survey of Oral Health in U.S. Employed Adults and Seniors: 1985–86.* NIH Publication Number 87-2868. Bethesda, MD. August 1987.

Head and Neck Cancer

Al-Joburi W, Clark DC, Fisher R. A comparison of the effectiveness of two systems for the prevention of radiation caries. *Clinical Preventive Dentistry* 1991; 13:15–19.

Allison PJ, Locker D, Feine JS. The relationship between dental status and health-related quality of life in upper aerodigestive tract cancer patients. *Oral Oncology* 1999; 35:138–143.

Bedwinek JM, Shukovsky LJ, Fletcher GH, Daley TE. Osteoradionecrosis in patients treated with definitive radiotherapy for squamous cell carcinomas of the oral cavity and naso- and oropharynx. *Radiology* 1976; 119:665–667.

Beumer III J, Silverman Jr S, Benak SB. Hard and soft tissue necroses following radiation therapy for oral cancer. *Journal of Prosthetic Dentistry* 1972; 27:640–644.

Beumer III J, Curtis T, Harrison RE. Radiation therapy of the oral cavity: Sequelae and management, part 1. *Head and Neck Surgery* 1979a; 1:301–312.

Beumer III J, Curtis T, Harrison RE. Radiation therapy of the oral cavity: Sequelae and management, part 2. *Head and Neck Surgery* 1979b; 1:392–408.

Beumer J, Harrison R, Sanders B, Kurrasch M. Osteoradionecrosis: Predisposing factors and outcomes of therapy. *Head and Neck Surgery* 1984; 6:819–827.

Brown RS, Miller JH, Bottonley WK. A retrospective oral/dental evaluation of 92 head and neck oncology patients, before, during and after irradiation therapy. *Gerodontology* 1990; 9:35–39.

Bruins HH, Koole R, Jolly DE. Pretherapy dental decisions in patients with head and neck cancer. A proposed model for dental decision support. *Oral Surgery, Oral Medicine, Oral Pathology, Oral Radiology and Endodontics* 1998; 86:256–267.

Bundgaard T, Tandrup O, Elbrond O. A functional evaluation of patients treated for oral cancer. A prospective study. *International Journal of Oral and Maxillofacial Surgery* 1993; 22:28–34.

Clayman L. Management of dental extractions in irradiated jaws: A protocol without hyperbaric oxygen therapy. *Journal of Oral and Maxillofacial Surgery* 1997; 55:275–281.

Coffin F. The incidence and management of osteoradionecrosis of the jaws following head and neck radiotherapy. *British Journal of Radiology* 1983; 56:851–857.

Curi MM, Dib LL. Osteoradionecrosis of the jaws: A retrospective study of the background factors and treatment in 104 cases. *Journal of Oral and Maxillofacial Surgery* 1997; 55:540–544.

De Graeff A, de Leeuw JRJ, Ros WJG, Hordijk GJ, Blijham GH, Winnubst JAM. A prospective study on quality of life of patients with cancer of the oral cavity or oropharynx treated with surgery with or without radiotherapy. *Oral Oncology* 1999; 35:27–32.

Dreizen S. Description and incidence of oral complications. U.S. Department of Health and Human Services, Public Health Service, National Institutes of Health. Consensus Development Conference on Oral Complications of Cancer Therapies: Diagnosis, Prevention, and Treatment. *National Cancer Institute Monographs* 1990; 9:11–15.

Dreizen S, Brown LR, Daly TE, Drane JB. Prevention of xerostomia-induced dental caries in irradiated cancer patients. *Journal of Dental Research* 1977; 56:99–104.

Epstein JB, Emerton S, Kolbinson DA, Le ND, Phillips N, Stevenson-Moore P, Osoba D. Quality of life and oral function following radiotherapy for head and neck cancer. *Head and Neck* 1999; 21:1–11.

Epstein JB, van der Meij EH, Emerton SM, Le ND, Stevenson-Moore P. Compliance with fluoride gel use in irradiated patients. *Special Care in Dentistry* 1995; 15:218–222.

Epstein JB, van der Meij EH, Lunn R, Stevenson-Moore P. Effects of compliance with fluoride gel application on caries and caries risk in patients after radiation therapy for head and neck cancer. *Oral Surgery, Oral Medicine, Oral Pathology, Oral Radiology and Endodontics* 1996; 82:268–275.

Epstein JB, van der Meij EH, McKenzie M, Wong F, Lepawsky M, Stevenson-Moore P. Postradiation osteonecrosis of the mandible. A long-term follow-up study. *Oral Surgery, Oral Medicine, Oral Pathology, Oral Radiology and Endodontics* 1997; 83:657–662.

Epstein JB, Wong FLW, Stevenson-Moore P. Osteoradionecrosis: Clinical experience and a proposal for classification. *Journal of Oral and Maxillofacial Surgery* 1987; 45:104–110.

Funegard U, Franzen L, Ericson T, Henriksson R. Parotid saliva composition during and after irradiation of head and neck cancer. *Oral Oncology, European Journal of Cancer* 1994; 30B:230–233.

Grant BP, Fletcher GH. Analysis of complications following megavoltage therapy for squamous cell carcinomas of the tonsillar area. *American Journal of Roentgenology* 1966; 96:28–36.

Health Care Financing Administration (HCFA). *Medicare Carrier's Manual, Part B.* Coverage and Limitations, Section 2136: Dental Services.

Horiot JC, Bone MC, Ibrahim E, Castro JR. Systemic dental management in head and neck irradiation. *International Journal of Radiation Oncology, Biology and Physics* 1981; 7:1025–1029.

Horiot JC, Schraub S, Bone MC, Bain Y, Ramadier J, Chaplain G, Nabid N, Thevenot B, Bransfield D. Dental preservation in patients irradiated for head and neck tumors: A 10-year experience with topical fluoride and a randomized trial between two fluoridation methods. *Radiotherapy and Oncology* 1983; 1:77–82.

Jansma J, Vissink A, Spijkervet FK, Roodenburg JL, Panders AK, Vermey A, Szabo BG, Gravenmade EJ. Protocol for the prevention and treatment of oral sequelae resulting from head and neck radiation therapy. *Cancer* 1992; 70:2172–2180.

Keys HM, McCasland JP. Techniques and results of a comprehensive dental care program in head and neck cancer patients. *International Journal of Radiation Oncology, Biology and Physics* 1976; 1:859–865.

Kluth EV, Jain PR, Stuchell RN, Frich JC Jr. A study of factors contributing to the development of osteoradionecrosis of the jaws. *Journal of Prosthetic Dentistry* 1988; 59:194–201.

Kumar HS, Bihani V, Kumar V, Chaundhary RK, Kumar L, Punia DP. Osteoradionecrosis of mandible in patients treated with definitive radiotherapy for carcinomas of oral cavity and oropharynx. A retrospective study. *Indian Journal of Dental Research* 1992; 3:47–50.

Lambert PM, Intriere N, Eichstaedt R. Management of dental extractions in irradiated jaws: A protocol with hyperbaric oxygen therapy. *Journal of Oral and Maxillofacial Surgery* 1997; 55:268–274.

Landis SH, Murray T, Bolden S, Wingo PA. Cancer statistics, 1999. *CA—A Cancer Journal for Clinicians* 1999; 49:8–31.

Liu RP, Fleming TJ, Toth BB, Keene HJ. Salivary flow rates in patients with head and neck cancer 0.5 to 25 years after radiotherapy. *Oral Surgery, Oral Medicine and Oral Pathology* 1990; 70:724–729.

Lockhart PB, Clark J. Pretherapy dental status of patients with malignant conditions of the head and neck. *Oral Surgery, Oral Medicine and Oral Pathology* 1994; 77:236–241.

Maier H, Zoller J, Herrmann A, Kreiss M, Heller W-D. Dental status and oral hygiene in patients with head and neck cancer. *Otolaryngology, Head and Neck Surgery* 1993; 108:655–661.

Makkonen TA, Kiminki A, Makkonen TK, Nordman E. Dental extractions in relation to radiation therapy of 224 patients. *International Journal of Oral and Maxillofacial Surgery* 1987; 16:56–64.

Manciani RD, Ownby HE. Osteoradionecrosis of the jaws. *Journal of Oral and Maxillofacial Surgery*. 1986; 44:218–223.

Manciani RD, Plezia RA. Osteoradionecrosis of the mandible. *Journal of Oral Surgery* 1974; 32:435–440.

Markitziu A, Zafiropoulos G, Tsalikis L, Cohen L. Gingival health and salivary function in head and neck-irradiated patients. A five-year follow-up. *Oral Surgery, Oral Medicine and Oral Pathology* 1992; 73:427–433.

Marx RE, Johnson RP, Kline SN. Prevention of osteoradionecrosis: A randomized prospective clinical trial of hyperbaric oxygen versus penicillin. *Journal of the American Dental Association* 1985; 111:49–54.

Maxymiw WG, Wood RE, Liu F-F. Postradiation dental extractions without hyperbaric oxygen. *Oral Surgery, Oral Medicine and Oral Pathology* 1991; 72:270–274.

Murray CG, Herson J, Daly TE, Zimmerman S. Radiation necrosis of the mandible: A 10-year study. Part I. Factors influencing the onset of necrosis. *International Journal of Radiation Oncology, Biology and Physics* 1980a; 6:543–548.

Murray CG, Herson J, Daly TE, Zimmerman S. Radiation necrosis of the mandible: A 10-year study. Part II. Dental factors; onset, duration and management of necrosis. *International Journal of Radiation Oncology, Biology and Physics* 1980b; 6:549–553.

Myers RAM, Marx RE. Use of hyperbaric oxygen in postradiation head and neck surgery. U.S. Department of Health and Human Services, Public Health Service, National Institutes of Health. Consensus Development Conference on Oral Complications of Cancer Therapies: Diagnosis, Prevention, and Treatment. *National Cancer Institute Monographs* 1990; 9:151–157.

National Institutes of Health (NIH). National Institutes of Health Consensus Development Conference Statement: Oral complications of cancer therapies: Diagnosis, prevention, and treatment. *Journal of the American Dental Association* 1989; 119:179–183.

Niewald M, Barbie O, Schnabel K, Engel M, Schedler M, Nieder C, Berberich W. Risk factors and dose–effect relationship for osteoradionecrosis after hyperfractionated

278 EXTENDING MEDICARE COVERAGE

and conventionally fractionated radiotherapy for oral cancer. *British Journal of Radiology* 1996; 69:847–851.

Pochanugool L, Manomaiudom W, Im-Erbsin T, Suwannuraks M, Kraiphibul P. Dental management in irradiated head and neck cancers. *Journal of the Medical Association of Thailand* 1994; 77:261–265.

Rahn AO, Drone JB. Dental aspects of the problems, care, and treatment of the irradiated oral cancer patient. *Journal of the American Dental Association* 1967; 74:957–966.

Rankow RM, Weissman B. Osteoradionecrosis of the mandible. *Annals of Otology* 1971; 80:603–611.

Ries LAG, Kosary CL, Hankey BF, Miller BA, Edwards BK (eds). *SEER Cancer Statistics Review, 1973–1996.* Bethesda, MD: National Cancer Institute, 1999.

Roos DE, Dische S, Saunders MI. The dental problems of patients with head and neck cancer treated with CHART. *Oral Oncology, European Journal of Cancer* 1996; 32B:176–181.

Schweiger JW. Oral complications following radiation therapy: A five-year retrospective report. *Journal of Prosthetic Dentistry* 1987; 58:78–82.

Shah JP, Karnell LH, Hoffman HT, Ariyan S, Brown GS, Fee WE, Glass AG, Goepfert H, Ossoff RH, Fremgen A. Patterns of care for cancer of the larynx in the United States. *Archives of Otolaryngology— Head & Neck Surgery* 1997; 123:475–483.

Shaha AR, Strong EW. Cancer of the head and neck. Pp. 355–377 in Murphy GP, Lawrence W Jr, Lenhard RE Jr. (eds). *American Cancer Society Textbook of Clinical Oncology*, 2nd ed. Atlanta: American Cancer Society, 1995.

Sonis ST, Woods PD, White BA. Pretreatment oral assessment. U.S. Department of Health and Human Services, Public Health Service, National Institutes of Health. Consensus Development Conference on Oral Complications of Cancer Therapies: Diagnosis, Prevention, and Treatment. *National Cancer Institute Monographs* 1990; 9:29–32.

Spaulding MB, Fischer SG, Wolf GT. Tumor response, toxicity, and survival after neoadjuvant organ-preserving chemotherapy for advanced laryngeal carcinoma. The Department of Veterans Affairs Cooperative Laryngeal Cancer Study Group. *Journal of Clinical Oncology* 1994; 12:1592–1599.

Surveillance, Epidemiology, and End Results (SEER) Program Public Use CD-ROM (1973–93). Washington, D.C.: National Cancer Institute, DCPC, Surveillance Program, Cancer Statistics Branch. 1993.

Teichgraeber J, Bowman J, Goepfert H. New test series for the functional evaluation of oral cavity cancer. *Head and Neck Surgery* 1985; 8:9–20.

Toljanic JA, Ali M, Haraf DJ, Vokes EE, Moran WJ, Graham L. Osteoradionecrosis of the jaws as a risk factor in radiotherapy: A report of an eight-year retrospective review. *Oncology Reports* 1998; 5:345–349.

U.S. Department of Health and Human Services, Public Health Service. *Healthy People 2000: National Health Promotion and Disease Prevention Objectives.* Washington, DC, 1991.

Valdez IH, Atkinson JC, Ship JA, Fox PC. Major salivary gland function in patients with radiation-induced xerostomia: Flow rates and sialochemistry. *International Journal of Radiation Oncology, Biology and Physics* 1992; 25:41–47.

Van Merkesteyn JPR, Bakker DJ, Porgmeijer-Hoelen AMMJ. Hyperbaric oxygen treatment of osteoradionecrosis of the mandible. Experience in 29 patients. *Oral Surgery, Oral Medicine, Oral Pathology, Oral Radiology and Endodontics* 1995; 80:12–16.

Wang CC. Management and prognosis of squamous-cell carcinoma of the tonsillar region. *Radiology* 1972; 104:667–671.

Widmark G, Sagne S, Heikel P. Osteoradionecrosis of the jaws. *International Journal of Oral and Maxillofacial Surgery* 1989; 18:302–306.

Wright WE. Pretreatment oral health care interventions for radiation patients. U.S. Department of Health and Human Services, Public Health Service, National Institutes of Health. Consensus Development Conference on Oral Complications of Cancer Therapies: Diagnosis, Prevention, and Treatment. *National Cancer Institute Monographs* 1990; 9:57–59.

Leukemia and Lymphoma

Ahmed T, Engelking C, Szalyga J, Helson L, Coombe N, Cook P, Corbi D, Puccio C, Chun H, Mittelman A. Propantheline prevention of mucositis from etoposide. *Bone Marrow Transplant* 1993; 12:131–132.

American Cancer Society (ACS). *Cancer Facts and Figures—1999: Selected Cancers.* Atlanta: ACS, 1999.

Anderson PM, Ramsay NK, Shu XO, Rydholm N, Rogosheske J, Nicklow R, Weisdorf DJ, Skubitz KM. Effect of low-dose oral glutamine on painful stomatitis during bone marrow transplantation. *Bone Marrow Transplant* 1998; 22:339–344.

Barasch A, Peterson DE, Tanzer JM, D'Ambrosio JA, Nuki K, Schubert MM, Franquin JC, Clive J, Tutschka P. Helium–neon laser effects on conditioning-induced oral mucositis in bone marrow transplantation patients. *Cancer* 1995; 76:2550–2556.

Bergmann OJ. Oral infections and septicemia in immunocompromised patients with hematologic malignancies. *Journal of Clinical Microbiology* 1988; 26:2105–2109.

Bergmann OJ. Oral infections and fever in immunocompromised patients with haematologic malignancies. *European Journal of Clinical Microbiology and Infectious Diseases* 1989; 8:207–213.

Bergmann OJ, Ellermann-Eriksen S, Mogensen SC, Ellegaard J. Acyclovir given as prophylaxis against oral ulcers in acute myeloid leukaemia: Randomised, double blind, placebo controlled trial. *British Medical Journal* 1995; 310:1169–1172.

Borowski B, Benhamou E, Pico JL, Laplanche A, Margainaud JP, Hayat M. Prevention of oral mucositis in patients treated with high-dose chemotherapy and bone marrow transplantation: A randomised controlled trial comparing two protocols of dental care. *European Journal of Cancer: B Oral Oncology* 1994; 30B:93–97.

Coda BA, O'Sullivan B, Donaldson G, Bohl S, Chapman CR, Shen DD. Comparative efficacy of patient-controlled administration of morphine, hydromorphone, or sufentanil for the treatment of oral mucositis pain following bone marrow transplantation. *Pain* 1997; 72:333–346.

Cohen G, Elad S, Or R; Galili D, Garfunkel AA. The use of tretinoin as oral mucositis prophylaxis in bone marrow transplantation patients: A preliminary study. *Oral Diseases* 1997; 3:243–246.

Cowen D, Tardieu C, Schubert M, Peterson D, Resbeut M, Faucher C, Franquin JC. Low energy helium–neon laser in the prevention of oral mucositis in patients undergoing bone marrow transplant: Results of a double blind randomized trial. *International Journal of Radiation Oncology, Biology, and Physics* 1997; 38:697–703.

Dreizen S, McCredie KB, Bodey GP, Keating MJ. Quantitative analysis of the oral complications of antileukemia chemotherapy. *Oral Surgery, Oral Medicine, Oral Pathology* 1986; 62:650–653.

Epstein JB, Vickars L, Spinelli J, Reece D. Efficacy of chlorhexidine and nystatin rinses in prevention of oral complications in leukemia and bone marrow transplantation. *Oral Surgery, Oral Medicine, Oral Pathology* 1992; 73:682–689.

Epstein JR. Infection prevention in bone marrow transplantation and radiation patients. *NCI Monographs* 1990; 9:73–85.

Ferretti GA, Ash RC, Brown AT, Parr MD, Romond EH, Lillich TT. Control of oral mucositis and candidiasis in marrow transplantation: A prospective, double-blind trial of chlorhexidine digluconate oral rinse. *Bone Marrow Transplant* 1988; 3:483–493.

Greenberg MS, Cohen SG, McKitrick JC, Cassileth PA. The oral flora as a source of septicemia in patients with acute leukemia. *Oral Surgery* 1982; 53:32–36.

Heimdahl A, Mattsson T, Dahllof G, Lonnquist B, Ringden O. The oral cavity as a port of entry for early infections in patients treated with bone marrow transplantation. *Oral Surgery, Oral Medicine, Oral Pathology* 1989; 68:711–716.

Hill HF, Chapman CR, Kornell JA, Sullivan KM, Saeger LC, Benedetti C. Self-administration of morphine in bone marrow transplant patients reduces drug requirement. *Pain* 1990; 40:121–129.

Karthaus M, Rosenthal C, Huebner G, Paul H, Elser C, Hertenstein B, Krauter J, Scharmann T, Geissler RG, Heil G, Ganser A. Effect of topical oral G-CSF on oral mucositis: A randomised placebo-controlled trial. *Bone Marrow Transplant* 1998; 22:781–785.

Labar B, Mrsic M, Pavletic Z, Bogdanic V, Nemet D, Aurer I, Radman I, Filipovic-Grcic N, Sertic D, Kalenic S, et al. Prostaglandin E2 for prophylaxis of oral mucositis following BMT. *Bone Marrow Transplant* 1993; 11:379–382.

Laine P, Meurman JH, Murtomaa H, Lindqvist C, Torkko H, Pyrhonen S, Teerenhovi L. One-year trial of the effect of rinsing with an amine fluoride–stannous fluoride-containing mouthwash on gingival index scores and salivary microbial counts in lymphoma patients receiving cytostatic drugs. *Journal of Clinical Periodontology* 1993; 20:628–634.

Lockhart PB, Schmidke MA. Antibiotic considerations in medically compromised patients. *Dental Clinics of North America* 1994; 38:381–402.

Lopez I, Goudou C, Ribrag V, Sauvage C, Hazebroucq G, Dreyfus F. Treatment of mucositis with vitamin E during administration of neutropenic antineoplastic agents. *Annales de Medecine Interne (Paris)* 1994; 145:405–408.

Meurman JH, Laine P, Murtomaa H, Lindqvist C, Torkko H, Teerenhovi L, Pyrhonen S. Effect of antiseptic mouthwashes on some clinical and microbiological findings in the mouths of lymphoma patients receiving cytostatic drugs. *Journal of Clinical Periodontology* 1991; 18:587–591.

Meurman JH, Pyrhonen S, Teerenhove L, Lindquist C. Oral sources of septicemia in patients with malignancies. *Oral Oncology* 1997; 33:389–397.

Overholser CD, Peterson DE, Williams LT, Schimpff SC. Periodontal infection in patients with acute nonlymphocytic leukemia. Prevalence of exacerbations. *Archives of Internal Medicine* 1982; 142:551–554.

Peterson DE. Pretreatment strategies for infection prevention in chemotherapy patients. *NCI Monographs* 1990; 9:61–71.

Pillitteri LC, Clark RE. Comparison of a patient-controlled analgesia system with continuous infusion for administration of diamorphine for mucositis. *Bone Marrow Transplant* 1998; 22:495–498.

Richard P, Amador Del Valle G, Moreau P, Milpied N, Felice MP, Daeschler T, Harousseau JL, Richet H. *Viridans* streptococcal bacteraemia in patients with neutropenia. *Lancet* 1995; 345:1607–1609.

Ries LAG, Kosary Cl, Hankey BF, Miller BA, Edwards BK (eds). *SEER Cancer Statistics Review, 1973–1996.* Bethesda, MD: National Cancer Institute, 1999.

Sonis ST, Fazio RC, Fang L (eds). *Principles and Practice of Oral Medicine,* 2nd ed. Philadelphia: WB Saunders, 1995.

Syrjala KL, Donaldson GW, Davis MW, Kippes ME, Carr JE. Relaxation and imagery and cognitive–behavioral training reduce pain during cancer treatment: A controlled clinical trial. *Pain* 1995; 63:189–198.

Toljanic JA, Bedard J-F, Larson RA, Fox JP. A prospective pilot study to evaluate a new dental assessment and treatment paradigm for patients scheduled to undergo intensive chemotherapy for cancer. *Cancer* 1999; 85:1843–1848.

Wahlin YB. Effects of chlorhexidine mouthrinse on oral health in patients with acute leukemia. *Oral Surgery, Oral Medicine, Oral Pathology* 1989; 68:279–287.

Weisdorf DJ, Bostrom B, Raether D, Mattingly M, Walker P, Pihlstrom B, Ferrieri P, Haake R, Goldman A, Woods W, et al. Oropharyngeal mucositis complicating bone marrow transplantation: Prognostic factors and the effect of chlorhexidine mouth rinse. *Bone Marrow Transplant* 1989; 4:89–95.

Wingard JR. Oral complications of cancer therapies. Infectious and noninfectious systemic consequences. *NCI Monographs* 1990; 9:21–26.

Organ Transplantation

Adams CK, Famili P. A study of the effects of the drug FK 506 on gingival tissues. *Transplant Proceedings* 1991; 23:3193–3194.

Antony SJ, Stratton CW, Dummer JS. Lactobacillus bacteremia: Description of the clinical course in adult patients without endocarditis. *Clinical Infectious Diseases* 1996; 23:773–778.

Bartold PM. Cyclosporine and gingival overgrowth. *Journal of Oral Pathology* 1987; 16:463–468.

Berry NJ, Burns DM, Wannamethee G, Grundy JE, Lui SF, Prentice HG, Griffiths PD. Seroepidemiological studies on the acquisition of antibodies to cytomegalovirus, herpes simplex virus and human immunodeficiency virus among general hospital patients and those attending a clinic for sexually transmitted diseases. *Journal of Medical Virology* 1988; 24:385–393.

Cohen SG. Renal disease. Chapter 15, pp. 487–509 in Lynch MA, Brightman VJ, Greenberg MS (eds). *Burket's Oral Medicine,* 9th ed. Philadelphia: JB Lippincott, 1994.

Colonna II JO, Winston DJ, Brill JE, Goldstein LI, Hoff MP, Hiatt JR, Quinones-Baldrich W, Ramming KP, Busuttil RW. Infectious complications in liver transplantation. *Archives of Surgery* 1988; 123:360–364

DeRossi SS, Glick M. Dental considerations for the patient with renal disease receiving hemodialysis. *JADA* 1996; 127:211–219.

Epstein JB, Sherlock CH, Wolber RA. Oral manifestations of cytomegalovirus infections. *Oral Surgery, Oral Medicine, Oral Pathology* 1993; 75:443–451.

Ferguson GA, Whyman RA. Dental management of people with renal disease and renal transplants. *New Zealand Dental Journal* 1998; 94:125–130.

Finberg R, Fingeroth J. Infections in transplant recipients. Chapter 136, pp. 840–846 in *Harrison's Principles of Internal Medicine,* 14th ed. New York: McGraw-Hill, 1998.

Fischel RJ, Payne WD, Gillingham KJ, Dunn DL, Sutherland DE, Matas AJ, Najarian JS. Long-term outlook for renal transplant recipients with one-year function. "Doctor, what are my chances?" *Transplantation* 1991; 51:118–122.

Fishman JA, Rubin RH. Infection in organ-transplant recipients. *New England Journal of Medicine* 1998; 338:1741–1750.

Genco RJ, Löe H. The role of systemic conditions and disorders in periodontal disease. *Periodontology 2000* 1993; 98:98–116.

Gruber SA, Gillingham K, Sothern RB, Stephanian E, Matas AJ, Dunn DL. De novo cancer in cyclosporine-treated and non-cyclosporine-treated adult primary renal allograft recipients. *Clinical Transplantation* 1994; 8:338–395.

Haffajee AD, Socransky SS. Microbial etiological agents of destructive periodontal diseases. *Periodontology 2000* 1994; 5:78–111.

Hanto DW. Transplantation. *Journal of the American College of Surgery* 1998; 186:232–239.

Health Care Financing Administration (HCFA). *Medicare Carrier's Manual, Part B.* Coverage and Limitations, Section 2136: Dental Services.

Jacobs C, Brunner FP, Brynger H, Chantler C, Donckerwolcke RA, Hathway RA, Kramer P, Selwood NH, Wing AJ. Malignant diseases in patients treated by dialysis and transplantation in Europe. *Transplant Proceedings* 1981; 13:729–732.

Jonas S, Rayes N, Neumann U, Neuhaus R, Bechstein WO, Guckelberger O, Tullius SG, Serke S, Neuhaus P. De novo malignancies after liver transplantation using tacrolimus-based protocols or cyclosporine-based quadruple immunosuppression with an interleukin-2 receptor antibody or antithymocyte globulin. *Cancer* 1997; 80:1141–1150.

Jorgensen MG. Prevalence of amlodipine-related gingival hyperplasia. *Journal of Periodontology* 1997; 68:676–678.

Katz MH, Greenspan D, Westenhouse J, Hessol NA, Buchbinder SP, Lifson AR, Shiboski S, Osmond D, Moss A, Samuel M, et al. Progression to AIDS in HIV-infected homosexuals and bisexual men with hairy leukoplakia and oral candidiasis. *AIDS* 1992; 6:95–100.

King GN, Thornhill MH. Dental attendance patterns in renal transplant recipients. *Oral Diseases* 1996; 2:145–147.

King GN, Fullinfaw R, Higgins TJ, Walker RG, Francis DM, Wiesenfeld D. Gingival hyperplasia in renal allograft recipients receiving cyclosporin-A and calcium antagonists. *Journal of Clinical Periodontology* 1993; 20:286–293.

King GN, Healy CM, Glover MT, Kwan JT, Williams DM, Leigh IM, Thornhill MH. Prevalence and risk factors associated with leukoplakia, hairy leukoplakia, erythematous candidiasis, and gingival hyperplasia in renal transplant recipients. *Oral Surgery, Oral Medicine, Oral Pathology* 1994; 78:718–726.

Kusne S, Manez R. Infectious complications. Chapter 11, pp. 315–332 in Shapiro R, Simmons RL, Starzl TE (eds). *Complications of Renal Transplantation*. Stamford, CT: Appleton & Lange, 1997.

Kusne S, Dummer JS, Singh N, Iwatsuki S, Makowka L, Esquivel C, Tzakis AG, Starzl TE, Ho M. Infections after liver transplantation. An analysis of 101 consecutive cases. *Medicine* (Baltimore) 1988; 67:132–143.

Lipkowitz GS, Madden RL. Transmission of Kaposi's sarcoma by solid organ donation. *Transplant Science* 1994; 4:9–11.

Löe H. Periondontal disease. The sixth complication of diabetes mellitus. *Diabetes Care* 1993; 16:329–334.

MacPhail LA, Hilton JF, Heinic GS, Greenspan D. Direct immunofluorescence vs. culture for detecting HSV in oral ulcers: A comparison. *JADA* 1995; 126:74–78.

Maier H, Zoller J, Herrmann A, Kreiss M, Heller W-D. Dental status and oral hygiene in patients with head and neck cancer. *Otolaryngology, Head and Neck Surgery* 1993; 108:655–661.

McCauley J. Medical complications. Chapter 11, pp. 299–313 in Shapiro R, Simmons RL, Starzl TE (eds). *Complications of Renal Transplantation*. Stamford, CT: Appleton & Lange, 1997.

Muzyka BC, Glick M. A review of oral fungal infections and appropriate therapy. *JADA* 1995; 126:63–72.

Naugle K, Darby ML, Bauman DB, Lineberger LT, Powers R. The oral health status of individuals on renal dialysis. *Annals of Periodontology* 1998; 3:197–205.

Naylor GD, Fredericks MR. Pharmacologic considerations in the dental management of the patient with disorders of the renal system. *Dental Clinics of North America* 1996; 40:665–683.

Naylor GD, Hall EH, Terezhalmy GT. The patient with chronic renal failure who is undergoing dialysis or renal transplantation: Another consideration for antimicrobial prophylaxis. *Oral Surgery, Oral Medicine, Oral Pathology* 1988; 65:116–121.

Okabe K, Nakagawa K, Yamamoto E. Factors affecting the occurrence of bacteremia associated with tooth extraction. *International Journal of Oral and Maxillofacial Surgery* 1995; 24:239–242.

Oliver RC, Tervonen T. Diabetes—A risk factor for periodontitis in adults? *Journal of Periodontology* 1994; 65:530–538.

Rateitschak-Pluss EM, Hefti A, Rateitschak KH. Gingival hyperplasia from cyclosporin A medication. *SSO Schweiz Monatsschr Zahnheilkd* 1983; 93:57–65.

Rees TD. Drugs and oral disorders. *Periodontology 2000* 1998; 18:21–36.

Reyna J, Richardson JM, Mattox DE, Banowsky LH, Nicastro-Lutton JJ. Head and neck infection after renal transplantation. *JAMA* 1982; 247:3337–3339.

Rose LF and Kaye D. *Internal Medicine for Dentistry,* 2nd ed. CV Mosby, St. Lewis, pp 567–570, 1990.

Rubin RH, Tolkoff-Rubin NE. Opportunistic infections in renal allograft recipients. *Transplant Proceedings* 1988; 20:12–18.

Ruskin JD, Wood RP, Bailey MR, Whitmore CK, Shaw BW. Comparative trial of oral clotrimazole and nystatin for oropharyngeal candidiasis prophylaxis in orthotopic liver transplant patients. *Oral Surgery, Oral Medicine, Oral Pathology* 1992; 74:567–571.

Sakurai K, Drinkwater D, Sutherland DE, Fleischmann J, Hage A, Yonemura C. Dental treatment considerations for the pre- and post-organ transplant patient. *Journal of the California Dental Association* 1995; 23:61–66.

Samaranayake LP, MacFarlane TW, Lamey PJ, Ferguson MM. A comparison of oral rinse and imprint sampling techniques for the detection of yeast, coliform and *Staphylococcus aureus* carriage in the oral cavity. *Journal of Oral Pathology* 1986; 15:386–388.

Schweitzer EJ, Matas AJ, Gillingham KJ, Payne WD, Gores PF, Dunn DL, Sutherland DE, Najarian JS. Causes of renal allograft loss. Progress in the 1980s, challenges for the 1990s. *Annals of Surgery* 1991; 214:679–688.

Seymour RA, Thomason JM , Nolan A. Oral lesions in organ transplant patients. *Journal of Oral Pathology and Medicine* 1997; 26:297–304.

Sheil AG, Disney AP, Mathew TH, Amiss N. De novo malignancy emerges as a major cause of morbidity and late failure in renal transplantation. *Transplant Proceedings* 1993; 25:1383–1384.

Strom BL, Albrutyn E, Berlin JA, Kinman JL, Feldman RS, Stolley PD, Levison ME, Korzeniowski OM, Kaye D. Dental and cardiac risk factors for infective endocarditis: A population-based, case-control study. *Annals of Internal Medicine* 1998; 129:761–769.

Svirsky JA, Saravia ME. Dental management of patients after liver transplantation. *Oral Surgery, Oral Medicine, Oral Pathology* 1989; 67:541–546.

Thomason JM, Seymour RA, Rice N. The prevalence and severity of cyclosporin and nifedipine-induced gingival overgrowth. *Journal of Clinical Periodontology* 1993; 20:37–40.

Thomason JM, Seymour RA, Ellis J. The periodontal problems and management of the renal transplant patient. *Renal Failure* 1994; 16:731–745.

Thomason JM, Seymour RA, Ellis JS, Kelly PJ, Parry G, Dark J, Wilkinson R, Ilde JR. Determinants of gingival overgrowth severity in organ transplant patients. An examination of the role of HLA phenotype. *Journal of Clinical Periodontology* 1996; 23:628–634.

Thomason JM, Ellis JS, Kelly PJ, Seymour RA. Nifedipine pharmacological variables as risk factors for gingival overgrowth in organ-transplant patients. *Clinical Oral Investigations* 1997; 1:35–39.

United Network for Organ Sharing (UNOS). 1998 Annual Report of the U.S. Scientific Registry for Transplant Recipients and the Organ Procurement and Transplantation Network—Transplant data: 1988–96. Richmond, VA, 1999.

Van der Meer, JTM, Thompson J, Valkenburg HA, Michel MF. Epidemiology of bacterial endocarditis in the Netherlands. II. Antecedent procedures and use of prophylaxis. *Archives of Internal Medicine* 1992; 151:1869–1873.

Varga E, Lennon M, Mair L. Pre-transplant gingival hyperplasia predicts severe cyclosporine-induced gingival overgrowth in renal transplant patient. *Journal of Clinical Periodontology* 1998; 25:225–230.

Westbrook P, Bednarczyk EM, Carlson M, Sheehan H, Bissada NF. Regression of ni-fedipine-induced gingival hyperplasia following switch to a same class calcium channel blocker, isradipine. *Journal of Periodontology* 1997; 68:645–650.

Wilson RF, Morel A, Smith D, Koffman CG, Ogg CS, Rigden PA , Ashley FP. Contri-bution of individual drugs to gingival overgrowth in adult and juvenile renal trans-plant patients treated with multiple therapy. *Journal of Clinical Periodontology* 1998; 25:457–464.

Wilson RL, Martinez-Tirado J, Whelchel J, Lordon RE. Occult dental infection causing fever in renal transplant patients. *American Journal of Kidney Diseases* 1982; 11:354–356.

Wondimu B, Dahllof G, Berg U, Modeer T. Cyclosporin-A-induced gingival overgrowth in renal transplant children. *Scandinavian Journal of Dental Research* 1993; 101:282–286.

Zeldin G, Magyars J, Klein PJ, Thuluvath J. Immunization, screening for malignancy, and health maintenance in the liver transplant recipient. *American Society of Trans-plant Surgeons*. Abstract 1998.

Ziccardi VB, Saini J, Demas PN, Braun TW. Management of the oral and maxillofacial surgery patient with end-stage renal disease. *Journal of Oral and Maxillofacial Sur-gery* 1992; 50:1207–1212.

Heart Valve Replacement and Repair

Drangsholt MT. A new causal model of dental diseases associated with endocarditis. *Annals of Periodontology* 1998; 3:184–196.

Roberts GJ. Dentists are innocent! "Everyday" bacteremia is the real culprit: A review and assessment of the evidence that dental surgical procedures are a principal cause of bacterial endocarditis in children. *Cardiology* 1999; 20:317–325.

Strom BL, Albrutyn E, Berlin JA, Kinman JL, Feldman RS, Stolley PD, Levison ME, Korzeniowski OM, Kaye D. Dental and cardiac risk factors for infective endocardi-tis: A population-based, case-control study. *Annals of Internal Medicine* 1998; 129:761–769.

Terezhalmy GT, Safadi TJ, Longworth DL, Muehrcke DD. Oral disease burden in pa-tients undergoing prosthetic heart valve implantation. *Annals of Thoracic Surgery* 1997; 63:402–404.

Van der Meer, JTM, Thompson J, Valkenburg HA, Michel MF. Epidemiology of bacte-rial endocarditis in the Netherlands. I. Patient characteristics. *Archives of Internal Medicine* 1992; 151:1863–1868.

APPENDIX D, PART 1

Immunosuppressive Therapy: The Scientific Basis and Clinical Practice of Immunosuppressive Therapy in the Management of Transplant Recipients

Robert S. Gaston, M.D.[*]

INTRODUCTION

The development and evolution of solid organ transplantation in the second half of the twentieth century is a unique achievement of modern medical technology. In 1964, Dr. Thomas E. Starzl noted that, to be considered a standard treatment, transplantation must ". . . first, be performed with an acceptably low mortality; second, the patient be restored to a reasonable state of health for a significant period of time; and finally, . . . the financial burden of care should be within the reach of the patient, the hospital, and the community."[1] Reflecting remarkable scientific and clinical progress, Starz's original criteria have now been fulfilled, as thousands of patients with previously fatal cardiac, hepatic, and renal diseases now routinely undergo transplantation, which affords complete or near-complete restoration of organ function. For the majority of allograft recipients, life is not only longer, but better. Current successes are the result of tireless efforts of transplant professionals to overcome the original hurdles of technical feasibility and immunological rejection. Now, the focus of transplantation is changing. As recently as 20 years ago, Rennie editorialized that ". . . even though it offers a much better quality of life while it works, a transplant in most cases (of kidney failure) can be considered only a temporary respite from the basic form of treatment, which is dialysis."[2] No longer is it practical to look at transplantation as a temporary intervention. For the kidney recipient, long-term graft survival is the best route to highly functional living; for the heart or liver recipient, survival of the allograft means life itself. Ensuring long-term success

---

[*]Associate Professor, Department of Medicine, Associate Professor, Department of Surgery, University of Alabama at Birmingham.

for as many transplant recipients as possible is the new challenge for the next century.

The interest of the federal government in solid organ transplantation dates back to 1972, when passage of the Social Security Amendments authorized Medicare entitlements for patients with end stage renal disease (ESRD) and included funding for kidney transplantation. At the time, for most patients, dialysis was considered optimal therapy.[3] Subsequent clinical developments led to a marked shift in the scientific underpinnings of the Medicare ESRD program, as data ever more convincingly confirmed the benefits of transplantation relative to dialysis. Medicare policies evolved to keep pace with these technological changes. However, recent clinical advances have again tilted the balance away from scientific and economic symmetry, particularly regarding issues related to long-term graft survival. In addition, funding considerations have previously focused only on kidney disease through the ESRD entitlements but in recent years, advances in transplantation of other solid organs have meant that recipients of other types of transplants are also affected by coverage policies. This changing environment challenges the rationale underlying current Medicare funding of transplantation. In this document, we will explore the scientific and clinical bases for current approaches to transplantation, and their relationship to other therapies (notably dialysis, for patients with ESRD). Successful transplantation has become inseparably linked to pharmacological immunosuppression that must be maintained for the life of the graft. By limiting payment for immunosuppressive drugs, current policies not only place a heavy burden on Medicare beneficiaries who have received transplants but continue to reflect the early impression that transplantation and pharmacological immunosuppression are temporary interventions.

THE SCIENTIFIC BASIS OF LONG-TERM ALLOGRAFT SURVIVAL

Expected Outcomes—Beyond Three Years

In 1963, future Nobel laureate Joseph Murray noted: "At present there is good evidence that chemical suppressive agents may be temporarily effective, [but] many questions remain unsolved. The eventual status of these homografted kidneys, the length of time for which the drug must be continued, whether or not the possibility for rejection diminishes with the passage of time and whether the original kidney disease will develop in the homograft are all unsolved problems. The total immunological potential of the host is not known when one is considering the course of his future lifetime. However, this report permits a note of cautious optimism in a problem that 10 years ago was considered almost insoluble."[4]

Transplantation has evolved in a very short time from a spectacular, experimental procedure to a commonplace event. Patients who previously faced near-certain death with cirrhosis, cardiomyopathy, or pulmonary hypertension now can return to functional, high-quality life with hepatic, cardiac, or pulmonary transplantation. Although challenges persist (particularly in lung transplantation), the overwhelming majority of transplant recipients can expect to be alive 1 year after transplantation, most with functioning grafts.[5,6] For patients with ESRD, transplantation from virtually any donor is now preferred over dialysis. In renal transplantation, graft losses for primary cadaver-donor renal transplants during the first year after transplantation declined from 26 percent in 1985 to 12 percent in 1995.[5] More recent data from single centers are reporting even fewer early losses.[7] Length of initial hospitalization has declined at many centers from several weeks to less than a week for live-donor transplantation and only incrementally longer for recipients of cadaver kidneys.[8] In the early days of transplantation, at least one episode of acute rejection was the norm for every patient, leading to prolonged initial hospitalization and frequent readmissions, with substantial infectious and other consequences of treating these episodes. Now, rejection rates of less than 50 percent are commonplace, and more than half of recipients are not readmitted to the hospital during the first posttransplant year.[7,9] In summary, these numbers reflect the ability to provide organs of ever-greater quality for recipients who have received better pretransplant care, coupled with the ability to reduce the impact of immunological rejection with less toxic and more specific immunosuppressive therapies. Murray's note of cautious optimism has evolved into a symphony of successful transplants.

Given these changes, the attention of the transplant community has also shifted and is now clearly focused on pursuing knowledge and interventions that facilitate long-term graft survival. Some investigators, citing a relatively stable attrition rate of functioning grafts over time, contend that improvement in short-term graft survival has not translated into a similar benefit in long-term graft survival.[10,11] Most data, however, document a steady, if not spectacular, increase in the "half-life" (the time at which 50 percent of grafts functioning at 1 year are lost) of both cadaveric-donor (from 5.4 to 8.5 years) and living-donor (from 10 to 14.7 years) transplants between 1986 and 1993.[5] If one excludes those graft losses due to death in a patient with a functioning allograft (death-censored survival), the half-life for cadaver-donor transplants rose from 11.1 to 16 years during the same period.[12] Data from the United Network for Organ Sharing (UNOS) Scientific Renal Transplant Registry indicate that 86 percent of kidney transplants performed between 1992 and 1994 were functional 1 year later, and 91 percent of those functioning at 1 year are still working at 3 years (actual 3-year graft survival of 78 percent).[6] More recent data, for transplants performed in 1995, indicate one-year graft survivals of 88 percent for recipients of first cadaveric kidneys and 93 percent for recipients of kidneys from living-related donors.[5] Since 1995, a watershed year for new transplant therapeutics (see below), it has not been unusual for single centers to report overall one-year graft survival in excess of 90 percent.[13] Thus, a reasonable projection for the next decade might be three-year renal allograft survival of 85 percent or better. Long-term graft survival is fast becoming the norm.

Transplant Immunology and Pharmacology

It is increasingly evident that the field of solid organ transplantation is entering a new era in which short-term success mandates greater attention to issues of long-term care. As noted elsewhere, this sea change is the result of the interplay of many scientific and clinical advances. When one views the improved outcomes against the backdrop of wider availability of the procedure with less selectivity of patients, the picture is even more dramatic. Although pretransplant medical care of potential candidates has improved significantly, transplantation is now offered to a greater percentage of older, high-risk ESRD patients.[5,14] Since many comorbid conditions worsen more rapidly in a patient on dialysis, lengthier waiting times may also negate the beneficial effect of better pretransplant care.[6] While techniques of organ procurement and preservation continue to improve, utilization of more and more organs from "extended-criteria donors" compromises quality, and an ever-greater percentage of organs is allocated to transplant centers beyond their area of procurement, resulting in longer preservation times[*,15,16] Organ allocation policies have resulted in a greater percentage of kidneys transplanted into extremely well-matched recipients.[15] However, fully 80 percent of cadaveric kidneys are transplanted despite significant HLA (human lymphocyte antigen) mismatches, and multicenter data document a progressively diminishing benefit of matching on outcome.[17] Better management of posttransplant medical and surgical complications (e.g., modern antibiotics and antivirals to treat the infectious complications of immunosuppression, effective prophylaxis of gastrointestinal hemorrhage) is not new. For each of these beneficial changes, there is a countervening variable with a potentially negative impact on graft survival—save one. The major factor contributing to dramatically improved outcomes is the ability to safely prevent and treat immunological rejection using newer and better immunosuppressant drugs.[18–20]

Human immune responses are complex, involving the interaction of cells, antibodies, and soluble proteins. These immune responses protect the body from injury and disease caused by bacteria, viruses, and malignant cell transformation. When non-self tissue (an allograft) is transplanted, the normal response of the immune system is to recognize the tissue as foreign and destroy it, a process known as rejection.[21] At this time, successful organ transplantation in humans is possible only by administration of pharmacological immunosuppressants that

---

[*]In an attempt to attenuate the imbalance between transplant candidates and available organs, many transplant centers now utilize organs from cadavers previously considered outside acceptable limits of age (6–55 years) and with limited comorbidity (well-controlled diabetes mellitus or hypertension). These are termed "extended-criteria donors."

prevent rejection. Preservation of long-term graft function requires ongoing treatment with these agents for the overwhelming majority of recipients.[22]

Immunosuppressive agents can be divided into four classes based on pharmacological characteristics and mode of action. The standard approach to long-term immunosuppressive therapy in this country is a multidrug protocol combining single agents from each class in order to maximize efficacy and minimize toxicity.[20,22,23]

Antibodies: Protein-Based Therapy

Antibodies are naturally occurring proteins whose function is to circulate in an animal, bind to specific tissues, and induce some immunological response as a consequence of the binding. These properties can be captured and manipulated for therapeutic benefit in transplantation (and other medical fields). In transplantation, antibodies are administered for short periods of time (usually 1–2 weeks) to achieve a specific goal. They may be utilized in the immediate post-transplant period to provide effective early immunosuppression, allowing time for institution and adjustment of maintenance therapy. They are also quite useful in treating episodes of acute rejection.[24] At most transplant centers, these agents are initially administered in an inpatient setting for a limited time. The newer monoclonal antibodies (daclizumab and basiliximab, approved by the Food and Drug Administration [FDA] in 1997 and 1998, respectively) have been genetically manipulated to confer low immunogenicity and long half-lives.[25,26] While it is conceivable that these (or other similar agents in development) may ultimately be used as a component of maintenance therapy for some outpatients, this is not current practice. Thus, although antibodies are quite expensive, reimbursement for their use in outpatients is rarely an issue.

Antiproliferative Agents (Azathioprine and Mycophenolate Mofetil)

The development of an effective oral immunosuppressant, azathioprine (Imuran®), resulted in the first long-term survivors of transplants between genetically nonidentical individuals (allografts) in the late 1950s and early 1960s.[4] Azathioprine is a thiopurine, the nitroimidazole derivative of 6-mercaptopurine.[27] As a purine analog, it blocks nucleic acid synthesis in rapidly dividing cells, preventing cellular differentiation and proliferation. The azathioprine dose is usually adjusted for body weight and reduced in the face of toxicity. Adverse effects of azathioprine are fairly predictable, reflecting the impact of an antimetabolite on rapidly dividing cells. These include marrow suppression (primarily neutrophils and platelets), hair loss, and stomatitis. Azathioprine may also cause hepatic dysfunction. All of these effects are typically dose related. Azathioprine is metabolized by xanthine oxidase; thus, allopurinol (a xanthine oxidase inhibitor indicated for the treatment of gout) inhibits degradation of azathioprine, and the combination is relatively contraindicated (an unfortunate circumstance given the prevalence of gout among transplant recipients). Over the long-term, the imidazole moiety of azathioprine may be an important factor contributing to the excess incidence of cutaneous malignancies in allograft recipients.

Azathioprine, administered in combination with low-dose corticosteroids, was the cornerstone of long-term immunosuppressive therapy from 1962 to1984. Almost all patients experienced at least one episode of acute rejection, and 1-year graft survival for recipients of cadaver kidneys was around 50 percent.[28] Infectious complications, related mostly to steroid administration, caused substantial morbidity, and one-year mortality was as high as 25 percent. Nonetheless, the effectiveness of such a regimen in some recipients of kidney transplants fueled ongoing work in cardiac and hepatic transplantation. Although such pioneering efforts allowed perfection of surgical techniques, they were rarely successful in inducing long-term survival among extrarenal recipients.

Mycophenolate mofetil (MMF) has been used clinically in the United States since its approval by the FDA in 1995. Its availability is a major reason that 1995 now appears to have been a watershed year in the advancement of transplant therapeutics. At most centers, MMF has supplanted azathioprine as the antiprolifcrative agent of choice, at least during the early posttransplant period (1–3 years).[13,18] While MMF inhibits purine synthesis, similar to azathioprine (albeit via a different mechanism), its effect is largely limited to lymphocytes (the key cells involved in rejection), imparting greater efficacy and less toxicity.[29, 30] MMF appears to be most effective in combination with a cytokine inhibitor (cyclosporine or tacrolimus, see below) and has shown efficacy in both preventing and reversing acute rejection episodes. Common adverse effects associated with MMF are primarily gastrointestinal in nature, consisting of dose-dependent nausea, vomiting, and diarrhea, with occasional mild marrow suppression. Despite a slight increase in viral infections (especially cytomegalovirus, or CMV) in MMF-treated patients, the drug is generally well tolerated.[31] Drug–drug interactions are uncommon. Unlike azathioprine, mycophenolate metabolism is unaffected by allopurinol, facilitating management of gout.

In three randomized, blinded multicenter trials (approximately 500 patients cach in the United States, Europe, Canada, and Australia), maintenance immunosuppression with MMF, cyclosporine, and prednisone reduced the risk of acute rejection (in comparison to three different cyclosporine-based protocols) by 50 percent, with 1-year survival of primary cadaveric transplants in excess of 90 percent.[32–34] Pooling data from all 1,500 patients demonstrated a benefit in overall graft survival as well.[18] The effect on graft survival of including MMF as part of long-term therapy is uncertain.[35,36] Likewise, the impact of discontinuing MMF after a defined period of time is unknown.

Corticosteroids

For over 40 years, corticosteroids have been a mainstay of pharmacological immunosuppression, despite early recognition of their association with significant adverse events. Early on, their use was restricted to a short course of high-dose therapy to reverse established acute rejection. Soon, it came to be recognized that ongoing administration of low doses of these agents (prednisone, methylprednisolone, etc.) might prevent rejection, making prednisone an essential part of maintenance therapy.[1,4] Currently, short courses of high-dose corticosteroids (2–7 mg/kg/d) are administered to treat or prevent acute rejection during the early posttransplant period, with rapid tapering of maintenance doses to 0.1–0.15 mg/kg/d.

The paradox of using corticosteroids in transplantation is that while they are effective and inexpensive, their use is limited by toxicity. Complications of steroid therapy are well documented and include weight gain, altered body habitus, moon facies, metabolic disturbances (hyperglycemia, hyperlipidemia), fluid retention, hypertension, bone disease, growth retardation, and depression. Sentiment within the transplant community has always favored steroid avoidance or withdrawal; with each advance in immunosuppression, the persistent preference of patients and physicians alike has been to do away with long-term steroid therapy.[1,37,38] However, given the immunological risks that accompany steroid withdrawal, current practice at most centers is to continue low-dose corticosteroid therapy for the duration of allograft function.

Calcineurin Phosphatase Inhibitors
(Cyclosporine, Tacrolimus)

The introduction of cyclosporine (CyA) in 1984 revolutionized solid organ transplantation, enhancing outcomes for recipients of kidney transplants and providing immunosuppression potent enough to support engraftment of hearts and livers. Although clinical practices have undergone substantial evolution over the last 15 years, CyA remains the cornerstone around which most immunosuppressive protocols are constructed. Early clinical trials in humans showed CyA to be effective in preventing rejection, but highly nephrotoxic. In combination with prednisone, CyA was further associated with an increased risk of infection and lymphoma.[39–42] Combination therapy evolved to capture the immunosuppressive benefits of cyclosporine, while minimizing the complications.[43–45] The attractiveness of combination therapy versus cyclosporine–prednisone dual therapy remains controversial, even as the agents used in combination continue to evolve.[*, 22,46]

---

[*]Many European centers and a few in the United States remain committed to dual CyA–prednisone therapy, attributing early difficulties with this regimen to inappropriate dosing of the drugs. Alternatively, most centers in this country add azathioprine or MMF,

Cyclosporine is a difficult drug to use. Its lipophilic nature makes absorption difficult, relatively unpredictable, and subject to widespread variability.[46] Neoral® is a new cyclosporine formulation, introduced in 1995, designed to improve absorption and reduce both inter- and intrapatient variability.[47,48] The therapeutic window for CyA is quite narrow, and blood levels demonstrate only rough correlation with clinical effect, making monitoring difficult.[49] CyA is metabolized by the P450 cytochrome system in the liver, and drug–drug interactions are common.[50] Adverse effects (including hypertension, nephrotoxicity, gingival hyperplasia, neurotoxicity, hirsutism, hyperuricemia, cholestasis, and hyperlipidemia) are ubiquitous. Thus, long-term management of cyclosporine-treated patients requires substantial familiarity with the drug.

Tacrolimus was approved by the FDA for use in transplantation of livers in 1994 and kidneys in 1997. Its immunosuppressive properties (inhibition of cytokine synthesis) are similar to CyA, although, on a milligram-for-milligram basis, it is 100-fold more potent.[19] The basic side-effect profile of tacrolimus is also similar to CyA (nephrotoxicity, hypertension, tremor, seizures, etc.), as are drug–drug interactions. However, tacrolimus appears to have a slight advantage in not causing gingival problems or hirsutism, and it may be less detrimental to lipid metabolism.[51] The chief disadvantage of tacrolimus is a greater tendency to elicit posttransplant glucose intolerance.[51,52] Some studies have reported enhanced efficacy of tacrolimus relative to CyA, while others find use of the two calcineurin inhibitors to result in similar outcomes.[51,52] Tacrolimus has also been used as rescue therapy for refractory rejection, with promising results in both single- and multicenter studies.[53,54] A remarkable clinical trend has emerged since tacrolimus was introduced: administered doses and desirable therapeutic levels of the agent have declined substantially, reducing both toxicity and cost without any apparent adverse impact on efficacy.[55] Currently, tacrolimus is the calcineurin inhibitor of choice in most liver transplant centers and is administered as well to 30–40 percent of de novo kidney transplant recipients.

Additional Agents

In the past 5 years, the FDA has approved seven new products for use in transplantation, including the Neoral® preparation of CyA, MMF, tacrolimus, daclizumab, basiliximab, and Thymoglobulin® (see Table D-1), and, most recently, sirolimus, which was approved in September 1999. At the time of this

---

along with a short-term course of prophylactic antibody administration, to the CyA–prednisone combination in order to enhance efficacy and reduce specific toxic effects of the two-drug combination. Experimental data exist to support both approaches.

294

TABLE D-1 Currently Available Immunosuppressants

Class	Drug Product	Dosage	Duration	Cost Per Year ($)[*]
Cytokine Inhibitors	Cyclosporine (Neoral®)	4–10 mg/kg/d	Long term	6,400
	Cyclosporine (SangCyA®)	4–10 mg/kg/d	Long term	4,800
	Tacrolimus (Prograf®)	0.1–0.3 mg/kg/d	Long-term	6,050
Antiproliferative Agents	Azathioprine (Imuran®)	1–2 mg/kg/d	Long term	900
	Mycophenolate (CellCept®)	1.5–3 g/d	Long term	4,800–9,700
Corticosteroids	Prednisone	0.1–0.15 mg/kg/d	Long term	200
Antilymphocyte agents	Atgam®	15 mg/kg/d	7–14 days	7,000
	Thymoglobulin®	1.5 mg/kg/d	7–14 days	6,300
	OKT3 (Orthoclone®)	5 mg/d	7–14 days	7,000
	Simulect® (basiliximab)	20 mg/dose	2 doses	2,500
	Zenapax® (daclizumab)	1 mg/kg/dose	5 doses	5,500

[*]Retail pharmacy costs in Birmingham, Alabama (May 1999) for average doses in a 70-kg patient.

writing, no other products appear close to approval, so the immunosuppressive armamentarium is likely to remain relatively unchanged for the next 5–10 years.

Sirolimus (rapamycin, RAD) is structurally similar to tacrolimus, binds to the same receptor, but inhibits immune responses via a different mechanism (interrupting lymphocyte function by blocking growth factor-driven proliferation).[30,56,57] The effects of sirolimus are not limited to T and B cells; it may also exert an inhibitory effect on proliferation of fibroblasts, endothelial cells, hepatocytes, and smooth muscle cells. Its immunosuppressive activity is synergistic with cyclosporine; proponents of sirolimus are hopeful that it will facilitate administration of significantly lower, less toxic doses of CyA.[56] Sirolimus also may have promise in preventing chronic rejection. Adverse effects associated with sirolimus include hyperlipidemia, neutropenia, and thrombocytopenia. Sirolimus appears not to be nephrotoxic but may exacerbate the nephrotoxicity of CyA.[56,58–60]

Current Uses and Future Trends

Currently, immunosuppressive therapy in the United States is in a state of flux. Before 1995, virtually all centers administered some combination of CyA, azathioprine, and steroids, with or without antibody "induction" in the early posttransplant period. Now, there is wide variability from center to center. Most still use "triple" therapy, with a calcineurin phosphatase inhibitor (CyA or tacrolimus), an antiproliferative agent (MMF or azathioprine), and steroids. The use of antibodies remains controversial, although the efficacy, side-effect profile, and relatively low cost of basiliximab and daclizumab have gained them rapid acceptance. Sirolimus is likely to be used as an adjunct, perhaps supplanting the antiproliferative agents from the protocol, although it may also have the potential of replacing either CyA or tacrolimus.[20,59]

The risk of acute rejection, and immunological graft loss, is greatest during the first 3 to 6 months after transplantation, requiring intense immunosuppression during this period.[61] Thereafter, most clinicians gradually reduce immunosuppressant doses or even discontinue a single agent (see below). This practice reflects "accommodation," or partial tolerance, between graft and host, a process initially described over 30 years ago.[4,62] In successful transplantation, there occurs over time a reduction in the intensity of anti-graft immunological responses that allows the transplant to function with lesser degrees of immunosuppression. Thus, patients are likely to be receiving substantially less pharmacological immunosuppression 3 or more years after their transplant than earlier in their course. Throughout the history of transplantation, investigators have pursued the "Holy Grail": complete and specific tolerance of host to graft without any chronic immunosuppression. Although recent developments seem ever more intriguing, no clinically successful approach allowing drug-free graft maintenance has yet emerged.[11,20,63]

COSTS OF ESRD THERAPY:
TRANSPLANTATION AND DIALYSIS

Recent data from the United States Renal Data System (USRDS) indicate that, in 1996, 27 percent of Medicare ESRD patients in this country had functioning renal allografts and consumed approximately 11 percent of a $9.6 billion Medicare ESRD budget.[5,64] The financial costs to Medicare of renal transplantation are well defined. During the year a transplant is performed, costs include the transplant hospitalization, organ acquisition, early readmissions (most commonly for acute rejection), outpatient labs and follow-up (which occur at more frequent intervals during the first year), and maintenance immunosuppressive therapy. In 1994, these initial costs amounted to $97,400 per patient.[64] After the first year, costs are much lower ($13,800 per patient-year), consisting primarily of payment for immunosuppressant drugs, along with less frequent laboratory studies and outpatient visits.[64] Relative to chronic dialysis (with 1994 per-patient costs of about $47,500 annually), transplant is significantly more expensive during the first year. However, after 3.1 years, the initial excess expenditure is recaptured. Thereafter, maintenance of a successful transplant is significantly less expensive than dialysis, with net savings of approximately $107,300 per patient over 10 years.[64]

Thus, the year-to-year financial costs of maintaining a successful allograft are substantially lower than those of maintenance dialysis, and the gap seems to be widening for at least two reasons. First, the improved outcomes of transplantation discussed above are enabling more recipients to become long-term survivors, able to recapture the initial investment and avoid the high costs of returning to dialysis or retransplantation. Currently, only 53 percent of successful transplant recipients have had their grafts for more than 3 years; based on recent advances in therapy, this percentage should grow rapidly.[5,65] Second, costs of dialysis have increased dramatically, at least in part due to the addition of coverage for pharmacological therapies administered during dialysis treatments, Calcijex® and erythropoietin (rHuEPO). Neither drug necessarily reduces dialysis-related mortality, but they may improve overall well-being and decrease morbidity. Calcijex® is an intravenous version of 1,25-dihydroxycholecalciferol, a necessary supplement for patients with ESRD. An oral version of this agent (Rocaltrol®) has been available for some time, but it is expensive, it is not covered by Medicare, and its use is subject to the vagaries of patient compliance. Administration of Calcijex®, though even more expensive, is covered by Medicare (indefinitely) and has proved more effective in slowing the progression of dialysis-related bone disease. Severe anemia (hemoglobin, 6–10 mg/dl) due to erythropoietin deficiency was a major contributor to the morbidity of chronic dialysis, causing fatigue, weakness, cardiovascular compromise, and at times, frequent transfusions. rHuEPO, usually administered subcutaneously and available to ESRD dialysis beneficiaries as an unlimited benefit, now costs Medicare

$1.2 billion annually, or $3,900 per patient per year.[66] It has achieved very high penetration in the dialysis community due to its relatively benign side-effect profile, its efficacy, and hopes of reduced morbidity among dialysis patients. Despite the absence of direct evidence that it improves survival in addition to quality of life, its benefits are deemed to exceed associated costs.[67,68] As these trends continue, with further improvement in transplant outcomes and increases in dialysis costs, the time necessary to recover the initial costs of transplantation will continue to decrease.

The cost of maintenance immunosuppressive therapy after the first post-transplant year can vary from $5,900 (generic cyclosporine, azathioprine, prednisone) to $13,000 (Neoral®, MMF, prednisone) annually. Based on currently available data, the most cost-effective approach to reduce rejection early after transplantation might be tacrolimus–azathioprine–prednisone ($7,000); however, in attempts to further reduce rejection rates, some prefer tacrolimus–MMF–prednisone, despite its higher cost.[51,69,70] Between 1994 and 1996, overall Medicare spending for immunosuppressive drugs doubled due to an increase in both the number of patients covered and the per-patient costs of therapy.[5] This increase coincides with the introduction of tacrolimus, Neoral®, and MMF into the U.S. market. As a potential offset to this expense are significant reductions in hospital readmissions and graft loss, which may ultimately reduce overall per-patient costs.[69,71] Indeed, a single-center report from the University of Alabama indicates that hospital readmissions in the first year after transplant have declined by 57 percent since 1995.[7] However, reliable long-term multicenter data concerning the impact of newer immunosuppressive therapies on overall costs do not yet exist.

At least three factors seem likely to keep long-term immunosuppressive costs at or below current levels for both renal and extrarenal transplant recipients. First, sirolimus, or other new agents, will not be *added to* regimens (as was the case with MMF in 1995) but will likely supplant an equally expensive agent (cyclosporine, tacrolimus, or MMF) from an immunosuppressive protocol. Second, given that some accommodation between patient and allograft underlies long-term graft survival, the practice of reducing immunosuppression over time is likely to continue. This means that, for each patient, overall immunosuppressive costs decrease over time, and the difference in cost between expensive and inexpensive regimens is minimized.* Finally, the introduction of quality generic

---

*As an example, a patient who receives Neoral®–MMF–prednisone ($13,000 per year) from the time of transplant will begin on full doses (and full costs) of each drug. Over time, due to dose reduction that is either purposeful or in response to adverse events, costs of all three drugs drop substantially such that annual costs after 3 years may be as low as $8,000 for effective immunosuppression. Conversely, a patient who receives Sang-CyA®, azathioprine, and prednisone begins therapy at a cost of $5,900. With similar dose reductions over time, costs are likely to remain in the $4,000–5,000 range.

equivalents for cyclosporine (of which SangCyA®, cyclosporine microemulsion, is the first), tacrolimus, and MMF will accelerate, with the potential to lower costs dramatically as the marketplace becomes more competitive.

ESSENTIALS OF LONG-TERM ALLOGRAFT SURVIVAL

Causes of Late Allograft Loss in Renal Transplantation

Under current therapies, early graft loss after solid organ transplantation is increasingly rare.[5-7,72,73] The majority of renal graft losses during the first year are due to either acute rejection of the transplanted organ or death of the patient from other causes while the graft is still functional. As improvements in the ability to manage the immune response have reduced the impact of rejection, the proportion of organs lost due to patient death has increased.[17] Beyond the first year, cadaveric grafts are lost at the relatively constant rate of 5–6 percent per year.[5,28] Death with function and chronic rejection account for roughly 70 percent of late losses, with recurrent kidney diseases (primarily glomerulonephritis) causing about 10 percent, and acute rejection even fewer.[74] Any strategy to improve long-term graft survival must address each of these causes.

Death with a functioning allograft, the ultimate in finite end points, is the most common cause of renal transplant failure after successful engraftment. The ultimate goal of renal transplantation is that every patient die with a functioning graft, just not prematurely. Currently, the death rate for transplanted patients is lower than for dialysis patients awaiting transplantation but higher than would expected for unaffected persons with a similar demographic background.[*,5,75] Although death with function is obviously the same finite end point, it reflects the impact of substantially different factors than before. In the early years of transplantation, death was most often a complication of the transplant procedure, commonly occurring during the first year after a transplant and many times the result of sepsis.[76,77] Of late, the demographics of those transplanted have changed dramatically. Diabetic patients account for a greater proportion of kidney recipients, increasing from 20 percent in 1986 to 25 percent in 1996. Fewer recipients are less than 45 years of age (69 percent in 1986 versus 53 percent in

---

*Mortality from any cause is significantly more common among dialysis patients than after renal transplantation. The death rate per 100 patient-years at risk in 1995 was 24.6 for dialysis patients versus 7.8 for cadaveric transplant recipients and 3.7 for recipients of live-donor transplants. However, older, sicker patients are not candidates for transplantation and remain clustered in the dialyis pool. The most meaningful group for comparison is dialysis patients who are wait-listed for transplantation and therefore thought to be physiologically similar. Beyond a year after transplant, relative risk of death is less than half for cadaveric transplant recipients compared to wait-listed dialysis patients.[5,75]

1996), and more are over age 64 (1 percent versus 5 percent).[5] Death is now most often caused by complications that are expected to be more common among these older individuals and diabetics (e.g., cardiovascular disease).[78] While long-term immunosuppressive therapy undoubtedly contributes to late mortality and better management of extrarenal comorbidity is highly desirable, it is difficult to envision significant declines in death rate without more restrictive transplant recipient selection.

Chronic rejection is undoubtedly a misnomer, implying a specific immunological event. In truth, chronic rejection is an amalgam of immunological and nonimmunological processes, resulting in gradual loss of allograft function over time. More accurate terminology would label the syndrome as chronic allograft nephropathy (CAN), defined as a state of impaired renal allograft function at least 3 months after transplantation, independent of acute rejection, overt drug toxicity, and recurrent or de novo specific disease entities, with supporting histological features on biopsy.[79,80] CAN is the main reason for returning to dialysis after transplantation and a major cause of ESRD in the Western world.[80,81] Its pathogenesis clearly has a strong underlying immunological basis, with previous episodes of acute rejection and degree of HLA incompatibility as strong predictive factors.[17,82,83] Late episodes of acute rejection and noncompliance with complicated medical regimens also are clearly associated with CAN.[83–85] However, the syndrome also reflects the impact of such nonimmunological factors as quality of implanted organ, size mismatch, hypertension, drug toxicity, and hyperlipidemia.[86–91] Nonetheless, the transplant community continues to focus on the underlying immunological basis of CAN and the provision of adequate immunosuppression to prevent graft loss.[80]

The first successful human renal transplants in the mid-1950s were isografts, performed between immunologically identical twins.[92] Rejection was not a problem, but over time, some of these transplants lost function due to recurrence of the recipient's original renal disease.[1,92] As effective immunosuppression became available, azathioprine and/or prednisone were administered even to identical-twin recipients in hopes of preventing recurrent disease. In the 1990s, with effective control of acute rejection in all transplants, recurrent diseases (including focal glomerulosclerosis, lupus, immunoglobulin [IgA] nephropathy, membranous nephropathy, and necrotizing vasculitis) account for approximately 10 percent of late allograft losses.[74] Evidence indicates that provision of adequate long-term immunosuppressive therapy may be critical in minimizing graft losses due to these diseases.[93,94] Finally, it seems likely that recurrence of some microangiopathic diseases, notably hemolyticuremic syndrome, may be potentiated by the vascular toxicities of cyclosporine and tacrolimus, emphasizing the need for ongoing surveillance of recipients by physicians experienced in the use of these drugs.[95]

Causes of Late Allograft Loss in Transplantation of Organs Other than Kidneys

Transplantation of each of the nonrenal organs is associated with a distinct constellation of long-term complications. Obviously, graft failure, in the absence of retransplantation, equates with death in recipients of heart, liver, and lung transplants. Although early rejection episodes are common in those receiving liver transplants, late rejection (episodes occurring beyond 6 months) is distinctly uncommon. Accordingly, chronic rejection is also uncommon, and most hepatic recipients require significantly less long-term immunosuppression than other transplanted patients. Late graft failure is a relatively rare event, resulting most commonly from recurrent disease (hepatitis B and C, autoimmune hepatitis).[72,96] In cardiac and pulmonary transplantation, late graft loss occurs more frequently. Chronic rejection (transplant coronary artery disease and bronchiolitis obliterans, respectively) is a significant long-term complication that requires substantial care and immunosuppressive monitoring.[97,98] Given the more potent immunosuppression required by those receiving thoracic transplants, infection and malignancy pose greater threats to long-term survival than in kidney and liver recipients.

Barriers to Long-Term Survival

Looking forward, advances in scientific understanding and clinical intervention for comorbid conditions, chronic allograft nephropathy, and recurrent disease are essential in prolonging allograft survival. However, evidence exists that substantial improvement may be possible with better use of currently available tools.

Providing Adequate Immunosuppression

Long-term allograft survival is impossible without adequate immunosuppression, but controversy exists regarding the precise definition of "adequate." Too little immunosuppression results in rejection and graft loss; too much in untoward complications. Transplant physicians and surgeons have always been trapped between these competing goals. Unfortunately, an accurate technique to assess how much immunosuppression is necessary for each individual patient does not exist. In the absence of an adequate measurement, those involved in monitoring immunosuppression have learned to negotiate narrow therapeutic limits with surprisingly little guidance from objective findings in clinical trials.

In the early days of transplantation, reduction and/or withdrawal of immunosuppression was almost always accompanied by rejection and graft loss.[4,99,100] Virtually all subsequent attempts to withdraw even a single drug from therapies have repeated this experience, at least to some degree in some patients. Because of their inherent toxicities, withdrawal of corticosteroids has been the goal of multiple trials. Most studies of complete steroid withdrawal document 10–40 percent risk of acute rejection depending on the patient population studied and the timing of withdrawal.[38,101–104] While this finding is relatively uniform, controversy exists regarding the ultimate impact of these rejection episodes on graft and patient survival. Some have found these rejections, despite requiring reinstitution of steroid therapy, to have little or no impact on graft survival.[105] Others have noted increased risk of CAN and graft loss among the steroid withdrawal group.[106,107] A recent randomized trial of steroid withdrawal (supported by the National Institutes of Health) using the most modern immunosuppressants available was terminated early due to increased incidence of acute rejection (19 percent versus 5 percent) in the withdrawal group, despite the absence of any differential effect on graft survival.[37]

Because of its toxicity and cost, CyA withdrawal has been attempted in multiple studies, again with very consistent results. The incidence of acute rejection rises after even gradual dose reduction and withdrawal, but with controversial implications.[108–111] A meta-analysis of 10 randomized and 7 nonrandomized trials of cyclosporine withdrawal found a 26 percent greater incidence of acute rejection in the withdrawal group, but without adverse impact on short-term graft loss or mortality.[110] In a nonrandomized trial of gradual CyA withdrawal for financial reasons in otherwise stable patients, there was substantial risk of late rejection and graft loss, particularly among African-American recipients.[111] When a similar group of socioeconomically disadvantaged recipients was provided cyclosporine indefinitely, outcomes were substantially improved.[112] Others have shown maintenance of therapeutic cyclosporine levels to be a critical factor in reducing the risk of chronic rejection and improving long-term graft survival.[113,114]

Since it has been difficult to document a beneficial effect of azathioprine in combination with CyA and prednisone, it should not be too surprising that azathioprine withdrawal, though poorly studied, appears to have little adverse impact. Studies of tacrolimus and MMF withdrawal are underway, but results as yet are unavailable. Thus, the preponderance of data concerning withdrawal of a single agent indicates that, while this feasible in some patients, adverse consequences may develop in others. As previously noted, to truly define the adequacy of immunosuppression, some reliable measurement of donor-specific immunological responsiveness is necessary.[115] Without such a measurement, it is obvious that across-the-board drug withdrawal is a hazardous approach for many patients. Thus, in the clinical arena, adequacy of immunosuppression will continue to be determined by laboratory and physical assessment of the recipient, performed at recurring intervals by providers familiar with the issues involved.

Avoiding Excessive Immunosuppression

Given that long-term graft survival requires ongoing immunosuppression, maximizing outcomes means minimizing complications of immunosuppressive therapies. Early after transplantation, when immunosuppression is most intense, risk of infectious complications is greatest.[116] In 1999, these infections are primarily viral, with bacterial and fungal infections posing life-threatening risk in only a limited number of patients. For long-term survivors, risk of infection diminishes with time, at least partially due to reduction in immunosuppressant drug dosages. However, risk of malignancy, itself often viral related, increases and remains substantially greater in transplant recipients than in the general population.[117] In addition, there are specific adverse effects of each immunosuppressive agent that require surveillance, such as cyclosporine nephrotoxicity and hypertension, steroid-induced bone disease, or hyperlipidemia.[118–120]

SUMMARY AND CONCLUSION

A common aphorism is that successful transplantation is not a cure, but rather substitutes the manageable disease of immunosuppression for the incurable and fatal disease of organ failure. Current clinical practice, with substantial scientific underpinnings, requires continual provision of adequate immunosuppression to ensure optimal outcomes for recipients. While future developments may change this paradigm, long-term survival of both graft and patient mandates ongoing access not only to a full complement of immunosuppressive agents, but also to requisite clinical expertise.

REFERENCES

1. Starzl TE. Experience in renal transplantation. Philadelphia: WB Saunders Co., 1964.
2. Rennie D: Home dialysis and the costs of uremia. N Engl J Med 298:399–400, 1978.
3. Friedman EA, Kountz SL: Impact of HR-1 on the therapy of end-stage uremia: How and where should uremia be treated? N Engl J Med 288:1286–1288, 1973.
4. Murray JE, Merrill JP, Harrison JH, Wilson RE, Dammin GJ: Prolonged survival of human-kidney homografts by immunosuppressive drug therapy. N Engl J Med 268: 1315–1323, 1963.
5. United States Renal Data System: Excerpts from USRDS 1998 Annual Data Report. Am J Kidney Dis 32(Suppl 1):S1–S162, 1998.
6. UNOS (United Network for Organ Sharing): 1997 Annual Report of the U.S. Scientific Registry for Transplant Recipients in the Organ Procurement and Transplantation Network: DHHS/HRSA, Richmond, Virginia, UNOS, 1997.
7. Gaston RS, Deierhoi MH, Hudson SL, Kew CE, Curtis JJ, Julian BA, Young CJ, Gallichio MJ, Diethelm AG: Sequential immunoprophylaxis in renal transplantation: Comparison of two doses of daclizumab to OKT3 induction (abstract). J Am Soc Nephrol 10 (in press), 1999.

8. Gaston RS, Kasiske BL, Tesi RJ, Danovitch GM, Bia MJ: Post-transplant management practices in renal allograft recipients in the United States. Submitted for publication, 1999.

9. Brennan DC, Flavin K, Lowell JA, Howard TK, Shenoy S, Burgess S, Dolan S, Kano JM, Mahon M, Schnitzler MA, Woodward R, Irish W, Singer GG: A randomized, double-blinded comparison of Thymoglobulin versus Atgam for induction immunosuppressive therapy in adult renal transplant recipients. Transplantation 67: 1011–1018, 1999.

10. Gjertson DW: Survival trends in long-term first cadaver-donor kidney transplants, in P.I. Terasaki and J.M.Cecka (eds), Clinical Transplants 1991. Los Angeles, UCLA Tissue Typing Laboratory, 1992, pp. 225–235.

11. Turka LA: What's new in transplant immunology: Problems and prospects. Ann Intern Med 128:946–948, 1998.

12. Hariharan S, Johnson CP, Bresnahan BA, Taranto S, Stablein D: Improved renal allograft survival from 1988–1996: An analysis from UNOS data (abstract). Transplantation 67:S269, 1999.

13. Gaston RS, Hudson SL, Curtis JJ, Julian BA, Kew CE, Young CJ, Gallichio MJ, Deierhoi MH, Diethelm AG: Treatment of acute rejection episodes in the 90s: Is there still an impact on outcome in renal transplantation (abstract). Transplantation 67:S157, 1999.

14. Rosansky SJ, Eggers PW: Trends in the US end-stage renal disease population: 1973–1983. Am J Kidney Dis 9:91–97, 1987.

15. Hata Y, Cecka JM, Takemoto S, Ozawa M, Cho YW, Terasaki PI: Effects of changes in the criteria for nationally shared kidney transplants for HLA-matched patients. Transplantation 65:208–212, 1998.

16. Gjertson DW: A multifactor analysis of kidney graft outcomes at one and five years posttransplantation: 1996 UNOS Update, in J.M. Cecka and P.I. Terasaki (eds), Clinical Transplants 1996. Los Angeles, UCLA Tissue Typing Laboratory, 1997, pp. 343–360.

17. Cecka JM: The UNOS Scientific Renal Transplant Registry, in J.M. Cecka and P.I. Terasaki (eds), Clinical Transplants 1996. Los Angeles, UCLA Tissue Typing Laboratory, 1997, pp. 1–14.

18. Halloran P, Mathew T, Tomlanovich S, Groth C, Hooftman L, Barker C: Mycophenolate mofetil in renal allograft recipients: A pooled efficacy analysis of three randomized, double-blind, clinical studies in prevention of rejection. Transplantation 63:39–47, 1997.

19. Peters DH, Fitton A, Plosker GL, Faulds D: Tacrolimus: A review of its pharmacology and therapeutic potential in hepatic and renal transplantation. Drugs 46:746–794, 1993.

20. Perico N, Remuzzi G: Prevention of transplant rejection: Current treatment guidelines and future developments. Drugs 54:533–570, 1997.

21. Suthanthiran M: Acute rejection of renal allografts: mechanistic insights and therapeutic options. Kidney Int 51:1289–1304, 1997.

22. Halloran PF, Batiuk TD, Goes NB, Campbell P: Strategies to improve the immunologic management of organ transplants. Clin Transplantation 9:227–236, 1995.

23. Suthanthiran M, Morris RE, Strom TB: Immunosuppressants: Cellular and molecular mechanisms of action. Am J Kidney Dis 28:159–172, 1996.

24. Ortho Multicenter Study Group: A randomized clinical trial of OKT3 monoclonal antibody for acute rejection of cadaveric renal transplants. N Engl J Med 313:337–340, 1985.

25. Nashan B, Moore R, Amlot P, et al.: Randomized trial of basiliximab versus placebo for control of acute cellular rejection in renal allograft recipients. Lancet 350:1193–1198, 1997.

26. Vincenti F, Kirkman R, Light S, Bumgardner G, Pescovitz M, Halloran P, Neylan J, Wilkinson A, Ekberg H, Gaston R, Backman L, Burdick J: Interleukin-2-receptor blockade with daclizumab to prevent acute rejection in renal transplantation. N Engl J Med 338:161–165, 1998.

27. d'Apice AJF: Non-specific immunosuppression: Azathioprine and steroids, in P.J. Morris (ed), Kidney Transplantation: Principles and Practice. Second Edition. London, Grune & Stratton, Inc., 1984, pp. 239–259.

28. Cook DJ: Long-term survival of kidney allografts, in P. I. Terasaki (ed), Clinical Transplants 1987, Los Angeles, UCLA Tissue Typing Laboratory, 1987, pp. 277–285.

29. Allison AC, Eugui EM: Mycophenolate mofetil, a rationally designed immunosuppressive drug. Clin Transplantation 7:96–112, 1992.

30. Morris RE: Mechanisms of action of new immunosuppressive drugs. Kidney Int 49(Suppl 53):S26–S38, 1996.

31. Birkeland SA, Andersen HK, Hamilton-Dutoit SJ: Preventing acute rejection, EBV infection, and posttransplant lymphoproliferative disorders after kidney transplantation: Use of acyclovir and mycophenolate mofetil in a steroid-free immunosuppressive protocol. Transplantation 67:1209–1214, 1999.

32. European Mycophenolate Mofetil Cooperative Study Group: Placebo-controlled study of mycophenolate mofetil combined with cyclosporin and corticosteroids for prevention of acute rejection. Lancet 345:1321–1325, 1995.

33. Sollinger HW, U.S. Renal Transplant Mycophenolate Mofetil Study Group: mycophenolate mofetil for the prevention of acute rejection in primary cadaveric renal allograft recipients. Transplantation 60:225–232, 1995.

34. Tricontinental Mycophenolate Mofetil Renal Transplantation Study Group: A blinded, randomized clinical trial of mycophenolate mofetil for the prevention of acute rejection in cadaveric renal transplantation. Transplantation 61:1029–1037, 1996.

35. Mathew TH, Tricontinental MMF Renal Transplantation Study Group: A blinded, long-term, randomized multicenter study of mycophenolate mofetil in cadaveric renal transplantation: Results at three years. Transplantation 65:1450–1454, 1998.

36. Vanrenterghem YFC: Impact of new immunosuppressive agents on late graft outcome. Kidney Int 52(Suppl 63):S81–S83, 1997.

37. Matas A, Ewell M, Cooperative Clinical Trials in Adult Transplantation: Prednisone withdrawal in kidney transplant recipients on CSA/MMF: A prospective, randomized study (abstract). Transplantation 67:S269, 1999.

38. Hricik DE, Whalen CC, Lautman J, Bartucci MR, Moir EJ, Mayes JT, Schulak JA: Withdrawal of steroids after renal transplantation—Clinical predictors of outcome. Transplantation 53:41–45, 1992.

39. Calne RY, White DJG, Thiru S, et al.: Cyclosporine in patients receiving renal allografts from cadaver donors. Lancet ii:1323–1327, 1978.

40. Calne RY, Rolles K, White DJG, et al.: Cyclosporin A initially as the only immuno-suppressant in 34 recipients of cadaveric organs: 32 kidneys, 2 pancreases and 2 livers. Lancet ii:1033–1036, 1979.

41. Canadian Multicentre Transplant Study Group: A randomized clinical trial of cyclosporine in cadaveric renal transplantation. New Engl J Med 309:809–815, 1983.

42. Harder F, Calne RY, Pichlmayr R, et al.: Cyclosporin A as sole immunosuppressive agent in recipients of kidney allografts from cadaver donors: Preliminary results of a European multicenter trial. Lancet ii:57–60, 1982.

43. First MR, Alexander JW, Wadhwa N, et al.: The use of low doses of cyclosporine, azathioprine and prednisone in renal transplantation. Transplant Proc 18:132–135, 1986.

44. Simmons RL, Canafax DM, Fryd DS, et al.: New immunosuppressive drug combinations for mismatched related and cadaveric renal transplantation. Transplant Proc 18:76–81, 1986.

45. Sollinger HW, Deierhoi M, Kalayoglu M, et al.: Sequential antilymphocyte globulin cyclosporine therapy: Cadaver renal transplantation. Transplant Proc 18:16–18, 1986.

46. Lindholm A, Kahan BD: Influence of cyclosporine pharmacokinetics, trough concentrations, and AUC monitoring on outcome after kidney transplantation. Clin Pharmacol Ther 54:205–218, 1993.

47. Keown P, Niese D: Cyclosporine microemulsion increases drug exposure and reduces acute rejection without incremental toxicity in de novo renal transplantation. International Sandimmun Neoral Study Group. Kidney Int 54:938–944, 1998.

48. Mueller EA, Kovarik JM, van Bree JB, et al.: Pharmacokinetics and tolerability of a microemulsion formulation of cyclosporine in renal allograft recipients—A concentration-controlled comparison with the commercial formulation. Transplantation 57:1178–1182, 1994.

49. Holt JW, Marsden JT, Johnston A, et al.: Blood cyclosporine concentrations and renal allograft dysfunction. Brit Med J 293:1057–1059, 1986.

50. Cockburn J: Cyclosporin A: A clinical evaluation of drug interactions. Transplant Proc 18:50–55, 1986.

51. Pirsch JD, Miller J, Deierhoi MH, Vincenti F, Filo RS: A comparison of tacrolimus and cyclosporine for immunosuppression after cadaveric renal transplantation. FK506 Kidney Transplant Study Group. Transplantation 63:977–983, 1997.

52. Jensik SC, FK506 Kidney Transplant Study Group: Tacrolimus in kidney transplantation: Three-year survival results of the U.S. multicenter, randomized comparative trial. Transplant Proc 30:1216–1218, 1998.

53. Jordan ML, Naraghi R, Shapiro R, Smith D, Vivas CA, Scantlebury VP, Gritsch HA, et al.: Tacrolimus rescue therapy for renal allograft rejection—Five year experience. Transplantation 63:223–228, 1997.

54. Woodle ES, Thistlethwaite JR, Gordon JH, Laskow D, Deierhoi MH, Burdick J, Pirsch JD, Sollinger H, et al.: A multicenter trial of FK506 (tacrolimus) therapy in refractory acute renal allograft rejection. Transplantation 62:594–599, 1996.

55. Laskow DA, Vincenti F, Neylan JF, Mendez R, Matas AJ: An open-label, concentration-ranging trial of FK506 in primary kidney transplantation: A report of the Uninte States Multicenter FK506 Kidney Transplant Group. Transplantation 62: 900–905, 1996.

56. Kahan BD: Emerging strategies for the clinical application of rapamycin. Clin Biochem 31:341–344, 1998.

57. Schuurman H-J, Cottens S, Fuchs S, Joergensen J, Meerloo T, Sedrani R, Tanner M, Zenke G, Schuler W: SDZ RAD, a new rapamycin derivative: Synergism with cyclosporine. Transplantation 64:32–35, 1997.

58. Andoh TF, Lindsley J, Franceschini N, Bennett WM: Synergistic effects of cyclosporine and rapamycin in a chronic nephrotoxicity model. Transplantation 63:311–316, 1996.

59. Groth CG, Backman L, Morales J-M, Calne R, Kreis H, Lang P, et al: Sirolimus-based therapy in human renal transplantation: Similar efficacy and different toxicity compared with cyclosporine. Transplantation 67:1036–1042, 1999.

60. Murgia MG, Jordan S, Kahan BD: The side effect profile of sirolimus: A phase I study in quiescent cyclosporine–prednisone-treated renal transplant patients. Kidney Int 49:209–216, 1996.

61. Gaston RS, Hudson SL, Deierhoi MH, Barber WH, Laskow DA, Julian BA, Curtis JJ, Barger BO, Shroyer TW, Diethelm AG: Improved survival of primary cadaveric renal allografts in blacks with quadruple immunosuppression. Transplantation 53:103–109, 1992.

62. Starzl TE, Marchioro TL, Waddell WR: The reversal of rejection in human renal homografts with subsequent development of homograft tolerance. Surg Gynecol Obstet 117:385, 1963.

63. Kirk AD, Burkly LC, Batty DS, Baumgartner RE, Berning JD, Buchanan K, Fechner JH, Germond RL, Kampen RL, Patterson NB, Swanson SJ, Tadaki DK, TenHoor CN, White L, Knechtle SJ, Harlan DM: Treatment with humanized monoclonal antibody against CD 154 prevents acute renal allograft rejection in nonhuman primates. Nature Medicine 5:686–693, 1999.

64. Eggers P, Milam R: Cost comparison of dialysis and transplantation. Abstract presented at the Immunosuppression Conference in Organ Transplantation: Patient Access to Long-Term Care. Philadelphia, American Society for Transplantation, December 4, 1998.

65. Evans RW: The economic impact of graft dysfunction. Graft 2(Suppl. 2):S144–S150, 1999.

66. Cotter DJ, Thamer M, Kimmel PL, Sadler JH: Secular trends in recombinant erythropoietin therapy among the U.S. hemodialysis population: 1990–1996. Kidney Int 54:2129–2139, 1998.

67. Muirhead N, Bargman J, Burgess E, Jindal KK, Levin A, Nolin L, Parfrey P: Evidence-based recommendations for the clinical use of recombinant human erythropoietin. Am J Kidney Dis 26(Suppl 1):S1–S24, 1995.

68. Powe NR, Eggers PW, Johnson CB: Early adoption of cyclosporine and recombinant human erythropoietin: Clinical, economic, and policy issues with emergence of high-cost drugs. Am J Kidney Dis 24:33–41, 1994.

69. Neylan JF, Sullivan EM, Steinwald B, Goss TF: Assessment of the frequency and costs of posttransplantation hospitalizations in patients receiving tacrolimus versus cyclosporine. Am J Kidney Dis 32:770–777, 1998.

70. Roth D, Colona J, Burke GW, Ciancio G, Esquenazi V, Miller J: Primary immunosuppression with tacrolimus and mycophenolate mofetil for renal allograft recipients. Transplantation 65:248–252, 1998.

71. Khosla UM, Martin JE, Baker GM, Schroeder TJ, First MR: One-year, single-center cost analysis of mycophenolate mofetil versus azathioprine following cadaveric renal transplantation. Transplant Proc 31:274–275, 1999.

72. Wiesner RH, Demetris AJ, Belle SH, Seaberg EC, Lake JR, Zetterman RK, Everhart J, Detre KM: Acute hepatic allograft rejection: Incidence, risk factors, and impact on outcome. Hepatology 28:638–645, 1998.

73. Keck BM, Bennett LE, Fiol BS, Daily OP, Novick RJ, Hosenpud JD: Worldwide thoracic organ transplantation: A report from the UNOS/ISHLT International Registry for Thoracic Organ Transplantation, in J.M. Cecka and P.I. Terasaki (eds), Clinical Transplants 1997, Los Angeles, UCLA Tissue Typing Laboratory, 1997, pp. 31–34.

74. Hariharan S, Peddi VR, Savin VJ, Johnson CP, First MR, Roza AM, Adams MB: Recurrent and de novo renal diseases after renal transplantation: A report from the renal allograft disease registry. Am J Kidney Dis 31:928–931, 1998.

75. Ojo AO, Port FK, Wolfe RA, Mauger EA, Williams L, Berling DP: Comparative mortality risks of chronic dialysis and cadaveric transplantation in black end-stage renal disease patients. Am J Kidney Dis 24:59–64, 1994.

76. Hill MN, Grossman RA, Feldman HI, Hurwitz S, Dafoe DC: Changes in causes of death after renal transplantation, 1966 to 1987. Am J Kidney Dis 17:512–518, 1991.

77. Schweitzer EJ, Matas AJ, Gillingham KJ, Payne WD, Gores PF, Dunn DL, Sutherland DE, Najarian JE: Causes of renal allograft loss. Progress in the 1980s, challenges for the 1990s. Ann Surg 214:679–688, 1991.

78. USRDS (United States Renal Data System): Exerpts from USRDS 1996 Annual Data Report. American Jounral of Kidney Disease 29(3 Suppl 2):S1–S165, 1996.

79. Matas AJ, Burke JF, DeVault GA, Monaco A, Pirsch JD: Chronic rejection. J Am Soc Nephrol 4:S23–S29, 1994.

80. Halloran PF, Melk A, Barth C: Rethinking chronic allograft nephropathy: The concept of accelerated senescence. J Am Soc Nephrol 10:167–181, 1999.

81. Paul LC: Chronic renal transplant loss. Kidney Int 47:1491–1499, 1995.

82. Matas AJ, Gillingham KJ, Payne WD, Najarian JS: The impact of an acute rejection episode on long-term renal allograft survival. Transplantation 57:857–859, 1994.

83. Leggat JE, Ojo AO, Leichtman AB, Port FK, Wolfe RA, Turenne MN, Held PJ: Long-term renal allograft survival: Prognostic implication of the timing of acute rejection episodes. Transplantation 63:1268–1272, 1997.

84. De Geest S, Borgermans L, Gemoets H, Abraham I, Vlaminck H, Evers G, Vanrenterghem Y: Incidence, determinants, and consequences of subclinical noncompliance with immunosuppressive therapy in renal transplant recipients. Transplantation 59:340–347, 1995.

85. Gaston RS, Hudson SL, Ward M, Jones P, Macon R: Late renal allograft loss: Noncompliance masquerading as chronic rejection. Transplant Proc 31(Suppl 4A):21S–23S, 1999.

86. Bia MJ: Nonimmunologic causes of late renal graft loss. Kidney International 47:1470–1480, 1995.

87. Brenner BM, Milford EL: Nephron underdosing: A programmed cause of chronic renal allograft failure. Am J Kidney Dis 21:66–72, 1993.

88. Opelz G, Wujciak T, Ritz E, for the Collaborative Transplant Study: Association of chronic kidney graft failure with recipient blood pressure. Kidney Int 53:217–222, 1998.

89. Massy ZA, Kasiske BL: Posttransplant hyperlipidemia: Mechanisms and management. J Am Soc Nephrol 7:971–977, 1996.

90. Matas AJ: Chronic allograft dysfunction: Clinical definitions and risk factors. Graft 1(Suppl. 2):48–51, 1998.

91. Naimark DMJ, Cole E: Determinants of long-term renal allograft survival. Transplant Reviews 8:93–113, 1994.

92. Merrill JP, Murray JE, Harrison JH, Guild WR: Successful homotransplantation of the human kidney between identical twins. JAMA 160:277–282, 1956.

93. Julian BA, Said M, Barker CV: Allograft loss in IgA nephropathy (abstract). J Am Soc Nephrol 9:91A, 1998.

94. Ramos EL: Recurrent diseases in the renal allograft. J Am Soc Nephrol 2:109–121, 1991.

95. Ruggenenti P, Remuzzi G: Malignant vascular disease of the kidney: Nature of the lesions, mediators of disease progression, and the case for bilateral nephrectomy. Am J Kidney Dis 27:459–475, 1996.

96. Weisner RH, Martin P, Stribling R: Post-transplant care/medical complications after liver transplantation, in D.J. Norman and W.N. Suki (eds), Primer on Transplantation, Thorofare, NJ, American Society of Transplant Physicians, 1998, pp. 343–362.

97. Lynch JP, Trulock EP: Expected clinical outcomes/analysis of risk factors in lung transplantion, in D.J. Norman and W.N. Suki (eds), Primer on Transplantation, Thorofare, NJ, Am Society of Transplant Physicians, 1998, pp. 555–560.

98. Costanzo MR, Cross AM, Haas GS: Post-transplant care/medical complications of cardiac transplantation, in D.J. Norman and W.N. Suki (eds), Primer on Transplantation, Thorofare, N.J., Am Society of Transplant Physicians, 1998, pp. 445–458.

99. Zoller KM, Cho SI, Cohen JJ, Harrington JT: Cessation of immunosuppressive therapy after successful transplantation: A national survey. Kidney Int 18:110–114, 1980.

100. Uehling Dt, Hussey JL, Weinstein AB, Wank R, Bach FH: Cessation of immunosuppression after renal transplantation. Surgery 79:278–282, 1976.

101. Hollander AAMJ, Hene RJ, Hermans J, Van Es LA, Van der Woude FJ: Late prednisone withdrawal in cyclosporine-treated kidney transplant patients: A randomized study. J Am Soc Nephrol 8:294–301, 1997.

102. Grinyo JM, Gil-Vernet S, Seron D, Cruzado JM, Moreso F, Fulladosa X, Castelao AM, Torras J, Hooftman L, Alsina J: Steroid withdrawal in mycophenolate mofetil-treated renal allograft recipients. Transplantation 63:1688–1690, 1997.

103. Kupin W, Venkat KK, Goggins M, Douzdjian V, Escobar F, Mozes M, Abouljoud M: Improved outcome of steroid withdrawal in mycophenolate Mofetil-treated primary cadaveric renal transplant recipients. Transplant Proc 31:1131–1132, 1999.

104. Schulak JA, Mayes JT, Moritz CE, Hricik DE: A prospective randomized trial of prednisone versus no prednisoone maintenance therapy in cyclosporine-treated and azathioprine-treated renal transplant patients. Transplantation 49:327–332, 1990.

105. Opelz G: Effect of the maintenance immunosuppressive drug regimen on kidney transplant outcome. Transplantation 58:443–446, 1994.

106. Ratcliffe PJ, Dudley CRK, Higgins RM, Firth JD, Smith B, Morris PJ: Randomized controlled trial of steroid withdrawal in renal transplant recipients receiving triple immunosuppression. Lancet 348:643–648, 1996.

107. St. Sinclair NR, Canadian Multicentre Transplant Study Group: Low-dose steroid therapy in cyclosporine-treated renal transplant recipients with well-functioning grafts. Can Med Assoc J 147:645–657, 1992.

108. Isoniemi HM, Ahonen J, Tikkanen MJ, von Willebrand EO, Krogerus L, Eklund BH, Hockerstedt KVA, Salmela KE, Hayry PJ: Long-term consequences of different immunosuppressive regimens for renal allografts. Transplantation 55:494–499, 1993.

109. Hall BM, Tiller DJ, Hardie I, Mahony J, Mathew T, Thatcher G, Miach P, Thomson N, Sheil AGR: Comparison of three immunosuppressive regimens in cadaver renal transplantation: Long-term cyclosporine, short-term cyclosporine followed by aza-thioprine and prednisolone, and azathioprine and prednisolone without cyclosporine. N Engl J Med 318:499–507, 1988.

110. Kasiske BL, Heim-Duthoy K, Ma JZ: Elective cyclosporine withdrawal after renal transplantation. A meta-analysis. JAMA 269:395–400, 1993.

111. Sanders CE, Curtis JJ, Julian BA, Gaston RS, Jones PA, Laskow DA, Deierhoi MH, Barber WH, Diethelm AG: Tapering or discontinuing cyclosporine for financial rea-sons—A single center experience. Am J Kidney Dis 21:9–15, 1993.

112. Sanders CE, Julian BA, Gaston RS, Deierhoi MH, Diethelm AG, Curtis JJ: Benefits of continued cyclosporine through an indigent drug program. Am J Kidney Dis 28:572–577, 1996.

113. Johnson EM, Canafax DM, Gillingham KJ, Humar A, Pandian K, Kerr SR, Najarian JS, Matas AJ: Effect of early cyclosporine levels on kidney allograft rejection. Clin Transplantation 11:552–557, 1997.

114. Almond PS, Matas A, Gillingham K, et al.: Risk factors for chronic rejection in renal allograft recipients. Transplantation 55:752–757, 1993.

115. Hricik DE: Withdrawal of immunosuppression: Implications for composite tissue allograft transplantation. Transplant Proc 30:2721–2723, 1998.

116. Rubin RH: Infectious disease complications of renal transplantation. Kidney Int 44: 221–236, 1993.

117. Penn I: Occurrence of cancers in immunosuppressed organ transplant recipients, in P.I. Terasaki and J.M. Cecka (eds), Clinical Transplants 1994. Los Angeles, UCLA Tissue Typing Laboratory, 1995, pp. 99–105.

118. Gaston RS, Curtis JJ: Hypertension following renal transplantation, in S.G. Massry and R.J. Glassock (eds), Textbook of Nephrology, Baltimore, Williams and Wilkins, Co., 1995, pp. 1694–1700.

119. Julian BA, Quarles LD, Niemann KMW: Musculoskeletal complications after renal transplantation: Pathogenesis and treatment. Am J Kidney Diseases 19:99–120, 1992.

120. Kobashigawa JA, Kasiske BL: Hyperlipidemia in solid organ transplantation. Transplantation 63:331–338, 1997.

Transplantation and Immunosuppressive Medications: Evolution of Medicare Policy Involving Transplantation and Immunosuppressive Medications— Past Developments and Future Directions

Robert S. Gaston, M.D.[*]

Medicare's policies for covering immunosuppressive drugs for recipients of renal and other solid organ transplants are unusual and often misinterpreted. They are unusual because they constitute one of the very few exceptions to Medicare's basic policy of excluding coverage of prescription drugs. This appendix reviews the history of Medicare coverage of both organ transplants and immunosuppressive drugs for transplant recipients. This review emphasizes the evolving relationship between technological advances and Medicare financing of transplantation. It also includes a section documenting the impact of Medicare policy on current beneficiaries, and, looking ahead, summarizes some possible future modifications.[†]

EVENTS IN THE EVOLUTION OF MEDICARE POLICY REGARDING TRANSPLANTATION

Medicare Policy and the Science of Transplantation: 1972

The 92nd Congress passed H.R.1 as section 299I of the Social Security Amendments of 1972 (PL 92-603).[1] This legislation created a new entitlement

---

[*]Associate Professor, Department of Medicine, Associate Professor, Department of Surgery, University of Alabama at Birmingham, Birmingham, Alabama.
[†]As the report of the IOM Committee on Extending Medicare Coverage was nearing completion and approaching public release, Congress was nearing action on a proposal to provide a limited extension of Medicare coverage of immunosuppressive drugs. The committee report provides a brief description but no additional analysis was possible.

for those (regardless of age) suffering from irreversible chronic kidney failure. Virtually all Americans, after a brief waiting period, would be eligible for Medicare benefits that included the costs of dialysis and/or renal transplantation. Senator Vance Hartke of Indiana, responding to the plight of those afflicted with the previously fatal disease of kidney failure, said, "How do we explain that the difference between life and death in this country is a matter of dollars?"[2] The legislation passed after 30 minutes discussion, part of a frenzy of legislative activity immediately preceding the 1972 election, and was signed by President Nixon on October 30. Proponents of the program were optimistic regarding costs, projected to be approximately $500 million annually to treat about 40,000 beneficiaries. This ultimately monumental miscalculation was but the first of many. Hartke also stated that, "Sixty percent of those on dialysis can return to work but require retraining and most of the remaining 40 percent need no retraining whatsoever."[2]

Subsection (f) of the bill authorized indefinite benefits for those remaining on dialysis, but terminated coverage for transplant recipients at 1 year following successful engraftment. At the time, it was generally accepted that for most end stage renal disease (ESRD) patients, chronic hemodialysis was the treatment of choice.[2,3] Only those patients fortunate enough to have a well-matched living donor might expect to derive greater benefit from transplantation than dialysis, a total of fewer than 500 patients nationally in 1972.[4] Receiving a cadaver kidney was associated with substantially greater mortality than remaining on dialysis, and only 40% of those transplanted maintained function 1 year later.[3,5]

In the early days of transplantation, a common assumption was that successfully engrafted patients were "cured," no longer subject to the unaffordable costs of maintenance dialysis therapy that had precipitated passage of the Social Security amendments in the first place. Some hoped that long-term allograft survival might be achieved without long-term immunosuppression.[6–8] However, seminal work in animals and early observations in humans during the 1960s established the necessity of ongoing immunosuppression to maintain stable allograft function.[9–13] Without chronic pharmacological immunosuppression, most grafts were lost to acute rejection, chronic rejection, or recurrent kidney disease.[14] The most commonly used immunosuppressants at the time were azathioprine and corticosteroids. Because these drugs were inexpensive, the cost of maintaining long-term allograft function was not an issue.[2,3,5,15] In 1974, transplantation accounted for 18% ($51 million) of total Medicare ESRD expenditures ($283 million).[1]

Medicare Policy and the Science of Transplantation: 1978

By 1978, 5 years after implementation of the Medicare ESRD program, the landscape had changed. The overall costs of the program had proved much greater than anticipated, having risen to an annual expenditure of $1 billion dollars to treat 47,000 ESRD patients (increased from 19,000 in 1974).[1] Projections that outlays might increase to $2.5 billion by 1985 and $4.5 billion by 1995 reflected fears that the program was "out of control."[2,16] The increased costs reflected substantial broadening of eligibility criteria for ESRD therapy.[2,17] It had become generally accepted that the Medicare ESRD program was essentially a dialysis entitlement, with transplant expenditures accounting for only nine percent of outlays.[1,18] Emerging experience indicated that the original hopes of rehabilitation were unlikely to be realized for chronic dialysis patients; over half of beneficiaries remained disabled.[2,15]

In response to these trends, the 95th Congress in 1978 modified the original ESRD legislation by passing PL 95-292, an act intended to control program costs, in part by allowing a more favorable reimbursement policy for the less expensive modalities of home dialysis and transplantation.[5] This legislation, among other provisions, extended time limits on Medicare benefits after kidney transplantation from 1 to 3 years but did not address the need for outpatient drugs.[1,19] Implicit in these modifications was the changing clinical perception that transplant recipients did indeed require ongoing care to ensure allograft function; transplant as "cure" was a fading notion.

Between 1974 and 1978, there had been only minor changes in the clinical practice of transplantation. The number of transplants performed annually grew slowly, from 3,000 to about 4,000, with the majority (80%) originating in cadaver donors and imparting 1- and 3-year graft survival of 54% and 42%, respectively.[20,21] However, the most notable change was an increase in patient survival for recipients of cadaver kidneys. Graft failure no longer equated with death.[4] Nonetheless, absent a living-related donor, an ESRD patient remained statistically better off on chronic dialysis.[2,15-17]

Medicare Policy and the Science of Transplantation: 1984–1986

By the mid 1980s, the Medicare ESRD program was again changing dramatically, particularly as regards transplantation. Medicare ESRD expenditures had increased to $2.1 billion (less than had been predicted 6 years earlier, and in constant 1974 dollars to $1 billion). There was a 300% increase in outlay for a 600% increase in patients covered, as per patient costs of therapy actually declined, even in the face of an ever older population of ESRD beneficiaries.[17,19] Transplant expenditures remained relatively small, accounting for only 6% of total Medicare ESRD outlays.

In previous years, there had been slow but steady improvement in graft survival for transplant recipients, but changes in immunosuppressive therapy in the mid-1980s revolutionized the field. Cyclosporine, first tested in humans in 1976, was approved for general use by the United States Food and Drug Administration in late 1983.[22,23] Graft survival improved: 75 percent of recipients of cadaver kidneys could now expect to have functioning allografts after 1 year.[20] In addition, cyclosporine use was accompanied by a dramatic decline in the morbidity associated with transplantation. This fact, in conjunction with improved clinical management of coexisting conditions, resulted in a corresponding increase in patient survival at 1 year, which rose significantly above the 90% level.[24-26]

These advances led to at least two dramatic changes regarding perceptions of transplantation. First, both cadaver- and live-donor transplantation could now be performed with sufficient hopes of success that, in terms of both patient outcome and cost, renal transplantation was now the optimal therapy for end stage renal disease.[21] The interests of both patient and government would be best served by promoting transplantation as much as possible vis-a-vis dialysis. For the first time, it became obvious that the availability of cadaver organs would become the key factor limiting access to transplantation.[19] Second, the relationship between adequate maintenance immunosuppression and a successful transplant was now well-enough established, and the cost of cyclosporine sufficiently high, to make access to immunosuppressants an issue.[19,27] Both were addressed by legislation passed in the mid-1980s. The National Organ Transplant Act of 1984 (PL 98-507) authorized:

- creation of a National Task Force on Organ Transplantation,
- assistance to organ procurement organizations,
- establishment of the Organ Procurement and Transplantation Network (OPTN), and
- creation of a scientific registry for organ transplantation.

In addition, provisions in the Omnibus Budget Reconciliation Act of 1986 (PL 99-509) authorized payment for immunosuppressive medications for 1 year after a Medicare-covered renal transplant, at least partially in response to the high cost of cyclosporine.

The final important change of the mid-1980s regarding Medicare and transplantation resulted from the increasing success noted in extrarenal transplantation after the advent of cyclosporine-based immunosuppression. In a series of policy changes occurring between 1986 and 1991, Medicare authorized coverage of cardiac and hepatic transplantation in beneficiaries, with immunosuppressant coverage subject to the same 1-year limitations as in the ESRD program.[28] However, unlike coverage for ESRD patients, these benefits were available only to patients who qualified for Medicare by reason of age or disability.

Medicare Policy and the Science of Transplantation: 1994

In the early 1990s, with broadening clinical experience and the introduction of new technologies, transplantation became even more successful. For recipients of cadaveric renal transplants, 80–85% graft survival at 1 year became the norm, and patient survival continued to rise well in excess of 95%, even as the procedure was offered to older and more complicated patients.[27] Outcomes for recipients of live-donor kidneys were also incrementally better.[29] These short-term improvements made long-term graft survival an increasingly important issue. Three-year cadaver graft survival for transplants performed in the early 1990s now approached 75% (in excess of what had been expected at 1 year only a decade earlier).[27] Even cadaveric transplantation was now clearly associated with improved longevity relative to dialysis.[30]

During this time, the cost-effectiveness of transplantation relative to dialysis became better defined. Transplantation accounted for 12% of Medicare ESRD outlays between 1991 and 1993, but annual costs per patient were roughly 40% of those associated with maintenance dialysis.[31] In an insightful analysis of transplants performed between 1987 and 1990, Paul Eggers of the Health Care Financing Administration (HCFA) noted that the high first-year costs of transplantation were recovered by Medicare within 4.9 years for recipients of cadaver kidneys, and even sooner (4 years) if the organ originated in a live donor.[32]

In the Omnibus Budget Reconciliation Act (OBRA) of 1987, Congress asked the Institute of Medicine (IOM) to evaluate the entire Medicare ESRD program. Subsequently, in a comprehensive analysis of ESRD in the United States, the IOM committee reaffirmed the benefits of renal transplantation, while acknowledging the financial burden even a successful transplant imposed on recipients in terms of need for lifelong medical supervision and pharmacologicaltherapy.[19] In its final report, published in 1991, the committee recommended that:

> . . . Congress eliminate the three-year Medicare eligibility limit for successful transplant patients and thereby authorize a lifetime entitlement comparable to that of dialysis patients. . . .

and that

> . . . coverage for payment of immunosuppressive medications for kidney transplant patients be made coterminous with the period of entitlement.[19]

Contemporaneously, the Senate Finance Committee asked the Office of Technology Assessment to address Medicare coverage of immunosuppressants.[33] The resulting document focused more closely on the issue of immunosuppressant coverage for all transplanted Medicare beneficiaries, without specifically endorsing any of several possible options for expansion. Despite strong support from the transplant community and patient advocacy groups for the IOM recommendations, the 102nd Congress in 1992 chose an intermediate approach.

They authorized a phased-in extension of the time limit for immunosuppressive drug coverage from 1 to 3 years posttransplant. They did not address extension of overall Medicare eligibility for kidney transplant recipients beyond the 3-year limit.

Thus, over a 27-year period, Medicare reimbursement policies and clinical transplantation evolved in tandem, with the government adjusting policy to address both the evolving clinical practice of transplantation and the changing needs of Medicare beneficiaries. Through these efforts, renal transplantation became available to virtually every American with ESRD via access to Medicare entitlements that continue for 3 years after the procedure. Renal transplants account for the majority of transplants and the majority of Medicare transplant spending. Extrarenal transplantation is also now covered, but only for those who were otherwise Medicare eligible. For all these beneficiaries, provision of immunosuppressive therapy is guaranteed for 3 years after transplant. As they were adopted, these policies represented a reasonable response to the realities of clinical transplantation. Even well into the 1990s, the focus was on the early posttransplant period, attempting to ensure successful engraftment of the transplanted organ.

Recent clinical and scientific advances (as described in Appendix D, Part 1) have made the inpatient components of care amazingly routine and highly successful. In pursuing the new goal of long-term graft survival (see Box D-1), the ultimate fate of the allograft is increasingly dependent on what happens beyond the early posttransplant period.

IMPACT OF CURRENT POLICIES ON MEDICARE BENEFICIARIES

As the committee considers the expected effectiveness and cost of expanding Medicare coverage, it seems helpful to review current payment options and their impact on transplant recipients.[‡] As previously noted (see Appendix D Part 1), maintaining an allograft requires ongoing access to medical care and pharmacological immunosuppression beyond the 3 years covered by Medicare. For some impoverished patients, Medicaid assistance may provide the necessary coverage for both services and drugs, although income eligibility requirements and payment restrictions vary by state.[47] For other transplant recipients, financial coverage for posttransplant care is a responsibility shared among private insurers, specifically developed state and pharmaceutical company programs, and individual patients and their families. Because the ongoing expenses of transplantation far exceed what most individuals can afford (with maintenance drug

---

[‡]The assistance of Cheryl Jacobs, Fairview University Transplant Services, Minneapolis, in preparing this discussion is gratefully acknowledged.

BOX D-1 Impact of Long-Term Transplant Survival

What does long-term graft survival mean to patients?

For recipients of hearts and livers, it means life itself.
For recipients of kidneys, it means:

• *Avoiding dialysis.*
"Persons who need continuing chronic dialysis may survive for years, but chances of significant rehabilitation are limited."[34]
• *Returning to work.*
The employment rate of transplant recipients is roughly twice that of demographically matched dialysis patients.[35–39]
• *Improved quality of life.*
Life on dialysis is, to put it mildly, onerous; to exist is possible, to thrive unusual, and to prosper almost unheard of.[40] Marcia Campbell Marden described her life on dialysis:

"A year ago I would not let you see me without mascara. Today you can view me three times a week without my pride. . . . I am dry, and always, always thirsty. . . . I smell old and sick. And even Shalimar cannot cover the odor of dialysate. . . I am afraid. . . . I am determined to escape this. I will not forget and I will not return."[41]

• *Avoiding retransplantation and an ever-lengthier waiting list.*
ESRD patients with failed grafts often ask to quickly be relisted for transplantation, but organ scarcity makes retransplantation less and less likely.[42]

What does long-term graft survival mean to payers?

For heart and liver transplants it means an ongoing commitment to ensure the heavy initial investment in the transplant procedure (often approaching $200,000) translates into the desired benefit.
For kidney transplants it means cost-savings relative to dialysis or retransplantation.

Most renal transplant candidates receive chronic dialysis, at a cost of $47,000 per patient/year. Although expenses in the transplant year average $92,000, lower costs associated with maintaining graft function result in net cost savings for individual recipients whose grafts function beyond 3 years.[43]

Continued

BOX D-1 *Continued*

What does long-term graft survival mean to physicians?

It means better patient outcomes, with reduction in morbidity and mortality relative to all other therapies.[44-46]

What does long-term graft survival mean to society?

It means preserving and protecting the transplanted organ, a very valuable resource. Given the scarcity of available organs, the length of waiting lists, and the patients who die awaiting transplantation, the donated organ is priceless.

It means honoring the sacrifice of families who have donated the organs of a loved one, confident that these organs will receive optimal care.

---

charges in excess of federal poverty guidelines for a family of two persons), financing has evolved into a creative dance among interested parties.

Current Medicare policies impose a substantial burden on a group of beneficiaries already heavily afflicted. For many recipients, these circumstances lead to what Lesley Sharp has called the "survival paradox": devoting the entirety of one's energies to a desperate battle for medical survival against enormous financial obstacles.[48,49]

For patients with cardiac or hepatic failure, transplantation is financed on the framework of preexisting coverage. For a Medicare beneficiary, cost of the procedure and 80 percent of immunosuppressant costs are covered expenses, subject to the usual deductible and copay requirements. However, fewer than 5% of heart and liver recipients are over 65 years of age.[50] Thus, many solid organ recipients establish Medicare coverage by qualifying for disability benefits during the illness preceding transplantation.[47] At times, the transplant occurs before a patient has established Medicare eligibility; the care is often provided gratis by the transplant center or paid by state Medicaid funds, with Medicare eligibility established during the posttransplant phase (personal communication, L. Lockett, University of Alabama at Birmingham). Benefits continue as long as the patient retains eligibility, except that coverage for immunosuppressive drugs ends 3 years after hospital discharge following the transplant.

Under current policies, Medicare reimburses approximately 24% of expenditures for extrarenal transplantation. Medicaid reimburses approximately 18%, and 58% comes from other sources.[51]

For patients with kidney failure, the system is more complex. First, ESRD is a disease most common in patients of lower socioeconomic status, often evolving on a background of inadequate care for glomerular disease, chronic infection, and hypertension. Thus, a large proportion of ESRD patients come to renal transplantation without any private insurance coverage. When patients begin ESRD therapy, regardless of age and including consideration of employment history, they become eligible for Medicare. For home dialysis or transplantation, coverage begins immediately, rewarding those choosing these less expensive therapies. For in-center dialysis, there is a 90-day waiting period before coverage is effective. If there is preexisting group health insurance, it remains primary for 30 months, with Medicare as secondary payer (paying for some expenses not paid by the group health plan). Medicare remains in force for the duration of dialysis therapy. Since dialysis confers almost certain eligibility for disability, most Medicare ESRD patients also receive Social Security disability benefits. If an ESRD Medicare beneficiary receives a transplant, coverage for medical care and immunosuppressive drugs continues for 3 years after transplantation, then ceases until the beneficiary establishes eligibility by reason of age or disability other than by ESRD status alone. In 1997, private insurance absorbed 29%, Medicaid 13%, and Medicare fully 58% of the overall costs of renal transplantation in the United States.[51]

As a transplant recipient progresses from short-term to long-term survivorship, the social worker, through whom comes knowledge and access to other resources, often becomes the key facilitator of Medicare, Medicaid, or other payment for services. Some centers have even hired "transplant financial coordinators" with the explicit task of helping patients navigate coverage complexities.[47,52] For ESRD beneficiaries of Medicare, the first challenge after coverage expires is dealing with the cost of physician visits, laboratory tests, and hospitalizations when necessary. One recipient noted,

> We're told, "Return to work to pay back your debt to society," and "Productivity is important.". . . You see, the doctors think we're cured. But we're not cured . . . we're seen as unreliable employees, and health insurance companies redline transplant patients. If they hire you they may refuse to let you join the health plan.[49]

An approach frequently chosen is to maintain or establish disabled status by whatever means necessary, although the specific number doing so solely to maintain Medicare coverage is unknown. As of December 31, 1995, there were 72,785 persons with a functioning kidney transplant, 38 percent of whom were disabled and continued to receive Medicare entitlements on that basis.[53] Many also receive Supplemental Security Income (SSI) and maintain Medicaid eligibility as well. In the current system, working enough to generate minimal income threatens all these benefits, a strong factor discouraging return to the workforce. The experience of many transplant social workers is that, due primarily to the high cost of health insurance, most small businesses and even many large corporations are reluctant to hire a transplant recipient, further discouraging return to work.

Eggers noted that, at the end of 1995, 26 percent of renal allograft recipients with functioning transplants had lost Medicare benefits due to time limitations on coverage.[53] Although the exact number is uncertain, as many as half of these patients face the daunting costs of posttransplant care beyond 3 years with no Medicaid or private insurance resources.

Having effectively negotiated some continued access to a medical provider, the next challenge for a recipient is ensuring an adequate supply of the immuno-suppressive drugs essential to sustaining long-term allograft function. Average retail costs for these drugs for most patients are between $7,000 and $14,000 annually, an amount greater than an average homeowner spends on mortgage payments.[48] In addition, many recipients are faced with the continued expenses for other drugs (which Medicare had not covered in the first place). Eighty per-cent require antihypertensive therapy, and many require care for hyperlipidemia and other comorbid conditions.[54,55]

Coping with these challenges requires efforts on the part of patients and providers to find alternatives to Medicare coverage. Even though Medicaid usu-ally covers immunosuppressive drug expenses, income limits for eligibility vary widely from state to state, and some states impose prescription limits. Twenty-eight states have high-risk insurance pools, again with varying eligibility, pre-mium, and coverage provisions. Twenty-eight also have financed State Kidney Programs, although only 19 of these programs assist with anti-rejection medica-tion costs.[47] For the recipient who does not have access to any of these programs (estimated by the Congressional Budget Office to represent 10% of all transplant recipients in 1996), payment options are limited.[56] These include paying out-of-pocket or seeking free medications by filing applications for indigent care from each individual pharmaceutical company. Applying directly to pharmaceutical companies for assistance is an onerous task made more complicated by the varying requirements imposed by each firm. Patient support groups, assisted at times by medical professionals, often become forums for illegal bartering of medications as the only way to acquire necessary drugs.[49]

For those patients who are unable to successfully negotiate these burden-some options and are unable to obtain needed drugs, the consequence at some point will be rejection and graft loss due to noncompliance. A recent survey found that 35% of Medicare-HMO patients, when faced with loss of drug cover-age, either reduced or discontinued their medications.[57] Most studies of non-compliance among renal transplant recipients find rates approximating 20%, with graft loss in perhaps 30–40% of those.[58–60] With recent dramatic reductions in acute rejection, and more transplanted organs surviving for longer periods of time, graft losses to noncompliance have become more visible. Given the in-creasing dependence of successful outcomes on advances in immunosuppressive therapy (see Appendix D Part 1), such losses have the potential to become more frequent as well.

Multicenter registries have not reliably collected data regarding noncompliance.[61] In some single center reports, noncompliance may be the most common cause of graft loss beyond the first posttransplant year.[60,62–64] Unfortunately, factors leading to noncompliance and the degree of noncompliance necessary to result in graft loss are highly variable, and the relative impact of financial limitations on outcome is uncertain.[65,66] Nonetheless, limited evidence and experience indicate that at least some portion of noncompliant behavior is attributable to recipients' inability to procure appropriate medication when Medicare coverage ends and no alternative resources are secured. Based on limited studies reviewed below and documented renal graft losses of 6% per year after the first year with somewhat higher loss rates for other organs, it is reasonable to estimate that perhaps a third to half of graft losses might reflect lack of financial access to immunosuppressive drugs.[46,60,70] Thus, ongoing provision of immunosuppressive drugs might save 2–3% of all grafts at risk each year.

Several investigators found low socioeconomic status to predict poorer long-term outcomes in renal transplantation.[64,67–69] At least two groups of investigators have found significant benefit to ongoing provision of immunosuppressant drugs for such patients. In the previously noted studies of Sanders and colleagues, a cohort of recipients whose Medicare benefits expired a year after transplantation was at significant risk of late rejection and graft loss after stopping cyclosporine.[69] When similar patients were furnished with maintenance cyclosporine via an indigent drug program, graft survival differences compared to a fully insured group of recipients disappeared.[71] In a recently completed study, Woodward and coworkers compared renal allograft survival at 1 and 3 years after transplant in two time periods, stratified by median family income for each patient's ZIP code.[70] For those transplanted in 1992–1993, when Medicare covered immunosuppressants for 1 year after transplantation, the researchers found no difference in graft survival at 1 year among recipients in different quartiles of income. By 3 years, however, transplant recipients in lower income groups had significantly lower graft survival (77 vs. 72%, $p < 0.001$). In contrast, since 1995, after 3 years of coverage had been completely phased in, differences in graft survival at 3 years by income grouping had disappeared (80% vs. 78%, p = n.s.), implying that ongoing access to medications made a significant impact on outcome for lower- and middle-income recipients.

POTENTIAL MODIFICATIONS TO THE MEDICARE PROGRAM

In 1972, Congress addressed the issue of ESRD care with the intention "to provide access to life-saving therapy for all who needed it where the costs of treatment were beyond the means of practically all individuals."[1] In the 1991 IOM report, it was noted that the Congress, via PL 95-292 in 1978, the National Organ Transplant Act of 1984, OBRA 1986, and the Transplant Amendments

Act of 1990, had consistently encouraged organ transplantation.[19] In the face of increasingly successful outcomes, and given that Medicare had made the commitment to fund the transplant procedure itself (with its substantial outlays during the first year), the previous committee saw no scientific basis supporting termination of access to care and immunosuppressant drugs at an arbitrarily defined time. They recognized that renal transplant recipients were not "cured," and that ongoing care was as essential to survival as the thrice-weekly dialysis treatments for non-transplanted ESRD patients. Now, almost a decade later, rapid advances in the science of transplantation have made current policy even less consistent with the original congressional intentions. As the issue of long-term care for Medicare-covered transplant recipients is revisited, what changes might restore equilibrium between policy and practice?

Option A: Indefinite Benefits for ESRD Recipients with Coterminous Immunosuppressant Coverage for All Other Medicare Beneficiaries

In 1991, the Institute of Medicine committee recommended:

> "that Congress eliminate the three-year limit on Medicare eligibility for ESRD patients who are successful transplant recipients and authorize an entitlement equal to that of ESRD patients who are treated by dialysis," and "that coverage of immunosuppressive medications for kidney transplant patients be made coterminous with the period of a patient's entitlement."[19]

This option would place renal transplant recipients on the same footing as ESRD patients receiving dialysis. Such a policy (especially if it came with no Medicare secondary payer requirements) would facilitate those able to return to the workforce doing so and would relieve potential employers of the burden of providing health insurance for this high-cost group. In the 1991 report, potential costs for such an approach, to include those recipients who had already lost benefits, was estimated to be $415 million–$500 million annually for 55,000 renal transplant beneficiaries by 1995.[19] Costs for indefinite immunosuppressant coverage alone were projected to have reached approximately $300 million annually by 1995. These cost estimates did not address any potential offsets, which might include the cost of graft failure and retransplantation due to noncompliance, reduced disability benefits, and reduction of Medicaid spending for those eligible for both Medicare and Medicaid.

The IOM recommendation also did not address coverage for extrarenal allograft recipients. In 1989–1991, Medicare covered such a small percentage of extrarenal transplants that these costs were not an issue. Since then, the number of such beneficiaries has grown.

The response of the Congress to the IOM report (as well as the concurrently prepared OTA report) was to extend coverage gradually for immunosuppressants from 1 year to 3 years, making immunosuppressive drug coverage and other Medicare benefits coterminous for renal transplant recipients.[19,33] Extrarenal transplant recipients saw their immunosuppressant coverage extended to 3 years as well.

In 1999, due to scientific and clinical advances, more recipients and allografts are surviving beyond 3 years. Even though the great majority of Medicare beneficiaries with transplants are renal recipients, needs of those with extrarenal grafts must be addressed as well.

Option B: Removing Limits on Immunosuppressant Coverage for Medicare Beneficiaries—H.R. 1115

H.R. 1115 was introduced in the 106th Congress on March 16, 1999, by Representatives Charles Canady and Karen Thurman of Florida, with 73 cosponsors. In essence, this bill would remove the 3-year limit on immunosuppressant coverage for all Medicare beneficiaries, without addressing the issue of loss of benefits at 3 years for ESRD recipients who do not qualify for Medicare by reason of age or disability. In 1996, the Congressional Budget Office projected Medicare costs for a similar proposal, which also did not address extension of other Medicare benefits for this group. The CBO projected savings of $166 million annually by reducing late graft loss; by 2002, these savings would mostly offset the additional $210 million to be spent on drugs, resulting in a projected net Medicare outlay of $44 million annually.[56] Total Medicare ESRD expenditures were projected to rise by less than 1% annually as a result of such a change.[46,56] Still, the quarter of renal allograft recipients who do not qualify for Medicare by reason of age or disability would continue to lose all benefits at 3 years and would have an even greater incentive to qualify for disability benefits and, thus, for Medicare. Given the original intent of the 1972 Social Security amendments to facilitate return of beneficiaries to productive life, the consequences of this legislation would appear to be counterproductive.

Option C: Creating a New Class of Medicare Beneficiary—S. 631

This legislation (the Immunosuppressive Drug Coverage Act of 1999) was introduced in the Senate by Senator Mike DeWine of Ohio, also on March 16, with six cosponsors. Like its House counterpart, it would remove the 3-year cap on immunosuppressant coverage for Medicare beneficiaries, while extending Medicare secondary payer requirements to shift some costs of long-term benefits to private insurers. Under the provisions of this legislative effort, all recipients whose transplant was financed by Medicare would receive immunosuppressive drug coverage for the life of the allograft, even after other Medicare entitlements were terminated.

The expected benefits of this proposal would be indefinite drug coverage for Medicare-eligible transplant recipients, ensuring access to necessary immunosuppressive support for the life of the allograft and reducing graft losses to financially related noncompliance. Incentives to remain disabled would be less than with H.R.1115, although the effect of this bill's secondary payer requirements is uncertain. Costs, as estimated by the Lewin Group, would be significantly greater than the House version but still less than 2% of the Medicare ESRD budget, and less than 20% of the annual costs of erythropoietin for dialysis beneficiaries.[72] A potential negative would be the vagaries of servicing a new class of beneficiaries not entitled to other Medicare benefits. These beneficiaries would thus not have Medicare coverage of visits to physicians/transplant centers for monitoring and other posttransplant care. Participating physicians would be placed in the unusual circumstance of supervising toxic immunosuppressive drugs without Medicare payment for blood monitoring or other care.

Option D: Other Potential Solutions and Modifiers

Several other initiatives and/or proposals might help transplant recipients pay for ongoing immunosuppressive therapy. Proposals to cover prescription drugs for all Medicare beneficiaries could help. However, circulating drafts of current proposals indicate an annual cap on benefits ($1,500–$2,000 per patient), which is far below the average cost of immunosuppressive drug regimens for transplant recipients (see Appendix D, Part 1).

At least two other options might be considered, both of which would offer Medicare benefits to all extrarenal transplant recipients, even if the transplant was not covered by Medicare. A first option would make virtually all solid organ transplant recipients eligible (with a suitable work history, regardless of age or disability status) for full Medicare benefits to include uninterrupted immunosuppressant drug costs. The second option would extend coverage only for immunosuppressive drugs for transplant recipients whose transplant was not covered by Medicare, as described in the OTA Report of 1991.[33] The potential drawback to either approach, apart from cost, is the absence of precedent for extending Medicare benefits to patients not otherwise eligible by reason of age, disability, or ESRD status.

In order to attenuate the financial costs of adopting one (or more) of the above options, several modifying provisions might be considered. First, the new benefit might be phased in gradually for new transplant recipients only. Second, a Medicare immunosuppressive benefit might remain secondary to group health coverage available to a recipient. Third, a financial "cap" on immunosuppressive drug coverage beyond 3 years might limit costs while ensuring access to medications for transplanted beneficiaries. For example, a limit of $8,000 per year (plus a 20% copay) would easily cover a year of therapy with a combination of tacrolimus, mycophenolate mofetil, and steroids for an averaged-sized person.

Given current knowledge, the least expensive maintenance protocol acceptable to most transplant physicians would include generic cyclosporine, azathioprine, and steroids, at a cost to Medicare of less than $5,000 per annum. The absolute amount of such a cap might be reevaluated on a year-to-year basis.

REFERENCES

1. Rettig RA, Marks EL: Implementing the end-stage renal disease program of Medicare (Rep. R-2505-HCFA/HEW). Santa Monica, California, the RAND Corporation, 1980.
2. Kolata BB: Dialysis after nearly a decade. Science 208:473–476, 1980.
3. Friedman EA, Kountz SL: Impact of HR-1 on the therapy of end-stage uremia: How and where should uremia be treated? N Engl J Med 288:1286–1288, 1973.
4. The 13th Report of the Human Renal Transplant Registry. Transplant Proc 9:9–26, 1977.
5. Stange PV, Sumner AT: Predicting treatment costs and life expectancy for end-stage renal disease. N Engl J Med 298:372–378, 1978.
6. Starzl TE: Experience in renal transplantation. Philadelphia, WB Saunders Co., 1964.
7. Hume DM: Kidney transplantation, in Human Transplantation, New York, Grune and Stratton, 1968, pp. 110–150.
8. Hume D, Merrill JP, Miller BF, Thorn GW: Experiences with renal homotransplantation in the human: Report of nine cases. J Clin Invest 34:327, 1955.
9. Alexandre GPJ, Murray JE, Dammin GJ, Nolan B: Immunosuppressive drug therapy in canine renal and skin homografts. Transplantation 1:432–461, 1963.
10. Calne RY, Alexandre GPJ, Murray JE: A study of the effects of drugs in prolonging survival of homologous renal transplants in dogs. Ann NY Acad Sci 99:1962.
11. Diethelm AG, Dubernard JM, Busch GJ, Murray JE: Critical re-evaluation of immunosuppressive therapy in canine renal allografts. Surg Gynecol Obstet 126:723–736, 1968.
12. Murray JE, Merrill JP, Harrison JH, Wilson RE, Dammin GJ: Prolonged survival of human-kidney homografts by immunosuppressive drug therapy. N Engl J Med 268:1315–1323, 1963.
13. Starzl TE, Marchioro TL, Waddell WR: The reversal of rejection in human renal homografts with subsequent development of homograft tolerance. Surg Gynecol Obstet 117:385, 1963.
14. Porter KA: Pathological changes in transplanted kidneys, in T. E. Starzl (ed), Experience in renal transplantation, Philadelphia, WB Saunders Co., 1964, pp. 299–359.
15. Friedman Ea, Delano BG, Butt KMH: Pragmatic realities in uremia therapy. N Engl J Med 298:368–371, 1978.
16. Rennie D: Home dialysis and the costs of uremia. N Engl J Med 298:399–400, 1978
17. Rosansky SJ, Eggers PW: Trends in the U.S. end-stage renal disease population: 1973–1983. Am J Kidney Dis 9:91–97, 1987.
18. Eggers PW: Health care policies/Economics of the geriatric renal population. Am J Kidney Dis 16:384–391, 1990.

19. Institute of Medicine. Kidney failure and the federal government. Washington, D.C., National Academy Press, 1991.
20. Cook DJ: Long-term survival of kidney allografts, in P. I. Terasaki (ed), Clinical Transplants 1987, Los Angeles, UCLA Tissue Typing Laboratory, 1987, pp. 277–285.
21. Eggers PW: Effect of transplantation on the Medicare end-stage renal disease program. N Engl J Med 318:223–229, 1988.
22. Calne RY, Rolles K, White DJG, et al.: Cyclosporin A initially as the only immunosuppressant in 34 recipients of cadaveric organs: 32 kidneys, 2 pancreases and 2 livers. Lancet ii:1033–1036, 1979.
23. Powe NR, Eggers PW, Johnson CB: Early adoption of cyclosporine and recombinant human erythropoeitin: Clinical, economic, and policy issues with emergence of high-cost drugs. Am J Kidney Dis 24:33–41, 1994.
24. Cho YW, Terasaki PI, Graver B: Fifteen-year kidney graft survival, in P. I. Terasaki (ed), Clinical Transplants 1989, Los Angeles, UCLA Tissue Typing Laboratory, 1989, pp. 325–334.
25. Hill MN, Grossman RA, Feldman HI, Hurwitz S, Dafoe DC: Changes in causes of death after renal transplantation, 1966 to 1987. Am J Kidney Dis 17:512–518, 1991.
26. Mickey MR: Kidney transplant mortality relationships, in P. I. Terasaki (ed), Clinical Transplants 1988, Los Angeles, UCLA Tissue Typing Laboratory, 1988, pp. 263–276.
27. Cecka JM, Terasaki PI: The UNOS Scientific Renal Transplant Registry, in J. M. Cecka and P. I. Terasaki (ed), Clinical Transplants 1995, Los Angeles, UCLA Tissue Typing Laboratory, 1996, pp. 1–18.
28. HCFA: Web Site www.hcfa.gov. 1999.
29. Ojo A, Port FK: Influence of race and gender on related donor renal transplantation rates. Am J Kidney Dis 22:835–841, 1993.
30. Cecka JM: The UNOS Scientific Renal Transplant Registry, in J. M. Cecka and P. I. Terasaki (ed), Clinical Transplants 1996, Los Angeles, UCLA Tissue Typing Laboratory, 1997, pp. 1–14.
31. UNOS (United Network for Organ Sharing): 1996 Annual Report of the U.S. Scientific Registry for Transplant Recipients in the Organ Procurement and Transplantation Network: DHHS/HRSA, Richmond, Virginia, UNOS, 1996.
32. Eggers PW: Comparison of treatment costs between dialysis and transplantation. Semin Nephrol 12:284–289, 1992.
33. U.S. Congress, Office of Technology Assessment: Outpatient immunosuppressive drugs under Medicare, OTA-H-452, Washington, D.C., U.S. Government Printing Office, 1991.
34. Tobe SW, Senn JS: Foregoing renal dialysis: A case study and review of ethical issues. Am J Kidney Dis 28:147–153, 1996.
35. Holley JL, Nespor S: An analysis of factors affecting employment of chronic dialysis patients. Am J Kidney Dis 23(5):681–685, 1994.
36. Ifudu O, Paul H, Mayers JD, Cohen LS, Brezsnyak WF, Herman AI, Avram MM, Friedman EA: Pervasive failed rehabilitation in center-based maintenance hemodialysis patients. Am J Kidney Dis 23:394–400, 1994.
37. Manninen DL, Evans RW, Dugan MK: Work disability, functinal limitations, and the health status of kidney transplantation recipients posttransplant, in P. I. Terasaki

and J. M. Cecka (ed), Clinical Transplants 1991, Los Angeles, UCLA Tissue Typing Laboratory, 1992, pp. 193–203.

38. Markell MS, DiBenedetto A, Maursky V, Sumrani N, Hong JH, Distant DA, Miles A-MV, Sommer BG, Friedman EA: Unemployment in inner-city renal transplant recipients: Predictive and sociodemographic factors. Am J Kidney Dis 29:881–887, 1997.

39. Matas AJ, Lawson W, McHugh L, Gillingham K, Payne WD, Dunn DL, Gruessner RWG, Sutherland DER, Najarian JS: Employment patterns after successful kidney transplantation. Transplantation 6a:729–733, 1996.

40. Laupacis A, Keown P, Pus N, Krueger H, Ferguson B, Wong C, Muirhead N: A study of the quality of life and cost-utility of renal transplantation. Kidney Int 50:235–242, 1996.

41. Marden MC: Kidney chronicles. Am J Kidney Dis 25:967–970, 1995.

42. Ojo AO, Wolfe RA, Agodoa LY, Held PJ, Port FK, Leavey SF, Callard SE, Dickinson DM, Schmouder RL, Leichtman AB: Prognosis after primary renal transplant failure and the beneficial effects of repeat transplantation: Multivariate analyses from the United States Renal Data System. Transplantation 66:1651–1659, 1998.

43. Eggers P, Milam R: Cost comparison of dialysis and transplantation, in Immunosuppression Conference in Organ Transplantation: Patient Access to Long-Term Care, Philadelphia, 1998.

44. Belle SH, Beringer KC, Detre KM: Recent findings concerning liver transplantation in the United States, in J. M. Cecka and P. I. Terasaki (ed), Clinical Transplants 1996, Los Angeles, UCLA Tissue Typing Laboratory, 1997, pp. 15–29.

45. Keck BM, Bennett LE, Fiol BS, Daily OP, Novick RJ, Hosenpud JD: Worldwide thoracic organ transplantation: A report from the UNOS/ISHLT International Registry for Thoracic Organ Transplantation, in J. M. Cecka and P. I. Terasaki (ed), Clinical Transplants 1997, Los Angeles, UCLA Tissue Typing Laboratory, 1997, pp. 31–45.

46. United States Renal Data System: Excerpts from USRDS 1998 Annual Data Report. Am J Kidney Dis 32(Suppl 1):S1–S162, 1998.

47. Jacobs C: Current national coverage of immunosuppression medication, in (ed), Immunosuppression Conference in Organ Transplantation: Patient Access to Long-Term Care, Philadelphia, 1998.

48. Sharp LA: A medical anthropologist's view on posttransplant compliance: The underground economy of medical survival. Transplant Proceedings 31(Suppl 4A):31S–33S, 1999.

49. Sharp LA: Organ transplantation as a transformative experience: Anthropological insights into the restructuring of the self. Medical Anthropology Quarterly 9:357–389, 1995.

50. UNOS (United Network for Organ Sharing): 1997 Annual Report of the U.S. Scientific Registry for Transplant Recipients in the Organ Procurement and Transplantation Network: DHHS/HRSA, Richmond, Virginia, UNOS, 1997.

51. Gorman K: The cost of immunosuppression and non-adherence, in Immunosuppression Conference in Organ Transplantation: Patient Access to Long-Term Care, Philadelphia, 1998.

52. Aguiar LJ: Role of the transplant financial coordinator and its effect on recipient compliance. Transplantation Proceedings 31(Suppl 4A):55S–56S, 1999.

53. Eggers PW: Memo-Functioning graft patients in the Medicare ESRD population. 1997.

54. Gaston RS, Curtis JJ: Hypertension following renal transplantation, in S. G. Massry and R. J. Glassock (ed), Textbook of Nephrology, Baltimore, Williams and Wilkins, Co., 1995, pp. 1694–1700.

55. Kobashigawa JA, Kasiske BL: Hyperlipidemia in solid organ transplantation. Transplantation 63:331–338, 1997.

56. Congressional Budget Office: Cost estimate-elimination of time limitation on Medicare benefits for immunosuppressive drugs, Letter dated July 3, 1996, from June O'Neill to Charles T. Canady, 1996.

57. Jernigan CL, Cox ER, Coons SJ, Draugalis JR: Medicare beneficiaries management of capped prescription benefits (abstract), in Academy of Managed Care Pharmacists, 1999.

58. Kory L: Nonadherence to immunosuppressive medications: A pilot survey of members of TRIO. Transplantation Proceedings 31(Suppl 4A):14S–15S, 1999.

59. Nevins T, Thomas W, Skeans M, Matas A: Medication compliance following renal transplantation: The natural history (abstract). Transplantation 67:S115, 1999.

60. Gaston RS, Hudson SL, Ward M, Jones P, Macon R: Late renal allograft loss: Noncompliance masquerading as chronic rejection. Transplant Proc 31(Suppl 4A):21S–23S, 1999.

61. Isaacs RB, Conners A, Nock S, Spencer C, Lobo P: Noncompliance in living-related donor renal transplantation: The UNOS experience. Transplantation Proceedings 31(Suppl 4A):19S–20S, 1999.

62. Dunn J, Golden D, Van Buren CT, Lewis RM, Lawen J, Kahan BD: Causes of graft loss beyond two years in the cyclosporine era. Transplantation 49:349–353, 1990.

63. De Geest S, Borgermans L, Gemoets H, Abraham I, Vlaminck H, Evers G, Vanrenterghem Y: Incidence, determinants, and consequences of subclinical noncompliance with immunosuppressive therapy in renal transplant recipients. Transplantation 59:340–347, 1995.

64. Schweizer RT, Rovelli M, Palmeri D, Vossler E, Hull D, Bartus S: Noncompliance in organ transplant recipients. Transplantation 49:374–377, 1990.

65. Cramer JA: Relationship between medication compliance and medical outcomes. Am J Health-Syst Pharm 52(Suppl. 3):S27–S29, 1995.

66. Urquhart J: Patient noncompliance with drug regimens: Measurement, clinical correlates, economic impact. Eur Heart J 17(Suppl. A):8–15, 1995.

67. Butkus DE, Meydrech EF, Raju SS: Racial differences in the survival of cadaveric renal allografts: Overriding effects of HLA matching and socioeconomic factors. N Engl J Med 327:840–845, 1992.

68. Kalil RSN, Heim-Duthoy KL, Kasiske BL: Patients with a low income have reduced renal allograft survival. Am J Kidney Dis 20:63–69, 1992.

69. Sanders CE, Curtis JJ, Julian BA, Gaston RS, Jones PA, Laskow DA, Deierhoi MH, Barber WH, Diethelm AG: Tapering or discontinuing cyclosporine for financial reasons—A single center experience. Am J Kidney Dis 21:9–15, 1993.

70. Woodward RS, Schnitzler MA, Lowell JA, Singer GG, Cohen DS, Spitznagel EL, Brennan DC: Medicare's extended immunosuppression coverage improved graft survival (abstract). J Am Soc Nephrol (in press) 1999.

71. Sanders CE, Julian BA, Gaston RS, Deierhoi MH, Diethelm AG, Curtis JJ: Benefits of continued cyclosporine through an indigent drug program. Am J Kidney Dis 28:572–577, 1996.

72. Lagnado, L. Transplant patients ply an illicit market for vital medicines. Wall Street Journal, 6/21/99, p. 1.

Cost Estimates for Expanded Medicare Benefits: Skin Cancer Screening, Medically Necessary Dental Services, and Immunosuppressive Therapy for Transplant Recipients

Allen Dobson, Ph.D.,[*] Joan DaVanzo, Ph.D., and Jesse Kerns, M.P.P.

INTRODUCTION

The Lewin Group was commissioned by the Institute of Medicine (IOM) Committee on Medicare Coverage Extensions to prepare cost estimates for selected expansions of Medicare benefits. Congress, in the Balanced Budget Act of 1997, requested that the IOM examine Medicare coverage for certain preventive and other benefits. The Lewin Group prepared cost estimates for the following services:

- skin cancer screening,
- medically necessary dental services (in connection with treatment of specific diagnoses), and
- elimination of the 3-year limit on immunosuppressive therapy.

The purpose of these cost estimates is to supplement the committee's analysis of the clinical evidence about the effectiveness of these services. For each topic, we consulted with the committee on specific coverage extension options to be examined.

The following sections summarize our cost estimates for these services, the data sources used for these estimates, and the key assumptions that underlie these estimates. The estimates are based on a series of assumptions, some of which have supporting evidence or data but others of which are best guesses based on committee and consultant judgment in the absence of such information. For each condition or service, the estimates are intended to suggest the order of

---

[*]Senior Vice President, Senior Manager, and Associate, The Lewin Group.

magnitude of the costs to Medicare of extending coverage, but they could be considerably higher or lower than what Medicare might actually spend were coverage policies changed. The text and tables in this appendix will allow readers to vary some of the assumptions and calculate alternative estimates.

We followed generic Congressional Budget Office (CBO) estimation practices such as not discounting future costs to present value. Our analytic process required estimations of both gross and net costs to Medicare for the 5-year period 2000–2004. Gross costs are the direct costs to Medicare of the services, and net costs are the gross costs minus the potential cost offsets (e.g., avoided hospitalization costs due to prevented infections) that Medicare would realize as a result of covering these services. Estimates of cost offsets are derived from the committee's analysis of the available research and expert judgement. We also reduced our cost estimates to account for cost-sharing offsets of 20% and premium offsets of 25% per CBO standards. [1] Numbers in the tables may not total exactly due to rounding.

Projections of the Medicare Part B population for the years 2000 through 2004, as well as other sources of Medicare Part A and Part B population statistics (such as race and sex), were provided by the Health Care Financing Administration (HCFA) Office of the Actuary.

The following sections discuss each of these estimates in detail.

SKIN CANCER SCREENING

For each of the coverage extension options considered here, Medicare would cover skin cancer screening for basal cell carcinoma, squamous cell carcinoma, and malignant melanoma. We assume skin cancer screening would be made available to all Medicare Part B beneficiaries.

Gross costs to Medicare of screening are built from estimates of the target population, and estimates of the costs of the services provided. Medicare net costs would be derived by offsetting Medicare savings from gross costs, but none were identified from the literature on skin cancer screening.

The major determinant of cost for Medicare coverage of skin cancer screening is the size of the target population. With more than 39 million enrollees in Medicare Part B, the costs depend on how many Medicare enrollees participate in skin cancer screenings.

We consider gross and net costs of three possible approaches to skin cancer screening:

---

[1] The Medicare Part B premium offset is set at 25% of Part B expenditures for the elderly Medicare population only. Because most transplant recipients qualify for Medicare based on disability or diagnosis of end-stage renal disease rather than age, premium offsets were not deducted from gross cost estimates for dental care or immunosuppressive therapy for transplant recipients.

• Approach 1: Single-step screening is covered for all Medicare Part B beneficiaries.

• Approach 2: Medicare Part B beneficiaries are identified as "high risk" during a visit to a primary care physician and then screened.

• Approach 3: Medicare Part B beneficiaries self-select themselves as high risk based on public outreach campaign and go to a dermatologist for screening.

Approaches 2 and 3 both require appraisal of patients as high risk. There are many indicators of high risk for skin cancer, including fair skin, light eyes, history of sunburns or sun exposure, multiple moles on body, and so forth. We assume approximately 10% of the Medicare-aged population fall into the high risk of skin cancer category. This estimate is based on an estimate of the relevant background paper author (Appendix B) and a study referenced in that paper.[2]

Each estimating approach yields a different volume of biopsies, skin cancer detection, and cost. The 5-year costs of the three approaches and the total biopsy yield are shown in Table E-1.

These cost estimates would be offset by premium increases for Medicare beneficiaries. The CBO uses a 25% reduction in direct costs due to these offsets. The costs of these three approaches taking the premium offset into account are shown in Table E-2.

The methodology of the cost per screen and cost per biopsy and a discussion of additional costs from induced demand for other Medicare services follow in the next section. Later sections discuss the three screening alternatives and the cost estimates for each.

Cost-per-Screen-and-Biopsy Methodology

Some basic cost assumptions underlie our gross cost estimates. All costs are determined for year 2000, then increased at 2% per year. We assume the cost of a screen as an add-on to physician visit is $20. This assumption is based on the average increase of one level in the Medicare non-facility-based reimbursement for a physician visit in 1998, which was $19. The cost of a screen as an independent physician visit is $50. This assumption is based on the weighted average reimbursement for a level 3 visit (one-third from new patient code 99203 and two-thirds from established patient code 99213) in 1998, which was $49. We use data from the Relative Value Unit (RVU) reimbursement rates for 1999 from the *Federal Register*.[3] The 1999 conversion factor was 34.7315. Because the RVU and conversion-factor derived values yield the "Medicare allowed"

---

[2]MacKie RM, Freudenberger T, Aitchison TC. Personal risk-factor chart for cutaneous melanoma, *Lancet* 2:487–490, 1989.

[3]*Federal Register*, Vol. 63, No. 211, November 2, 1998.

TABLE E-1 Estimated Total Cost (in millions) and Total Number of Biopsies Resulting from Three Approaches to Skin Cancer Screening

	2000	2001	2002	2003	2004	Total	Total No. of Biopsies
Approach 1	$225.9	$232.6	$239.4	$246.8	$254.8	$1,199.4	1,422,090
Approach 2	96.8	99.4	102.0	104.8	107.8	510.8	1,486,674
Approach 3	37.8	38.8	39.8	40.9	42.1	199.5	660,744

TABLE E-2 Estimated Cost (in millions) with Offset Due to 25% Part B Premium Increases for Three Approaches to Skin Cancer Screening

	2000	2001	2002	2003	2004	Total	Total No. of Biopsies
Approach 1	$169.4	$174.4	$179.6	$185.1	$191.1	$899.5	1,422,090
Approach 2	72.6	74.5	76.5	78.6	80.8	383.1	1,486,674
Approach 3	28.4	29.1	29.9	30.7	31.6	149.6	660,744

charge, which customarily includes a 20% copay from the Medicare enrollee, the Medicare cost per screen is reduced by 20%. Therefore, the add-on cost is reduced to $16 from $20, and the independent visit cost is reduced to $40 from $50. These figures reflect the actual cost to Medicare for these services. The cost of a biopsy is assumed to be $90, a figure supplied by a dermatologist on the committee.

Case-Finding Approach 1: All Medicare Part B Beneficiaries Are Screened

Under this approach, Medicare Part B beneficiaries may be screened during any visit to a primary care physician. We estimate a total 5-year net cost of $1.12 billion for case-finding approach 1, as detailed in Table E-3. The 5-year gross cost estimate is also $1.12 billion because there was no evidence of cost offsets substantiated by the current literature.

Methodology

We assume a majority of Medicare Part B beneficiaries visit a primary care physician each year. Health services research and Medicare data indicate that (1) not all patients will be offered screening due to physician time pressures, lack of familiarity or agreement with recommendations for screening, or other factors; and (2) some beneficiaries will decline screening due to time pressure, modesty, or other factors. Based on information summarized in Chapter 3 of this report, we assume that 30% of Medicare Part B beneficiaries will be screened each year.[4]

We then assume that those found with suspicious lesions will be referred to a dermatologist for a second screen. We assume 5% of those screened will be referred to and see a dermatologist, and 50% of those referred will receive a biopsy.

Case-Finding Approach 2: Only Those Identified as High Risk Are Screened

Under this approach, Medicare Part B beneficiaries may be identified as high risk during any visit to a primary care physician. We estimate a total 5-year net cost of $510.8 million for case-finding approach 2, as detailed in Table E-4. The 5-year gross cost estimate is also $510.8 million because there was no evidence of cost offsets substantiated by the current literature.

---

[4]Projections of the annual number of screens are calculated as 30% of total Medicare Part B enrollment projections for 2000–2004 by the HCFA Office of the Actuary.

TABLE E-3 Estimated Total Cost of Approach 1 to Skin Cancer Screening

	2000	2001	2002	2003	2004	Total
Annual number of "high-risk" screens	11,153,400	11,259,000	11,363,400	11,485,200	11,622,600	NA
Cost of initial screen	$16	$16	$17	$17	$17	NA
Total cost of initial screens (millions)	$178.5	$183.7	$189.2	$195.0	$201.3	$947.7
Proportion receiving referral	5%	5%	5%	5%	5%	NA
Number receiving referrals	557,670	562,950	568,170	574,260	581,130	2,844,180
Cost per referred screen	$40	$41	$42	$42	$43	NA
Total cost of referred screens (millions)	$22.3	$23	$23.6	$24.4	$25.2	$118.5
Proportion who receive biopsy	50%	50%	50%	50%	50%	NA
Number who receive biopsy	278,835	281,475	284,085	287,130	290,565	1,422,090
Cost per biopsy	$90	$92	$94	$96	$97	NA
Total cost of biopsy (millions)	$25.1	$25.8	$26.6	$27.4	$28.3	$133.3
Total cost, Approach 1 (millions)	$225.9	$232.6	$239.4	$246.8	$254.8	$1,199.4

TABLE E-4 Total Cost of Approach 2 to Skin Cancer Screening

	2000	2001	2002	2003	2004	Total
Annual number of "high-risk" screens	2,933,460	2,952,630	2,970,810	2,992,320	3,017,520	NA
Cost of initial screen	$16	$16	$17	$17	$17	NA
Total cost of initial screens (millions)	$46.9	$48.2	$49.5	$50.8	$52.3	$247.6
Proportion receiving referral	20%	20%	20%	20%	20%	NA
Number receiving referrals	586,692	590,526	594,162	598,464	603,504	2,973,348
Cost per referred screen	$40	$41	$42	$42	$43	NA
Total cost of referred screens (millions)	$23.5	$24.1	$24.7	$25.4	$26.1	$123.8
Proportion who receive biopsy	50%	50%	50%	50%	50%	NA
Number who receive biopsy	293,346	295,263	297,081	299,232	301,752	1,486,674
Cost per biopsy	$90	$92	$94	$96	$97	NA
Total cost of biopsy (millions)	$26.4	$27.1	$27.8	$28.6	$29.4	$139.3
Total cost, Approach 2 (millions)	$96.8	$99.4	$102.0	$104.8	$107.8	$510.8

Methodology

We assume a majority of the aged Medicare part B population visits a primary care physician each year but that not all physicians will assess patients for skin cancer risk. We assume that 10% of the aged Medicare Part B population will be identified as high risk, be offered screening, and accept it. (Some additional beneficiaries who are at high risk due to past diagnosis of cancerous or precancerous skin lesions will have yearly skin examinations as a part of usual follow-up care.) We then assume that those found with suspicious lesions are referred to a dermatologist for a second screen. We assume 20% of those screened will be referred, and 50% of those referred to a dermatologist will receive a biopsy.

Screening Approach 3: Mass Screening, Beneficiaries at High Risk Self-Select

Under this approach, a public information campaign targets the 10% of the Medicare population who are at high risk for skin cancer for a direct screen by a dermatologist. We estimate a total 5-year net cost of $199.5 million for this mass screening approach, detailed in Table E-5. The 5-year gross cost estimate is also $199.5 million because there was no evidence of cost offsets substantiated by the current literature.

Methodology

We assume that self-identification of risk is reasonably accurate and that 20% of those who identify themselves as at high risk will elect to seek clinical screening. Of the group who elect screening, 20% are assumed to have a biopsy.

Some high-risk individuals already self-identify warning signs of cancer (rather than just a risk factor such as fair skin) and seek physician examination, which Medicare now covers. Also, other individuals with a past diagnosis of a cancerous or precancerous skin lesion will see physicians for examinations as part of covered follow-up care. The assumption for this scenario is that an additional 20% of high-risk people will seek screening who would not have done so in the absence of a new mass screening program. To the extent, however, that a mass screening program brings in those who would have sought an examination anyway, then estimated new costs to Medicare would be lower than presented here.

MEDICALLY NECESSARY DENTAL SERVICES

The cost estimates considered here assume that Medicare would cover certain dental services determined to be medically necessary in connection with treatment of the following specific conditions:

- cancer of the head or neck,
- leukemia,

TABLE E-5 Estimated Total Cost of Approach 3 to Skin Cancer Screening

	2000	2001	2002	2003	2004	Total
All Medicare Part B aged population	32,594,000	32,807,000	33,009,000	33,248,000	33,528,000	NA
Proportion "high risk"	10%	10%	10%	10%	10%	NA
Proportion of "high risk" who elect screen	20%	20%	20%	20%	20%	NA
Number screened	651,880	656,140	660,180	664,960	670,560	3,303,720
Cost per screen	$40	$41	$42	$42	$43	NA
Total cost of screens (millions)	$26.1	$26.8	$27.5	$28.2	$29.0	$137.6
Proportion who receive biopsy	20%	20%	20%	20%	20%	NA
Number who receive biopsy	130,376	131,228	132,036	132,992	134,112	660,744
Cost per biopsy	$90	$92	$94	$96	$97	NA
Total cost biopsies (millions)	$11.7	$12.0	$12.4	$12.7	$13.1	$61.9
Total cost, Approach 3 (millions)	$37.8	$38.8	$39.8	$40.9	$42.1	$199.5

- lymphoma,
- organ transplantation, and
- congenital or acquired valvular and heart disease.

The basis for selecting the medical conditions listed above is H.R. 1288 (introduced April 1997). Medically necessary dental care is defined in H.R. 1288 "as a direct result of, or will have a direct impact on" treatment of these conditions. The portion of H.R. 1288 that states, "Dental services shall be considered to be cost-effective if furnished in connection with treatment of an individual with . . ." any of the above four conditions is disregarded because the focus here is on cost estimates not cost-effectiveness.

In our construction of cost estimates for dental services associated with the specified medical conditions, we reviewed previous cost estimates of these benefits developed by the HCFA Office of the Actuary (produced by the Actuarial Research Corporation), the CBO, and the Federation of Special Care Organizations in Dentistry. Our estimates are only for coverage of dental services in the year of the procedure. If services after the intervention are covered by Medicare in years following surgery, radiation, chemotherapy, or other treatment, the cost estimates could be substantially higher.

Total Five-Year Gross and Net Costs for All Conditions

We estimate a total 5-year net cost of $207.7 million for the total dental benefits under consideration, as detailed in Table E-6. The 5-year gross cost estimate is $213.3 million, less a $5.6 million offset from cost savings for one condition. A Medicare premium offset of 25% would reduce the 5-year net costs to $155.8 million. The CBO regularly reduces cost estimates by 25% to account for this premium offset. We determined there was evidence of cost savings of $5.6 million for radiation therapy of the head or neck preventive dental services. There was no other evidence of cost offsets substantiated by the current literature.

Our cost estimate for medically necessary dental services is substantially lower than comparable estimates conducted by the CBO and the HCFA Office of the Actuary. These estimates are the first to estimate the number of Medicare beneficiaries likely to be affected by the policy based on incidence data for each condition. The HCFA Office of the Actuary estimated costs for the five conditions, but it estimated that a fixed percentage of all dental visits of Medicare beneficiaries would be covered under this benefit, essentially a "top-down" approach. In contrast, the cost estimates in this report constitute a "bottom-up" approach, beginning with incidence data for each condition and building the estimate based on these data.

The methodology for our "cost-per-case" estimate, an essential element of each estimate, follows. Subsequent sections discuss the individual cost estimates for each condition and the underlying methodology for each estimate.

TABLE E-6 Estimated Cost (in millions) of Dental Care for Five Selected Conditions with Offset Due to 25% Part B Premium Increases

	2000	2001	2002	2003	2004	Total
Radiation therapy for head or neck cancer with savings from prevented ORN	$2.1	$2.3	$2.5	$2.6	$2.8	$12.9
Leukemia	3.7	3.9	4.2	4.4	4.6	20.9
Lymphoma	5.8	6.1	6.4	6.8	7.2	32.3
Organ transplantation	4.1	4.4	4.8	5.2	5.6	24.2
Heart valve repair or replacement	18.4	20.7	23.2	26.0	29.2	117.5
Total net cost for five conditions	32.1	35.2	38.6	42.4	46.6	207.7
Medicare premium offset (25%)	8.0	8.8	9.6	10.6	11.7	51.9
Total net cost less premium offset	24.1	26.4	28.9	31.8	35.0	155.8

Cost-per-Visit Methodology

A standardized dental "cost per visit" to Medicare was constructed from the best available data, and is displayed in Table E-7. The Medicare cost per dental visit is built from 1987 (National Medical Expenditure Survey [NMES]) cost-per-case data for the aged population. This value is inflated by the Consumer Price Index for dental services (CPI-U Dental) to 1997, and inflated for 2000–2004 by the average CPI-U Dental increase for 1993–1997 (4.8% annual). The 1987 NMES cost per case is based on the average cost per dental visit adjusted with a 33% increase for greater acuity (similar to an earlier Actuarial Research Corporation adjustment for "medically necessary" dental services). This figure was then adjusted downward to account for a Medicare "discount" and cost sharing. A Medicare Part B copayment of 20% was deducted, and a Medicare discount of 30% is deducted. The Medicare premium offset of 25% is discounted from the estimated total cost for all conditions in the earlier overview section. The yield of the cost per visit is outlined in the following table.

Five-Year Gross and Net Cost Estimate for Dental Care Prior to Radiation Therapy of Head or Neck Cancer

We estimate a 5-year net cost of $12.9 million for dental care prior to radiation therapy for head or neck cancer. The 5-year gross cost estimate for this benefit is $18.6 million.

We have projected potential cost offsets (savings) of $5.6 million over the period 2000–2004. This reduces our 5-year estimate to a net cost of $12.9 million. The results are displayed in Tables E-8 and E-9.

Methodology

Only patients receiving radiation therapy for head and neck cancer were considered. We applied incidence rates for larynx and pharynx cancer, and rates of radiation therapy, for these groups, from the Surveillance, Epidemiology, and End-Results (SEER) database to Medicare Part B population projections. There was a further modification to these incidence rates based on trends in the annual change of incidence rates over time.

- *Larynx cancer:* Incidence 45 per 100,000 over 65; 6.5 per 100,000 under 65; 74.2% receive radiation therapy, annual change in incidence rate of –0.4% (source: SEER database).
- *Oral cavity and pharynx cancer:* Incidence 19.7 per 100,000 over 65; 3.7 per 100,000 under 65; 49.7% receive radiation therapy, annual change in incidence rate of +0.4% (source: SEER database).

TABLE E-7 Estimated Cost per Dental Visit for Years 2000–2004

	2000	2001	2002	2003	2004
Medicare dental cost per visit	$169	$177	$185	$194	$204

TABLE E-8 Estimated Gross Cost (in millions) of Dental Care for Patients Receiving Radiation Therapy for Head and Neck Cancer

	2000	2001	2002	2003	2004	Total
Oral cavity and pharynx cancer cases	15,011	15,105	15,197	15,314	15,415	NA
Larynx cancer cases	5,924	6,009	6,094	6,190	6,296	NA
Total number of cases	20,934	21,114	21,291	21,504	21,746	NA
Radiation therapy cases	11,856	11,966	12,075	12,204	12,350	NA
Cost per visit	$169	$177	$185	$194	$204	NA
Cost per patient	$279	$292	$306	$321	$336	NA
Total gross cost (millions)	$3.3	$3.5	$3.7	$3.9	$4.2	$18.6

An average of 1.65 dental visits per patient was applied. This includes two visits per patient with teeth (approximately 65% of Medicare population) and one visit per patient without teeth (approximately 35% of Medicare population). This estimate is based on consultation with committee members and relevant background paper authors.

Cost Offsets (Savings) for Radiation Therapy

We have projected potential cost offsets of $5.6 million over the period 2000–2004. This reduces our 5-year estimate to a net cost of $12.9 million. These offsets are derived from evidence in the literature concerning hyperbaric oxygen (HBO) treatment for osteoradionecrosis (ORN). HBO treatment, one procedure available to treat this condition, is very costly, therefore, precluding ORN and HBO treatment can produce substantial cost savings. Data in the background paper suggest that 26.4% of ORN patients receive HBO treatment. ORN occurs in 10.2% of radiation therapy patients, and we estimated (based on Appendix C) that with tooth-preserving services, this rate would be reduced to 2.25%. The reduction in ORN cases would lead to a reduction in HBO treatment cases. Therefore our net cost estimate includes these offsets.

The resultant cost savings and total net costs for these preventive services are shown in Table E-10.

The cost per case of HBO treatment is based on an assumed average cost of $24,000 per patient in 1999 (figure supplied by background paper author). We have reduced the cost to Medicare for HBO treatment by 25% to account for the premium offset and by 20% to account for beneficiary cost sharing. Costs are assumed to increase at 2% per year. Cost savings are derived form the number of avoided ORN cases that would have been treated with HBO.

Five-Year Gross and Net Cost Estimate for Leukemia and Lymphoma Conditions

We estimate a 5-year net cost of $20.9 million for leukemia dental services and $32.3 million for lymphoma dental services. The 5-year gross cost estimates are also $20.9 million and $32.3 million, respectively. There were no cost offsets identified from evidence in the literature review, therefore, our gross cost estimate is equivalent to our net cost estimate, as displayed in Tables E-11 and E-12.

Methodology

Assumptions for gross cost estimate of leukemia and lymphoma dental services are built from incidence rates of leukemia and lymphoma in the aged (65 and over) and nonaged (below 65) populations. Leukemia and lymphoma incidence rates (all derived from the SEER database) are

TABLE E-9 Estimated Total Net Cost (in millions) of Dental Care for Patients Receiving Radiation Therapy for Head or Neck Cancer

	2000	2001	2002	2003	2004	Total
Total gross cost	$3.3	$3.5	$3.7	$3.9	$4.2	$18.6
Cost savings	1.1	1.1	1.1	1.2	1.2	5.6
Total net cost	2.2	2.4	2.6	2.8	3.0	12.9

TABLE E-10 Estimated Savings Resulting from Preventing Services ORN in Patients Receiving Radiation Therapy for Head or Neck Cancer

	2000	2001	2002	2003	2004	Total
No. of ORN cases without preventive dental services (10.2%)	363	366	370	374	379	1,852
No. of ORN cases with preventive dental services (2.25%)	89	90	91	92	93	454
No. of ORN cases prevented	274	277	279	282	286	1,398
No. of ORN cases that receive HBO (26.4%)	72	73	74	75	75	369
Average cost to Medicare per ORN case	$14,688	$14,982	$15,281	$15,587	$15,899	NA
Total savings from prevented ORN (millions)	$1.1	$1.1	$1.1	$1.2	$1.2	$5.6

TABLE E-11 Estimated Total Cost of Dental Services for Leukemia (without premium offset)

	2000	2001	2002	2003	2004	Total
Leukemia cases	17,019	17,137	17,249	17,382	17,536	NA
Cost per visit	$169	$177	$185	$194	$204	NA
Total cost per patient	$220	$230	$241	$253	$265	NA
Total cost (millions)	$3.7	$3.9	$4.2	$4.4	$4.6	$20.9

TABLE E-12 Estimated Total Costs of Dental Services for Lymphoma (without premium offset)

	2000	2001	2002	2003	2004	Total
Lymphoma cases	26,323	25,508	26,685	26,893	27,136	NA
Cost per visit	$169	$177	$185	$194	$204	NA
Total cost per patient	$220	$230	$241	$253	$265	NA
Total cost (millions)	$5.8	$6.1	$6.4	$6.8	$7.2	$32.3

- Leukemia—51.4 per 100,000 applied to aged Medicare Part B population, 5.8 per 100,000 applied to disabled Medicare Part B population; and
- Lymphoma—79.1 per 100,000 applied to aged Medicare Part B population, 11.8 per 100,000 applied to disabled Medicare Part B population.

These incidence rates are applied to the Medicare Part B population projections for the years 2000 through 2004. An average of 1.3 dental visits per patient was then applied. This includes two visits for patients with teeth (approximately 65% of the Medicare population) and no visits per patient without teeth (the remaining 35%). This estimate is based on consultation with committee members and relevant background paper authors.

Five-Year Gross and Net Cost Estimate for Organ Transplantation

We estimate a 5-year net cost of $24.2 million for this dental care benefit. The 5-year gross cost estimate is also $24.2 million. There were no cost offsets identified from evidence in the literature review, therefore, our gross cost estimate is equivalent to our net cost estimate, as displayed in Table E-13.

Methodology

We assume an average of 1.6 dental visits per patient per year, two per patient with teeth (assumed to be 80% of the transplant patients) and none per patient without teeth (the remaining 20%). The source of this estimate is the relevant background paper author. Transplant incidence is assumed to increase at 3.2% per year, the average annual kidney transplant increase from 1993 to 1998.

If Medicare were to cover dental services indefinitely after transplant surgery, this will increase the costs to the Medicare program. If we assume the average number of dental visits posttransplant is two per patient per year, the 5-year gross cost for transplant-related dental care increases to $157.5 million. This estimate would further increase if coverage were retroactive and included current transplant survivors. Likewise, if patients who spend a long time on a waiting list for transplantation have to be reexamined, this will add somewhat to costs.

Five-Year Gross and Net Cost Estimate for Heart Valve Repair and Replacement

We estimate a 5-year net cost of $117.5 million for this dental care benefit. The 5-year gross cost estimate is also $117.5 million. There were no cost offsets identified from evidence in the literature review. Therefore, our gross cost estimate is equivalent to our net cost estimate, as displayed in Table E-14.

TABLE E-13 Estimated Total Cost of Dental Care for Organ Transplant Recipients

	2000	2001	2002	2003	2004	Total
Total kidney transplants	13,797	14,239	14,694	15,164	15,650	NA
Total other transplants for >65 population	470	485	501	517	533	NA
Total other transplants for disabled population	940	970	1,001	1,033	1,066	NA
Total transplant incidence	15,207	15,694	16,196	16,714	17,249	NA
Cost per visit	$169	$177	$185	$194	$204	NA
Total cost per patient	$270	$283	$297	$311	$326	NA
Total cost (millions)	$4.1	$4.4	$4.8	$5.2	$5.6	$24.2

Methodology

The annual number of cases is estimated based on Medicare-covered heart valve diagnosis-related group (DRG)[5] discharge volume from 1990 to 1995 projected for the years 2000–2004. Medicare-covered heart valve DRGs increased by approximately 7% annually from 1990 through 1995; this rate of growth is assumed to continue through 2004.

An average of 1.3 dental visits per patient was then applied. This includes two visits for patients with teeth (approximately 65% of the Medicare population) and no visits per patient without teeth (the remaining 35%). This estimate is based on consultation with committee members and relevant background paper authors.

EXTENDED IMMUNOSUPPRESSIVE DRUG COVERAGE

In this section we estimate costs for eliminating Medicare's current 3-year limit on immunosuppressive drug therapy for kidney, heart, liver, and lung transplant recipients. (Pancreas transplants are not considered separately because they are covered by Medicare only in conjunction with a kidney transplant.) Medicare gross costs are built from estimates of the population with graft survival greater than 3 years and estimates of the costs of the immunosuppressive therapy.

Our analysis considers kidney transplants separately from all other transplants for two reasons:

1. Kidney transplants represent the substantial majority of covered transplants and associated immunosuppressive therapy.
2. Kidney transplants have clearly associated cost offsets.

However, extended coverage for immunosuppressive drugs in terms of kidney transplants could apply in at least two ways. First, extended coverage could apply to the two-thirds of transplant recipients who remain Medicare eligible after 3 years (due to either disabled or aged status). Second, extended coverage of immunosuppressive drugs could apply to the entire Medicare transplant population including those kidney transplant recipients who are not classified as either aged or disabled and currently lose all Medicare coverage 3 years following a transplant. Because these two alternatives produce different cost estimates, we have developed estimates of both the costs and the cost savings for each approach.

---

[5]See Appendix C.

TABLE E-14 Estimated Total Cost of Dental Care for Heart Valve Surgery Patients

	2000	2001	2002	2003	2004	Total
Heart valve repair or replacement cases	83,997	89,877	96,169	102,900	110,103	NA
Cost per visit	$169	$177	$185	$194	$204	NA
Total cost per patient	$220	$230	$241	$253	$265	NA
Total cost (millions)	$18.4	$20.7	$23.2	$26.0	$29.2	$117.5

We estimate a total 5-year net cost for all organs of $778 million for the extension of immunosuppressive therapy coverage for transplant recipients limited to the "Medicare-eligible" kidney population (Table E-15). We estimate a total 5-year net cost for all organs of $1.06 billion for the extension of immunosuppressive therapy coverage for transplant recipients that includes the "entire" population of Medicare kidney transplants (Table E-16). We determined cost savings of between $550 million to $830 million from coverage of kidney transplant recipients (depending on the extent of extended coverage), primarily due to the avoidance of graft removal and continued dialysis. We found no evidence of cost offsets for other organ transplants substantiated by the current literature and discussions with the committee and consultant who authored Appendix D.

As part of our cost estimate, a Medicare Part B copayment of 20% is deducted from the cost of immunosuppressive drugs. We do not apply a 25% premium offset to the gross costs because Medicare Part B premiums are based on treatment costs for the elderly and only a small proportion of covered tranplants recipients are elderly.

There are several key assumptions that underlie our cost estimates:

• *Key assumption 1*: As noted above, the proposed coverage could take the form of either a *coverage* extension or an *entitlement* extension. A coverage extension would apply to the two-thirds of transplant recipients who maintain Medicare eligibility after 3 years. Under an entitlement extension, all prior eligible transplant recipients (including those eligible by reason of ESRD status) with graft survival greater than 3 years will be eligible for coverage of immunosuppressive therapy costs. In such a case, if the transplant recipient is not otherwise Medicare eligible by virtue of age or disability status, other Medicare services are not covered under this entitlement. Thus, only costs for immunosuppressive drugs are estimated as new costs from extending coverage for both alternatives. We produce cost (and cost-savings) estimates for extended coverage both for the Medicare-eligible population (either disabled or aged) and for the entire population of Medicare kidney transplant recipients.

• *Key assumption 2:* Regardless of the assumptions above, the proposed coverage will be offset somewhat by Medicare Secondary Payer (MSP) provisions. We recognize that the elimination of coverage limits could result in substantial or total "crowd-out" of private insurance coverage (i.e., private insurance will transfer all coverage costs to the Medicare program whenever possible). However, we assume that Congress will extend Medicare's secondary payer requirements for ESRD beneficiaries from 30 months to indefinitely. We therefore reduce the number of eligible graft recipients by 25% for both the Medicare-eligible estimates and the entire population estimates. According to the United Network for Organ Sharing (UNOS), more than 36% of 3-year-plus kidney transplant recipients are employed full time. If we assume that approximately 75% of this group have employer-sponsored health

TABLE E-15 Estimated Total Net Cost (in millions) of Extending Coverage for Immunosuppressants, All Organs (assuming coverage limited to Medicare-eligible kidney transplant population)

	2000	2001	2002	2003	2004	Total
Gross cost (kidney, limited)	$173.1	$195.5	$220.8	$249.3	$281.6	$1,120.2
Gross cost (other organs)	31.4	36.9	42.6	47.8	53.4	212.1
Total gross (all organs)	204.5	232.3	263.4	297.1	335.0	1,332.3
Cost savings (kidney)	57.2	108.9	116.0	129.0	142.8	553.9
Total net cost (all organs)	147.2	123.4	147.4	168.2	192.2	778.4

TABLE E-16 Estimated Total Net Cost (in millions) of Extending Coverage for Immunosuppressants, All Organs (assuming coverage for "entire" kidney transplant population)

Net Costs	2000	2001	2002	2003	2004	Total
Gross cost (kidney, entire)	$260.9	$293.9	$331.0	$372.8	$419.9	$1,678.0
Gross costs (other organs)	31.4	36.9	42.6	47.8	53.4	212.1
Total gross (all organs)	292.3	330.7	373.6	420.6	473.3	1,890.0
Cost savings (kidney)	86.3	163.9	174.1	193.0	213.1	830.4
Total net cost (all organs)	206.0	166.8	199.5	227.6	260.1	1,060.1

insurance,[6] we can assume that the resultant 25% will be subject to MSP. We then assume that MSP will affect the Medicare-eligible and total population groups equally. Therefore, we have reduced the populations for both the Medicare-eligible and total population estimates by this 25%. For purposes of this estimate, we assume that Medicare picks up no costs as secondary payer.

• *Key assumption 3:* The cost to Medicare of immunosuppressive therapy is assumed to be $5,400 per patient per year in the year 2000, increasing at 4% per year in subsequent years. This cost reflects a 20% Medicare cost-share and a 5% Medicare discount from the "average wholesale price" of the drugs.[7] Adjusting back up for these reductions yields a per-patient cost of approximately $7,100 in 2000.[8] This figure applies to kidney, heart, liver, and lung transplant recipients. As shown in Appendix D, the range of cost for immunosuppressive therapy in 1999 is between approximately $5,000 and $13,000. If we assume that 75% of beneficiaries receive coverage on the low end of this spectrum, while 25% receive coverage at the high end, this produces a weighted average cost of $7,000 per member per year.[9]

Additional Discussion: Potential Savings to the Medicaid Program

Savings to the Medicaid program are not specifically included in our cost estimate. However, the government would realize savings from the Medicaid program as a result of this coverage. In 1996, the CBO estimated total savings to the Medicaid program of $6 million per year, for the years 2000 and 2001, for extended coverage for Medicare-eligible transplant patients. The CBO estimate considered the pool of transplant recipients that would still be Medicare eligible 3 years after transplant, whereas our estimate considers both this subgroup and all Medicare-covered transplants. For the Medicare-eligible extension, this would produce 5-year savings to the federal share of the Medicaid program of approximately $32.5 million.[10] Current figures suggest that 66% of Medicare-covered transplants who survive beyond 3 years retain Medicare eligibility (i.e., are either disabled or over 65), while 34% are no longer Medicare eligible.[11] If we adjust the CBO-calculated Medicaid program savings by a comparable ratio, savings to the Medicaid program in the case of a total population would produce

---

[6]EBRI issue brief: *Sources of Health Insurance and Characteristics of the Uninsured,* an analysis of March 1998 Current Population Survey.

[7]As provided in the Balanced Budget Act of 1997.

[8]This estimate of the average cost of immunosuppressive therapy was provided by the HCFA Office of the Actuary and the author of Appendix D.

[9]$(0.75 \times \$5,000) + (0.25 \times \$13,000) = \$7,000$

[10]Assumes immunosuppressive drug costs increase at 4% per year.

[11]Population distribution data courtesy of Dr. Paul Eggers, HCFA.

352

EXTENDING MEDICARE COVERAGE

5-year savings to the federal share of the Medicaid program of approximately $49 million.[12]

The following sections detail gross and net costs for both Medicare-eligible kidney transplants and total population kidney transplants and other organ costs.

Kidney Immunosuppressive Gross and Net Cost Estimates

We have produced two cost estimates for kidney immunosuppressive coverage:

1. *Medicare-eligible kidney population:* an estimate of costs and savings associated with extended coverage for kidney recipients who retain Medicare eligibility beyond 3 years (approximately two-thirds of this population).

2. *Entire population:* an estimate of costs and savings associated with extended coverage for all kidney recipients originally covered by Medicare (under the ESRD program, the entire population that receives a Medicare-covered transplant receives immunosuppressive coverage regardless of other Medicare eligibility status).

Our rationale for producing both estimates is the possibility that extended coverage could apply to either the subset of this population that remains Medicare eligible after 3 years (due to either disabled or aged status) or the entire Medicare transplant population (as the whole ESRD kidney transplant population receives coverage for 3 years).

Total Net Costs of Medicare-Eligible and "Entire" Kidney Transplant Population Coverage Extension

We estimate a total 5-year net cost of $566 million for extending immunosuppressant coverage for the Medicare-eligible kidney transplant population. This estimate incorporates a 5-year gross cost estimate of $1.12 billion, and a 5-year cost savings offset estimate of $554 million, as shown in Table E-17.

We estimate a total 5-year net cost of $848 million for a coverage extension for the "entire" kidney transplant population. This estimate incorporates a 5-year gross cost estimate of $1.68 billion and a 5-year cost savings offset estimate of $830 million, as shown in Table E-18.

---

[12]This value is produced by the equation [0.66X = $6 million] and solving for X. It assumes Medicaid immunosuppressant costs increase at 4% per year.

TABLE E-17 Estimated Net Cost (in millions) for Medicare-Eligible Kidney Transplant Population Only

	2000	2001	2002	2003	2004	Total
Gross cost	$173.1	$195.5	$220.8	$249.3	$281.6	$1,120.2
Cost savings	57.2	108.9	116.0	129.0	142.8	553.9
Net cost	115.8	86.6	104.8	120.4	138.8	566.3

TABLE E-18 Estimated Net Cost (in millions) for "Entire" Kidney Transplant Population

	2000	2001	2002	2003	2004	Total
Gross cost	$260.9	$293.9	$331.0	$372.8	$419.9	$1,678.4
Cost savings	86.3	163.9	174.1	193.0	213.1	830.4
Net cost	174.6	129.9	156.9	179.8	206.7	848.0

The methodology and assumptions that underlie both the gross cost estimates and the cost offset estimates for each level of coverage are discussed below. The cost savings for each coverage scenario differ because the potential savings from avoided graft failure are based on different initial population estimates (i.e., there are more greater-than-3-year grafts in the overall transplant population than in the Medicare-eligible population, therefore, a greater number of failed grafts could be prevented with extended coverage).

Gross and Net Cost Estimates for Medicare-Eligible Kidney Transplant Population

In this section we consider the gross and net costs of extended coverage for the Medicare-eligible kidney transplant population. Gross costs are the annual costs of immunosuppressive therapy for all Medicare-eligible kidney transplant recipients with graft survival greater than 3 years, and net costs are the gross costs less the avoided costs due to this extended coverage. The 5-year gross cost estimate of this coverage is $1.12 billion, as shown in Table E-19.

We estimated potential 5-year cost savings of $553 million attributable to extended immunosuppressive coverage of kidney transplant recipients. These cost savings yield a total estimated 5-year net cost of $566 million as already shown in Table E-17.

Methodology

The numbers of kidney transplant recipients with grafts longer than 3 years, and of the subset of this population that retains Medicare eligibility after 3 years, were supplied by Dr. Paul Eggers, Director, Division of Beneficiaries Research, HCFA. We assume the Medicare-eligible greater-than-3-year kidney graft population will grow at an 8.6% annual rate. This rate is derived from the 3-year average growth rate from 1995 through 1997. This figure is also consistent with historical trends data, increasing patient and graft survival, and the limited pool of donor organs.

This population estimate is then reduced by 25% to account for graft recipients who receive coverage through other insurance (see discussion above).

Cost savings are derived from assumed reductions in:

• the number of grafts that fail due to noncompliance with drug regimen associated with cost pressure;
  • the resultant costs of surgery to remove failed grafts;
  • the cost of dialysis for these patients; and
  • the cost of retransplantation for those who lose their graft and subsequently receive a new transplant.

355

TABLE E-19 Estimated Gross Cost (in millions) of Extended Immunosuppressive Drug Therapy for Medicare-Eligible Kidney Transplant Population

	2000	2001	2002	2003	2004	Total
Kidney graft patient > 3 years, Medicare eligible (less secondary payer)	32,048	34,804	37,797	41,048	44,578	NA
Cost per year of immunotherapy	$5,400	$5,616	$5,841	$6,074	$6,317	NA
Gross cost	$173.1	$195.5	$220.8	$249.3	$281.6	$1,120.2

We assume an annual graft failure rate due to cost pressure of 2.5%. This assumption is based on the weighted average failure rate of kidney grafts after 3 years of 7% (cadaveric donor 8%, living donor 5%).[13] We then assume that one-third of these failures are due to noncompliance with immunosuppressive therapy due to cost pressure. This figure was agreed upon by the consultant who authored Appendix D and Dr. Eggers, and informed by some cited evidence from "natural" experiments as described in Appendix D.

The "cost-of-loss" measure incorporates all costs in the year of failure, including surgery, treatment, hospitalization, and dialysis costs for that year. The failed-graft population returns to dialysis. The "cost of dialysis" includes all direct medical costs associated with dialysis.

Certain factors remove patients from the failed-graft–returned-to-dialysis pool. Data suggest 12% annual mortality after graft failure, so the failed graft population is reduced by this rate annually. Because approximately 10% of all renal transplants are retransplants, we assume 10% of the failed-graft pool receive new transplants each year. Since the cost of retransplantation would have been avoided if the graft had not failed, the associated costs of retransplantation for these patients are also potential cost savings. The cost-of-loss, dialysis, and retransplantation values were provided by Dr. Eggers, HCFA. The results are displayed in Table E-20.

We estimated potential 5-year cost savings of $553 million attributable to extended immunosuppressive coverage of kidney transplant recipients. These cost savings would offset gross costs.

Gross and Net Costs of "Entire" Population Kidney Transplants

In this section we consider the gross and net costs of extended coverage for the entire kidney transplant population, shown in Table E-21. Gross costs are the annual costs of immunosuppressive therapy for all kidney transplant recipients with graft survival greater than 3 years; net costs are gross costs less the avoided costs due to extending coverage. The 5-year gross cost estimate of this coverage is $1.68 billion.

We estimated potential 5-year cost savings of $830 million attributable to extended immunosuppressive coverage of kidney transplant recipients. These cost savings yield a total estimated 5-year net cost of $848 million, as shown already in Table E-18.

---

[13]UNOS database.

TABLE E-20 Estimated Cost (in millions) Due to Loss of Renal Grafts Attributed to Cost Pressure on Beneficiaries, Medicare-Eligible Population Only

	2000	2001	2002	2003	2004	Total
Graft failure rate from cost pressure	2.5%	2.5%	2.5%	2.5%	2.5%	NA
Annual >3-year failed grafts	801	870	945	1,026	1,114	NA
Prior number of >3-year failed grafts	—	625	616	675	733	NA
Total >3-year failed grafts	801	1,495	1,561	1,702	1,847	NA
Cost of loss	$61,057	$62,278	$63,523	$64,794	$66,090	NA
Total annual cost of removal (millions)	$48.9	$93.1	$99.2	$110.3	$122.1	$473.5
Per unit cost of dialysis	$53,042	$54,103	$55,185	$56,289	$57,415	NA
Total cost of dialysis (millions)	—	$68.0	$129.1	$185.7	$239.3	$622.1
Number retransplanted (10% of total)	80	150	156	170	185	NA
Cost per retransplantation	$103,607	$105,679	$107,793	$109,949	$112,148	NA
Total costs of retransplantations (millions)	$8.3	$15.8	$16.8	$18.7	$20.7	$80.4
Total cost due to graft loss	$57.2	$108.9	$116.0	$129.0	$142.8	**$553.9**

TABLE E-21 Estimated Gross Cost of Immunosuppressive Drug Therapy for "Entire" Kidney Transplant Population

	2000	2001	2002	2003	2004	Total
Kidney graft patient > 3 years, total population (less secondary payer)	48,315	52,325	56,668	61,372	66,466	NA
Cost per year of therapy	$5,400	$5,616	$5,841	$6,074	$6,317	NA
Total gross cost (millions)	$260.9	$293.9	$331.0	$372.8	$419.9	$1,678.4

Methodology

The numbers of kidney transplant recipients with grafts longer than 3 years, and of the subset of this population that retains Medicare eligibility after 3 years, were supplied by Dr. Paul Eggers, Director, Division of Beneficiaries Research, HCFA. We assume the Medicare-eligible greater than 3-year kidney graft population will grow at an 8.6% annual rate. This rate is derived from the 3-year average growth rate from 1995 through 1997. This figure is also consistent with historical trends data, increasing patient and graft survival, and the limited pool of donor organs. This population estimate is then reduced by 25% to account for graft recipients who receive coverage through other insurance (see discussion above).

Cost savings are derived from assumed reductions in:

- the number of grafts that fail due to noncompliance with drug regimen associated with cost pressure;
- the resultant costs of surgery to remove failed grafts;
- the cost of dialysis for these patients; and
- the cost of retransplantation for those who lose their graft and subsequently receive a new transplant.

We assume an annual graft failure rate due to cost pressure of 2.5%. This assumption is based on the weighted average failure rate of kidney grafts after 3 years of 7% (cadaveric donor 8%, living donor 5%).[14] We then assume that one-third of these failures are due to noncompliance with immunosuppressive therapy due to cost pressure. This figure was agreed upon by the consultant who authored Appendix D and Dr. Eggers, and informed by some evidence described in Appendix D.

The cost of loss measure incorporates all costs in the year of failure, including surgery, hospitalization, and dialysis for that year. The failed-graft population returns to dialysis. The cost of dialysis includes all direct medical costs associated with dialysis.

Certain factors remove patients from the failed-graft–returned-to-dialysis pool. Data suggest 12% annual mortality after graft failure, so the failed-graft population is reduced by this rate annually. Because approximately 10% of all renal transplants are retransplants, we assume 10% of the failed graft pool receive new transplants each year. Since the costs of retransplantation would have been avoided if the graft had not failed, the associated cost of retransplantation for these patients are also potential cost savings. The cost-of-loss, dialysis, and retransplantation values were provided by Dr. Eggers, HCFA. We estimated potential 5-year cost savings of $830 million attributable to extended immuno-

---

[14]UNOS database.

suppressive coverage of kidney transplant recipients. These cost savings would offset gross costs. The results are displayed in Table E-22.

Heart, Liver, and Lung Gross and Net Cost Estimates

We estimate a total 5-year gross cost of $212 million for the extension of immunosuppressive therapy coverage for heart, liver, and lung transplant recipients. There were no cost offsets, therefore, the 5-year net cost estimate is also $212 million. These costs, displayed in Table E-23, apply to all immunosuppressive therapy for Medicare-eligible heart, liver, and lung transplant recipients with graft survival greater than 3 years.

Methodology

We estimated the number of grafts with greater-than-3-year survival by combining historical Medicare covered transplants (MEDPAR data) and graft survival rates from UNOS. These estimates were determined in conjunction with Dr. Eggers.

We estimated a projected rate of increase for each organ population (heart, liver, and lung), based on historical rates of population growth and transplant trends:

- heart: estimated to grow at rates from 17% (2001) to 10% (2004),
- liver: estimated to grow at rates from 20% (2001) to 10% (2004), and
- lung: estimated to grow at rates from 40% (2001) to 10% (2004).

The only viable cost offset found due to heart, liver, and lung extended coverage is retransplantation, which is an expensive procedure (often costing as much as $300,000, according to the background paper author). However, virtually all retransplants of these organs occur within the first year following the transplant; therefore few cost offsets can be attributed to a greater-than-3-year coverage extension. Also, graft failure due to chronic rejection is low in liver transplant patients, the most common category after kidney transplants.

TABLE E-22 Estimated Cost (in millions) Due to Loss of Renal Grafts Attributed to Cost Pressure on Patients, "Entire" Transplant Population

Avoided Costs	2000	2001	2002	2003	2004	Total
Graft failure rate from cost pressure	2.5%	2.5%	2.5%	2.5%	2.5%	NA
Annual >3-year failed grafts	1,208	1,308	1,417	1,534	1,662	NA
Prior number of >3-year failed grafts	—	942	926	1,012	1,096	NA
Total >3-year failed grafts	1,208	2,250	2,343	2,547	2,757	NA
Cost of loss	$61,057	$62,278	$63,523	$64,794	$66,090	NA
Total annual cost of removal (millions)	$73.7	$140.1	$148.8	$165.0	$182.2	$709.9
Per unit cost of dialysis	$53,042	$54,103	$55,185	$56,289	$57,415	NA
Total cost of dialysis (millions)	—	$68.0	$129.1	$185.7	$239.3	$622.1
Number retransplanted (10% of total)	121	225	234	255	276	NA
Cost per retransplantation	$103,607	$105,679	$107,793	$109,949	$112,148	NA
Total costs of retransplantations (millions)	$12.5	$23.8	$25.3	$28.0	$30.9	$120.5
Total cost due to graft loss	$86.3	$163.9	$174.1	$193.0	$213.1	$830.4

TABLE E-23 Estimated Gross Cost of Immunosuppressive Therapy for Heart, Liver, and Lung Transplant Patients

	2000	2001	2002	2003	2004	Total
Annual heart > 3 years	1,863	2,179	2,506	2,757	3,032	NA
Annual liver > 3 years	1,735	2,082	2,395	2,634	2,897	NA
Annual lung > 3 years	217	304	395	474	521	NA
Total graft patient > 3 years	5,815	6,566	7,297	7,867	8,455	NA
Cost per year of immunosuppressive therapy	$5,400	$5,616	$5,841	$6,074	$6,317	NA
Gross cost in millions	$31.40	$36.87	$42.62	$47.79	$53.41	$212.1

APPENDIX F

Committee Biographies

ROBERT LAWRENCE, M.D. (*Chair*), is the associate dean for professional education and programs and professor of health policy at Johns Hopkins University School of Hygiene and Public Health. Dr. Lawrence is a member of the Institute of Medicine (IOM). Prior IOM committee memberships have included the following: Guidelines on Thyroid Cancer Screening Committee (chair); Committee on Health Care Services in the U.S.-Associated Pacific Basin (chair); Committee on Priorities for Vaccine Development (chair); Committee on Health and Human Rights (chair); Committee on Human Rights of the National Academy of Sciences, National Academy of Engineering, the Institute of Medicine, and the Board on Health Promotion and Disease Prevention (chair). Other memberships include the U.S. Preventive Services Task Force. His expertise and research interests include community and social medicine, human rights, health promotion and disease prevention, evidence-based decision rules for prevention policy, and international health.

JACK EBELER, M.P.A., is senior vice president and director of the Health Care Group at the Robert Wood Johnson Foundation. In 1995 and 1996, he served in the U.S. Department of Health and Human Services as deputy assistant secretary for Planning and Evaluation/Health and then as acting assistant secretary for Planning and Evaluation. Previous positions include principal, Health Policy Alternatives, Inc., vice president at Group Health, Inc. (now HealthPartners), and senior staff associate focusing on Medicare and the budget at the Subcommittee on Health and the Environment of the House Committee on Energy and Commerce (1981–1983). Mr. Ebeler has a Master's in Public Administration from the John F. Kennedy School of Government at Harvard University, and a B.A. from Dickinson College in Carlisle, PA. He is a principal in the Council for Excellence in Government, and a member of the National Academy of Social Insurance.

ROBERT J. GENCO, D.D.S., Ph.D. (through May 15, 1999), is distinguished professor and chairman, Department of Oral Biology, and distinguished professor of microbiology, Schools of Dentistry and Medicine, State University of New York (SUNY) at Buffalo. A member of the IOM, Dr. Genco has served on the faculty at SUNY, Buffalo, since 1967. He has also been on staff at Buffalo General Hospital since 1969. Previous memberships include IOM Committee on Career Paths for Clinical Research, and the National Institute of Dental Research Scientific Advisory Panel and Board of Scientific Counselors. He currently chairs the Food and Drug Administration Dental Products Panel and is past chair of the Over-the-Counter Products Subcommittee. His teaching has been in the areas of epidemiology and community dentistry, periodontal biology, microbiology, clinical periodontology, and molecular and cellular bases of immunology. Dr. Genco holds seven patents, is the author of numerous publications, and is the current recipient of several research grants and contracts from the U.S. Public Health Service. Dr. Genco is a member and past president of the International and American Associations for Dental Research (IADR), and a member of the American Association of Immunologists, the American Association for the Advancement of Science (past chair of the Dental Section), and the American Academy of Periodontology. He is presently the editor-in-chief of the *Journal of Periodontology* and *Annals of Periodontology,* and is on the editorial boards of several other journals. He was awarded the Gold Medal for Research by the American Dental Association, and the Basic Research in Oral Sciences Award and the Periodontal Research Award from the IADR.

MARTHE R. GOLD, M.D., M.P.H. is the Arthur C. Logan Professor and chair of the Department of Community Medicine and Social Medicine at the City University of New York Medical School. Previous positions were held with the University of Rochester Medical School and the Office of the Assistant Secretary for Health. Dr. Gold served on the Task Force for Health Care Reform in 1993 and the Panel on Cost-Effectiveness in Health and Medicine. She was a consultant and coeditor for the IOM report *Summarizing Population Health* (1998). Dr. Gold's scholarship and publications are in the areas of community-oriented primary care, socioeconomic predictors of health, cost-effectiveness analysis, and measurement of health outcomes. Her teaching, at the medical undergraduate and resident levels, has been in the areas of evidenced-based medicine, cost-effectiveness analysis, population health, and clinical preventive services.

BERTRAM L. KASISKE, M.D., is director, Division of Nephrology, Hennepin County Medical Center, and professor of medicine, University of Minnesota. Memberships include the American Society of Transplant Physicians (Board of Directors) and Clinical Practice Guidelines Committee (cochair); Review Committee for National Institute of Allergy and Infectious Diseases Immunopathogenesis of Chronic Graft Rejection (chair); Juvenile Diabetes Foundation International Grant Peer Review Committee; and American Society of Transplant Physicians Patient Care and Education Committee (cochair 1991–1993, chair 1993–1994). Dr. Kasiske is a fellow of the American College of Physicians. He is the recipient of more than five substantial research support grants and the author of numerous articles. Research interests include evidence-based medicine, immunosuppressive drugs and other therapies for transplant patients, and other topics related to transplantation and renal disease.

LAUREN L. PATTON, D.D.S. (from May 20, 1999), is associate professor of dental ecology in the School of Dentistry of the University of North Carolina (UNC) in Chapel Hill. Dr. Patton also served previously as the director of hospital dentistry in that institution. Prior to joining the faculty at UNC in 1990, Dr. Patton served as a clinical staff fellow at the National Institutes of Health (NIH). Dr. Patton is board-certified in oral medicine. Memberships include the American Dental Association, American Association of Hospital Dentists, American Academy of Oral Medicine, and the American Association of Dental Research, among others. She is a fellow of the American Association of Hospital Dentists. Her teaching has been in the area of management of dental patients with systemic disease. She is the author of many peer-reviewed articles and has contributed chapters and monographs to the field. Her major research interests include the oral manifestations of HIV and periodontal disease in persons with HIV/AIDS, oral complications of head and neck cancer therapy, and salivary gland function and dysfunction in patients with systemic disease.

STEPHEN G. PAUKER, M.D., is vice chairman for clinical affairs, Department of Medicine, New England Medical Center, and Sara Murray Jordan Professor of Medicine, Tufts University. Dr. Pauker is a member of the Institute of Medicine. Prior committee memberships have included IOM's Guidelines on Thyroid Cancer Screening; the Committee to Evaluate the Artificial Heart Program of the National Heart, Lung, and Blood Institute; and Workshops on the National Institutes of Health Consensus Development Process and the Use of Drugs in the Elderly, both within the IOM. His publications and research have focused on screening for cancer and other conditions, applications of clinical decision theory and medical informatics to health policy, technology assessment and the individualization of patient care, cost-effectiveness analysis, clinical cardiology, telemedicine, ethics of various reimbursement models, and efficiency of care delivery.

ROBERT S. STERN, M.D., is professor of dermatology, Harvard Medical School at the Beth Israel Deaconess Medical Center in Boston. His postgraduate and fellowship training includes a residency in dermatology at Harvard-Massachusetts General Hospital and fellowships at the NIH (epidemiology-clinical genetics) and the Harvard Center for Community Health and Medical Care (health services). He has served on the Harvard Medical School faculty since 1976. His research focuses on epidemiology of skin disease with special focus on nonmelanoma skin cancers, psoriasis, and cutaneous drug eruptions. He is particularly interested in risk factors for the development of nonmelanoma skin cancer, the relative cost-effectiveness of alternative therapies, and the assessment of treatment based on patient-oriented outcomes. He is the author of numerous original peer-reviewed publications.

Index

AAD. *See* American Academy of Dermatology (AAD)

ACPM. *See* American College of Preventive Medicine (ACPM)

Acquired immune deficiency syndrome/human immunodeficiency virus (AIDS/HIV), 90, 96, 113, 250
See also Infectious agents

ACS. *See* American Cancer Society (ACS)

Actinic keratoses (AK), 190, 201

Actuarial Research Corporation, 338, 340

ADA. *See* American Dental Association (ADA)

Africa
Burkitt's lymphoma in, 250

Age and aging
melanoma incidence/mortality and, 173–174
nonmelanoma skin cancer and, 176
population aged 65 and older, 228–231
preventive services for, U.S. Preventive Services Task Force recommendations, 130
preventive services for, U.S. Preventive Services Task Force recommendations/Medicare coverage comparison, 9, 128–131
skin cancer and, 172, 173

teeth (natural), population 65 and older retaining, 228–231
transplant recipients aged 65 and older, statistics, 258
See also Population

Agency for Health Care Policy and Research (AHCPR), 6, 20, 95, 98, 131, 132, 135.
See also Evidence-Based Practice Centers (EPCs)

AHA. *See* American Heart Association (AHA)

AIDS/HIV. *See* Acquired immune deficiency syndrome/human immunodeficiency virus (AIDS/HIV)

AK. *See* Actinic keratoses (AK)

Alabama. *See* University of Alabama

Albuquerque, New Mexico
basal cell cancer incidence, 176

Allograft. *See* Organ transplantation

American Academy of Dermatology (AAD), 38, 210
Melanoma/Skin Cancer Screening Programs, 203
skin cancer screening recommendations, 57

American Cancer Society (ACS), 38, 234
Department of Epidemiology and Surveillance Research, 233

367